FIRST AID FOR THE

USMLE ~

STEP 2

SECOND EDITION

A STUDENT TO *COMPLETELY REVISED AND EXPANDED* STUDENT GUIDE

FIRST AID FOR THE

USMLE STEP 2

SECOND EDITION

A STUDENT TO REVISED STUDENT GUIDE

COMPLETELY REVISED AND EXPANDED

TAO LE, MD
University of California, San Francisco, Class of 1996
Yale–New Haven Hospital, Resident in Internal Medicine

CHIRAG AMIN, MD
University of Miami, Class of 1996
Orlando Regional Medical Center, Resident in Orthopaedic Surgery

VIKAS BHUSHAN, MD
University of California, San Francisco, Class of 1991
Diagnostic Radiologist

ROSS BERKELEY, MD
University of Pittsburgh Medical Center
Resident in Emergency Medicine

ROSS LEVINE
Johns Hopkins School of Medicine
Class of 1999

DIEGO RUIZ
University of California, San Francisco
Class of 1999

APPLETON & LANGE
STAMFORD, CT

Copyright © 1999 by Appleton & Lange
First edition copyright © 1996 by Appleton & Lange

Information, tables and images from the following Appleton & Lange titles were incorporated into Section II: Database of High-Yield Facts with permission: Bondi, *Dermatology: Diagnosis and Therapy*, 1st ed, 1991; Vaughan, *General Ophthalmology*, 14th ed, 1995; Saunders, *Current Emergency Diagnosis & Treatment*, 4th ed, 1992; Tierney, *Current Medical Diagnosis & Treatment*, 37th ed, 1998; Way, *Current Surgical Diagnosis & Treatment*, 10th ed, 1994; Aminoff, *Clinical Neurology*, 3rd ed, 1996; Crawford, *Current Diagnosis & Treatment in Cardiology*, 1st ed, 1995; Grendell, *Current Diagnosis & Treatment in Gastroenterology*, 1st ed, 1996; DeCherney, *Current Obstetrics and Gynecology Diagnosis and Treatment*, 8th ed, 1994; Skinner, *Current Diagnosis & Treatment in Orthopedics*, 1st ed, 1995; Chandrasoma, *Concise Pathology*, 3rd ed, 1998; Ochs, *Recognition & Interpretation of ECG Rhythms*, 3rd ed, 1997; Stites, *Basic & Clinical Immunology*, 8th ed, 1994; Stobo, *The Principles and Practice of Medicine*, 23rd ed, 1996; Cogan, *Fluid and Electrolytes*, 1st ed, 1991; Goldfrank, *Toxicologic Emergencies*, 6th ed, 1998; Tanagho, *Smith's General Urology*, 13th ed, 1992; Benson, *Handbook of Obstetrics & Gynecology*, 8th ed, 1983; Rudolph, *Rudolph's Fundamentals of Pediatrics*, 1st ed, 1994; Milikowski, *Color Atlas of Basic Histopathology*, 1st ed, 1997; Hurwitz, *Pathology of the Skin*, 2nd ed, 1998. Additional images were provided courtesy of Vincent Piscitelli (Yale–New Haven Hospital Microbiology Services), Dr. Peter McPhedran, Nancy Wachuk, MT, (Yale University School of Medicine), Dr. Henry Shih (UCLA School of Medicine), the Yale Department of Dermatology, and the Washington University Department of Ophthalmology.

99 00 01 02 03 / 10 9 8 7 6 5 4 3 2 1

Prentice Hall International (UK) Limited, *London*
Prentice Hall of Australia Pty. Limited, *Sydney*
Prentice Hall of Canada, Inc., *Toronto*
Prentice Hall Hispanoamericana, S.A., *Mexico*
Prentice Hall of India Private Limited, *New Delhi*
Prentice Hall of Japan, Inc., *Tokyo*
Simon & Schuster Asia Pte. Ltd., *Singapore*
Editora Prentice Hall do Brasil Ltda., *Rio de Janeiro*
Prentice Hall, *Upper Saddle River, New Jersey*

Acquisitions Editor: Robin Lazrus
Production: Rainbow Graphics, LLC
Editorial Consultant: Andrea Fellows
Cover Design: Design Group Cook
Interior Design: Elizabeth Sanders

0-8385-2604-7

90000

9 780838 526040

PRINTED IN THE UNITED STATES OF AMERICA

To our families, friends, and loved ones, who endured
and assisted in the task of assembling this guide.

&

To the contributors to this and future editions, who took
time to share their knowledge, insight, and
humor for the benefit of students.

Contributors

MICHELLE PINTO
Contributing Author, High-Yield Facts
Yale University, Class of 1999

STEVEN BROWN, MD
Contributing Author, High-Yield Facts
University of California, San Francisco
Resident in Family Practice

ANTONY CHU
Contributing Author, Exam Guide
Yale University, Class of 2001

GREGORY RASKIN, MD
Contributing Author, High-Yield Facts
New York University Medical Center
Resident in Internal Medicine

Reviewers

EDWARD MCNULTY, MD
Chief Resident in Internal Medicine
Yale-New Haven Hospital

THAO PHAM, MD
Resident in Pediatrics
Yale-New Haven Hospital

NUTAN SHARMA, MD
Resident in Neurology
Yale-New Haven Hospital

ANN VU, MD
Resident in Dermatology
Yale-New Haven Hospital

Contents

Preface to the Second Edition

With the second edition of *First Aid for the USMLE Step 2*, we continue our commitment to providing students with the most useful and up-to-date preparation guide for the USMLE Step 2. The second edition represents a thorough revision in many ways and includes:

- A completely revised and updated exam preparation guide for the new computerized USMLE Step 2. Includes detailed analysis as well as all new study and test-taking strategies for the new computer-based testing (CBT) format.
- Revisions and new material based on student experience with the 1998 administrations of the USMLE Step 2.
- Concise summaries of over 240 heavily tested clinical topics.
- A basic science primer which features clinically relevant high-yield basic science facts from *First Aid for the USMLE Step 1*.
- Expanded USMLE advice for international medical graduates.
- A new collection of over 120 high-yield glossy photos similar to those appearing on the USMLE Step 2 exam.
- Useful reference links to prototypical clinical cases from the popular *Underground Clinical Vignette* series (S2S Medical Publishing).
- A completely revised, in-depth guide to clinical science review and sample examination books.

The second edition would not have been possible without the help of the hundreds of students and faculty members who contributed their feedback and suggestions. We invite students and faculty to continue sharing their thoughts and ideas to help us improve *First Aid for the USMLE Step 2*. (See How to Contribute, p. xvii, and User Survey, p. xxv.)

New Haven	Tao Le
Orlando	Chirag Amin
Los Angeles	Vikas Bhushan
Pittsburgh	Ross Berkeley
Baltimore	Ross Levine
San Francisco	Diego Ruiz

March 1999

Acknowledgments

This has been a collaborative project from the start. We gratefully acknowledge the thoughtful comments, corrections, and advice of the many medical students, international medical graduates, and faculty who have supported the authors in the continuing development of *First Aid for the USMLE Step 2*.

For significant contributions to the second edition, we would like to thank Andrew Weiss, Lawrence Etter, Dr. Vladimir Coric, Drs. Archana and Sanjay Bindra, Aminah Bliss, Brad Spellberg, Ryan Crowley, Vipal Soni, Vishall Pall, Jose Fierro, and Henry Nguyen.

Thanks to Melanie Nelson (NBME) for providing updated USMLE Step 2 information. For helping us obtain information concerning review books, we thank Barnes & Noble medical bookstore (New York City) and Yale Co-op medical bookstore. Thanks Elizabeth Sanders and Ashley Pound for the interior design and Design Group Cook for the cover design.

For support and encouragement throughout the process, we are grateful to Thao Pham, Jonathan Kirsch, Esq., Cindy Andrien, and the Yale University School of Medicine Office of Student Affairs.

Thanks to our publisher, Appleton & Lange, for the valuable assistance of their staff. For enthusiasm, support, and commitment for this challenging project, thanks to our editors, Robin Lazrus and Marinita Timban. We would also like to thank Lisa Guidone, John Williams, Deborah King, Cheryl Mehalik, Eve Siegel, and Lynne Vail-Nagle at Appleton & Lange for keeping the project on track. For personal and last-minute production support, thanks to our able administrative assistant, Gianni Le Nguyen, and our copy editors, Andrea Fellows and Erica Simmons. A special thanks to Jimmy and Bennie Sauls (Rainbow Graphics) for remarkable production work.

For contributions, corrections and surveys we thank Chris Aiken, Ken Baum, James Borin, Vapjista Broumand, Shaina Bull, Scotty Cardoni, Deanna Chin, Matt Cooperberg, Dan Coghlin, Elly Falzarano, Tanya Froelich, Mark Hamill, Jason Klenoff, Mary Grey Maher, JoAnne McDonough, Rod J. Oskouian, Shilpa Pai, Joshua Pierce, Jeff Reynolds, Adam Schaffner, Samir Shah, Seth Schwartz, Sudavadee Supanwanid, Darcy Thompson, Patricia Vherova, Amit Sarma, Rahul Pandit, Stephen Eigles, Cindy Nguyen, Daniel Carlic, Vanessa Oppenlander, Margaret Gourlay, Chandon Devireddy, Constance Fung, Jeffrey Horowitz, Chad Coleman, Blake Weathersby, Simon Trubek, Frank Winton, David Byerbach, Tanya Smith, Ashraf Zamin, Kaushal Shah, Betty Lee, Linda Russo, Diana Aung, and Alex Grimm. Our apologies if we accidentally omitted or misspelled your name.

New Haven	Tao Le
Orlando	Chirag Amin
Los Angeles	Vikas Bhushan
Pittsbrugh	Ross Berkeley
Baltimore	Ross Levine
San Francisco	Diego Ruiz

How to Contribute

This version of *First Aid for the USMLE Step 2* incorporates hundreds of contributions and changes suggested by faculty and student reviewers. We invite you to participate in this process. We also offer **paid internships** in medical education and publishing ranging from three months to one year (see next page for details).

Please send us your suggestions for:

- Study and test-taking strategies for the new computerized USMLE Step 2
- New facts, mnemonics, diagrams, and illustrations
- High-yield topics that may reappear on future Step 2 exams
- Personal ratings and comments on review books that you have examined

For each entry incorporated into the next edition, you will receive $10 cash per entry, as well as personal acknowledgment in the next edition. Diagrams, tables, partial entries, updates, corrections, and study hints are also appreciated, and significant contributions will be compensated at the discretion of the authors. Also let us know about material in this edition that you feel is low yield and should be deleted.

The preferred way to submit entries, suggestions, or corrections is via electronic mail. Please include name, address, school affiliation, phone number, and e-mail address (if different from address of origin). Please send submissions to:

taotle@aol.com
chiragamin@aol.com
vbhushan@aol.com

Otherwise, please send entries, neatly written or typed or on disk (Microsoft Word), to: First Aid for the USMLE Step 1, 1015 Gayley Ave., #1113, Los Angeles, CA 90024, Attention: Contributions. Please use the contribution and survey forms on the following pages. Each form constitutes an entry. (Attach additional pages as needed.)

Another option is to send in your entire annotated book. We will look through your additions and notes and will send you cash based on the quantity and quality of any additions that we incorporate into the next edition. Books will be returned upon request.

Internship Opportunities

The author team of Bhushan, Le, and Amin is pleased to offer part-time and full-time paid internships in medical education and publishing to motivated medical students and physicians. Internships may range from three months (e.g., a summer) up to a full year. Participants will have an opportunity to author, edit, and earn academic credit on a wide variety of projects, including the popular First Aid series. Writing/editing experience, familiarity with Microsoft Word, and Internet access are desired. For more information, e-mail a résumé or a short description of your experience along with a cover letter to the authors at their e-mail addresses above.

Note to Contributors

All entries become property of the authors and are subject to editing and reviewing. Please verify all data and spellings carefully. In the event that similar or duplicate entries are received, only the first entry received will be used. Include a reference to a standard textbook to facilitate verification of the fact. Please follow the style, punctuation, and format of this edition if possible.

Contribution Form I

Contributor Name: ______________________

School/Affiliation: ______________________

Address: ______________________

____

Telephone: ______________________

E-mail: ______________________

Topic:

Signs and Symptoms:

Diagnosis:

Management:

Notes, Diagrams, Tables, and Mnemonics:

Reference:

You will receive personal acknowledgment and $10 cash for each entry that is used in future editions.

Please seal with tape only.
No staples or paper clips.

- - - - - - - - - - - - - - (fold here) -

BUSINESS REPLY MAIL
FIRST-CLASS MAIL PERMIT NO. 74036 LOS ANGELES CA

POSTAGE WILL BE PAID BY ADDRESSEE

MSC 1113
FIRST AID FOR THE USMLE STEP2
1015 GAYLEY AVE
LOS ANGELES CA 90024-8980

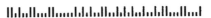

- - - - - - - - - - - - - - (fold here) -

Contribution Form II

Contributor Name: _____

School/Affiliation: _____

Address: _____

_____

Telephone: _____

E-mail: _____

Please place the clinical topic (e.g., ulcerative colitis) on the first line and the high-yield vignette or topic on the following two lines.

1. Subject: _____

   Vignette: _____

   _____

2. Subject: _____

   Vignette: _____

   _____

3. Subject: _____

   Vignette: _____

   _____

4. Subject: _____

   Vignette: _____

   _____

5. Subject: _____

   Vignette: _____

   _____

6. Subject: _____

   Vignette: _____

   _____

7. Subject: _____

   Vignette: _____

   _____

8. Subject: _____

   Vignette: _____

   _____

9. Subject: _____

   Vignette: _____

   _____

10. Subject: _____

    Vignette: _____

    _____

You will receive personal acknowledgment and $10 cash for each entry that is used in future editions.

Please seal with tape only.
No staples or paper clips.

- (fold here) -

BUSINESS REPLY MAIL
FIRST-CLASS MAIL PERMIT NO. 74036 LOS ANGELES CA

POSTAGE WILL BE PAID BY ADDRESSEE

MSC 1113
FIRST AID FOR THE USMLE STEP2
1015 GAYLEY AVE
LOS ANGELES CA 90024-8980

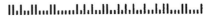

- (fold here) -

Contribution Form III

Contributor Name: _____

School/Affiliation: _____

Address: _____

_____

Telephone: _____

E-mail: _____

We welcome additional comments on review resources rated in Section III as well as reviews of resources not rated in Section III. Please fill out each review entry as completely as possible. Please do not leave "Comments" blank. Rate texts using the letter grading scale provided on p. 355, taking into consideration current ratings of other books on that subject.

1. *Title/Author:* _____   Days needed to read: _____

   Publisher/Series: _____   ISBN Number: _____

   Rating: _____   *Comments:* _____

   _____

   _____

2. *Title/Author:* _____   Days needed to read: _____

   Publisher/Series: _____   ISBN Number: _____

   Rating: _____   *Comments:* _____

   _____

   _____

3. *Title/Author:* _____   Days needed to read: _____

   Publisher/Series: _____   ISBN Number: _____

   Rating: _____   *Comments:* _____

   _____

   _____

   _____

4. *Title/Author:* _____   Days needed to read: _____

   Publisher/Series: _____   ISBN Number: _____

   Rating: _____   *Comments:* _____

   _____

   _____

5. *Title/Author:* _____   Days needed to read: _____

   Publisher/Series: _____   ISBN Number: _____

   Rating: _____   *Comments:* _____

   _____

   _____

You will receive personal acknowledgment and $10 cash for each entry that is used in future editions.

Please seal with tape only.
No staples or paper clips.

- (fold here) -

**NO POSTAGE
NECESSARY
IF MAILED
IN THE
UNITED STATES**

BUSINESS REPLY MAIL
FIRST-CLASS MAIL PERMIT NO. 74036 LOS ANGELES CA

POSTAGE WILL BE PAID BY ADDRESSEE

MSC 1113
FIRST AID FOR THE USMLE STEP2
1015 GAYLEY AVE
LOS ANGELES CA 90024-8980

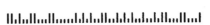

- (fold here) -

User Survey

Contributor Name: _____

School/Affiliation: _____

Address: _____

_____

Telephone: _____

E-mail: _____

What student-to-student advice would you give someone preparing for the computerized USMLE Step 2?

What commercial review courses have you been enrolled in, and what were your overall assessments of the courses?

What would you change about the study and test-taking strategies listed in Section I: Guide to Efficient Exam Preparation?

Were there any high-yield facts, topics, or vignettes in Section II that you think were inaccurate or should be deleted? Which ones and why? What would you change or add?

What review resources for the USMLE Step 2 are not covered in Section III? Would you change the rating of any of the review resources in Section III? If so, which one(s) and why?

What other suggestions do you have for improving *First Aid for the USMLE Step 2*? Any other comments or suggestions? What did you dislike most about the book? What did you like most?

You will receive personal acknowledgment and $10 cash for each entry that is used in future editions.

Please seal with tape only.
No staples or paper clips.

- (fold here) -

BUSINESS REPLY MAIL
FIRST-CLASS MAIL PERMIT NO. 74036 LOS ANGELES CA

POSTAGE WILL BE PAID BY ADDRESSEE

MSC 1113
FIRST AID FOR THE USMLE STEP2
1015 GAYLEY AVE
LOS ANGELES CA 90024-8980

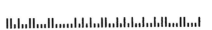

- (fold here) -

Guide to Efficient Exam Preparation

Introduction
USMLE Step 2 - The CBT Basics
Defining Your Goal
Study Resources
Practice Tests
Test-Taking Strategies
Testing Agencies

The goal of Step 2 is to examine your ability to apply your knowledge of medical facts to actual situations that you may encounter as a resident.

INTRODUCTION

For many US medical graduates, the United States Medical Licensing Examination (USMLE) Step 2 is often looked upon as an afterthought, shoved somewhere in between residency applications, "away" rotations, and matching. Nevertheless, the clinical approach of the questions allows you to pull together your clinical experience on the wards with the numerous "factoids" and classical disease presentations that you have memorized over the years.

USMLE STEP 2 - THE CBT BASICS

The USMLE Step 2 is the second of three examinations that you must pass in order to become a licensed physician in the United States. It is a joint endeavor of the National Board of Medical Examiners (NBME) and the Federation of State Medical Boards (FSMB). Previously, Step 2 was administered twice annually in a paper-and-pencil format over two days. The year 1999, however, marks a year of tremendous change in the administration of the USMLE. For the first time, all three Steps of the USMLE will be administered on computer.

The new computerized version of the Step 2 exam will be a one-day (nine-hour, 400-question) multiple-choice exam. It will include test questions in internal medicine, obstetrics and gynecology, pediatrics, preventive medicine, psychiatry, and surgery. The first computerized versions of the USMLE Step 2 exam are currently scheduled to begin in mid-August of 1999. Although relatively new, computer-based testing (CBT) is by no means without precedent; in fact, national standardized exams such as the Graduate Records Examination (GRE) and the Graduate Management Admissions Test (GMAT) have used this format for years.

There are several reasons for the NBME's move to CBT. Above all, CBT allows a large number of tests to be easily administered and processed. In addition, the limited human contact involved and increased test security features (such as software encryption) are aimed at reducing the incidence of cheating.

The NBME has contracted with a company called Sylvan Learning Systems to administer the new computer-based format of the USMLE Step 2. The exam will be administered both domestically and internationally by a special division known as Sylvan Prometric.

Currently there are 309 Sylvan sites in the United States and Canada, as well as 199 sites outside these two countries, where examinees can take Step 2. These numbers are expected to increase in the future. Examinees will have the option of taking the new CBT USMLE at any of the Sylvan Technology Centers (STCs) in the United States and Canada as well as at any STC internationally. For a list of center locations nearest you, contact http://www.sylvanprometric.com.

The most significant changes expected with the computerized version of Step 2 are as follows:

- **Shorter test.** In contrast to the former two-day, 720-question marathon, the CBT format will consist of 400 questions given in one day. The test will consist of eight question "blocks" of 50 questions timed at 60 minutes each (Fig. 1). During the time allotted to complete each block, the examinee will be able to answer test questions in any order as well as to review responses and change answers. Once the allotted block time has expired, however, further review of test questions or changing of answers within that block will not be possible. Expect to spend nine hours at the STC.

- **No more grid-ins.** The countless little black circles and number-2 pencils once required for processing standardized exams will be a thing of the past. Examinees will instead use a mouse to "point and click" on answers.

- **Shorter test blocks.** As noted above, the CBT exam is divided into 60-minute blocks. These blocks were designed to reduce eye strain and fatigue during the exam. Once an examinee finishes a particular block, he or she must click on a screen icon to continue to the next block. Examinees will not be able to go back and change answers from any previous block.

- **Year-round testing.** Step 2 will now be offered year-round (except for the first two weeks of January) rather than only twice a year. In the US and Canada, the exam will be offered Monday through Saturday. Weekly schedules can vary, however, at international test centers. Some schools will eventually be able to administer the exam on their own campuses (see p. 8).

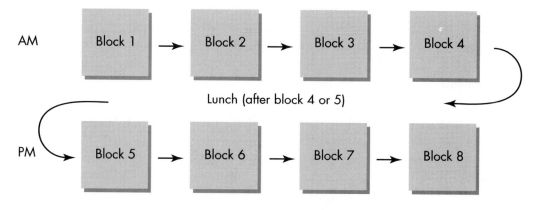

FIGURE 1. Schematic of CBT Exam

Testing Conditions

Because of the unique environment of the CBT, it's important that you familiarize yourself ahead of time with your test-day conditions. For this reason, the NBME has included a five-minute full-motion video on its free CD-ROM, which will be included with your application materials. Here's what the walk-through tour on the CD-ROM describes:

- The examinee will enter a waiting room and sign in.
- The examinee will wait in that room until the proctor calls him or her for "check-in."
- The examinee will place personal belongings in a locker and will follow the proctor into an office for official check-in festivities. This includes showing the proctor one's scheduling permit along with a signed photo identification. Next, the proctor will take a picture or "image capture" of the examinee with a digital camera. The examinee will then receive two laminated boards and ink markers for scratch work. Earplugs will also be offered at this time.
- The examinee will next be led into the testing area by the proctor. The testing workstation includes a computer, a monitor, a desk lamp, and an adjustable chair. The monitor can be adjusted for contrast. (In fact, a color calibration preceding the exam will be necessary to ensure accurate presentation of images.)
- Examinees will be required to sign out with the proctor for breaks. At this time, the examinee will be able to remove personal items from their locker, but these items must be replaced before the examinee returns to the testing area.
- Questions that arise during the exam period will be answered by the proctor as soon as the examinee raises his or her hand.
- After the examinee completes the exam, test information will be transmitted electronically to the NBME. The examinee will then be required to check out and return laminated boards and markers, after which he or she will receive a written confirmation of exam completion.

For security reasons, examinees will not be allowed to bring any personal electronic equipment into the testing area. This includes digital watches (although the student in the Sylvan video is erroneously wearing a digital watch), watches with computer communication and/or memory capability, cellular telephones, and electronic paging devices. Food and beverages are prohibited. The testing centers are monitored by audio and video surveillance equipment.

The following information is based on software previews from the NBME and on student experiences with the trial testing of the computerized field test at Sylvan Prometric Learning Centers throughout the country. Check the USMLE website (http://www.usmle.org) or with your medical school for updates.

The typical question screen (Fig. 2) has a question followed by a number of

To mark item for review

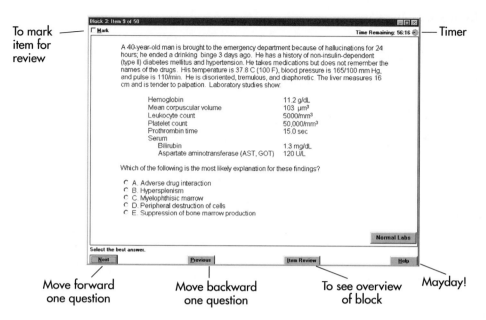

Timer

Move forward one question

Move backward one question

To see overview of block

Mayday!

FIGURE 2. Typical Question Screen

choices on which an examinee can click, along with navigational buttons at the bottom of the screen. There is also a button that allows the examinee to mark the question for review. A countdown timer is placed in the upper right-hand corner of the screen. If the question happens to be longer than the screen, a scroll bar will appear on the right, allowing the examinee to see the rest of the question. Regardless of whether the examinee clicks on an answer or leaves it blank, he or she must click the "Next>>" button in order to advance to the next question.

Some questions contain figures or color illustrations (Fig. 3). These are typically situated to the right of the question. Although the contrast and bright-

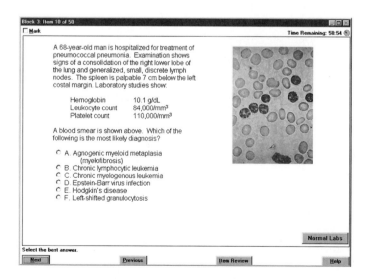

FIGURE 3. Question Screen with Illustration

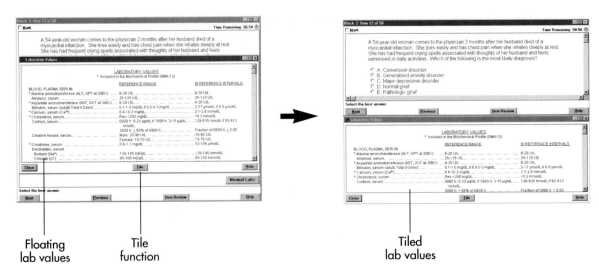

Floating
lab values

Tile
function

Tiled
lab values

FIGURE 4. Lab Values Screen—Floating and Tiled

ness of the screen can be adjusted, there are no other ways to manipulate the picture (e.g., zooming or panning).

The examinee can also call up a window displaying normal lab values (Fig. 4). However, if he or she does not click on "Tile" in the normal-values screen, the normal-values window will often obscure the question. In addition, the examinee will have to scroll down for most laboratory values.

There exists an option to mark a question for review at a later time. Clicking "Item Review" at the bottom of the screen will access a screen (Fig. 5) that gives an over-

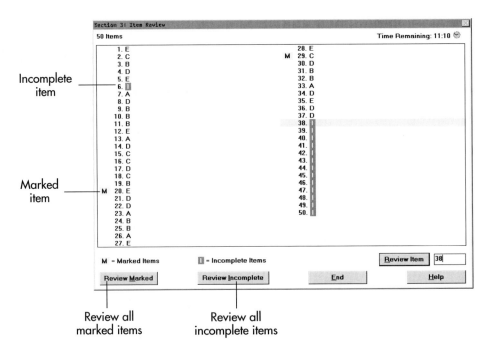

Incomplete
item

Marked
item

Review all
marked items

Review all
incomplete items

FIGURE 5. Item Review Screen

view of the block, allowing the examinee to pinpoint questions marked for review as well as unanswered questions. This also serves as a quick way of navigating to any question in the block, regardless of whether that question has been answered.

How Do I Register to Take the Exam?

Application packets are available at your student affairs office or from the NBME at (215) 590-9700. International medical graduates (IMGs) can receive a packet by calling the Educational Commission for Foreign Medical Graduates (ECFMG) at (215) 386-5900 (see "Testing Agencies," p. 23, for full contact information). Applicants will select one of 12 overlapping three-month blocks in which to be tested. In mid-August of 1999, when CBT begins, the fee will be $280. Upon receipt of your application materials, the NBME will contact your medical institution to verify your eligibility for taking the exam, and you will receive a "scheduling permit."

The scheduling permit you receive from the NBME will contain your USMLE identification number, the eligibility period in which you can take the exam, and two unique numbers, one of which is known as your "scheduling number." You will need this number to make your exam appointment with Sylvan. The other number is known as the "candidate identification number." Examinees must enter this candidate identification number at the Sylvan workstation in order to access their exam. Sylvan has no access to the codes in advance and will not be able to supply these numbers. Do not lose this permit! You will not be allowed to take the boards unless you present this permit along with a photo identification with your signature.

Once you receive your scheduling permit, you must call the Sylvan toll-free number to arrange a time to take the exam. Although requests for taking the exam may be made more than six months before the test date, examinees will not receive their scheduling permits earlier than six months before the eligibility period. The eligibility period is the three-month period you have chosen to take the exam. Because exam scheduling is given on a "first-come, first-serve" basis, it is recommended that you telephone Sylvan as soon as you have received your permit. Be sure to read the 1999 USMLE *Bulletin of Information on Computer-Based Testing* for further details.

Because the exam is scheduled on a "first-come, first-serve" basis, call Sylvan as soon as you receive your scheduling permit!

When Should I Register for the Exam?

Although there are no deadlines for registering for Step 2, you should plan to register at least nine months ahead of your desired test date. This will ensure that you will get either your STC of choice or one within a 50-mile radius of your first choice. You should also be able to schedule a date within two weeks of your desired test date.

Because of the limited number of computers available, only a certain number of examinees will be able to take the computer exam on any given day. With over 300 sites in Canada and the US, as many as 6000 exams could be administered per day. Of course, precisely how difficult it will be to schedule an exam will depend on the location of the STC and on the number of test takers (both US students and IMGs) in the region. Some areas may have more test takers than available STCs.

Where Can I Take the Exam?

There are two general locations available for taking the new computerized exam:

- **Sylvan Testing Centers.** If you register early, you can take the exam at your preferred site or at the next-closest testing center within a 50-mile radius. Note that there is a difference between Sylvan Learning Centers (SLCs) and Sylvan Testing Centers (STCs). Sylvan Testing Centers are add-on centers to Sylvan Learning Centers. The USMLE will be offered only at SLCs with an STC. Call 1-800-EDUCATE (800-338-2283) to find an STC near you.

- **Medical schools.** The NBME is authorizing a limited number of medical schools to serve as non-Sylvan testing centers. This means that some medical schools will choose to dedicate some of their own computer resources for the administration of the new computer exam. Owing to costs and limited resources, these sites will be limited (especially initially). Check with your student affairs office to see if your school is planning to participate.

Your testing location is arranged with Sylvan when you call for your test date.

How Long Will I Have to Wait Before I Get My Scores?

Initially, examinees may not receive their scores for six to eight weeks. Eventually, however, this time will be reduced to two weeks. The initial delay in reporting scores will be due to the various statistical analyses that will be carried out to ensure that the pass/fail rate has not changed and that the standard is equivalent to that of the former paper exam.

What Did Other Students Like/Dislike About the CBT Format?

Students participating in field trials noted that the feature they most enjoyed was the point-and-click simplicity of the new format.

What did students dislike most about the test? The main complaint was having to access lab-values data as a cumbersome floating screen (Fig. 4). In addition, students noted that the inability to mark questions and answers was inconvenient. Some students also cited difficulties with images and text quality. Some of the images were reportedly of poor quality or too small. Some images could not be viewed along with the corresponding question text. Some students complained of eye strain and fatigue as a result of small text.

What About Time?

The most critical time change in the CBT exam is the consolidation of the exam into one day. Here's a breakdown of the exam schedule:

Tutorial	15 minutes
60-minute question blocks (50 questions per block)	8 hours
Break time (includes time for lunch)	45 minutes
Total test time	9 hours

The computer will keep track of how much time has elapsed. However, the computer will show you only how much time you have remaining in a given block. Therefore, it is up to you to determine if you are pacing yourself properly (at a rate of approximately one question per 60–72 seconds).

The computer will not warn you if you are spending more than your allotted time for a break. Thus, taking long breaks between early question blocks or for lunch may mean that you will not be able to take breaks later in the day. You should budget your time so that you can take a short break when you need it but still have time to eat.

Be especially careful not to waste too much time in between blocks (you should keep track of how much time elapses from when you finish a block of questions to when you start the next block). After you finish one question block, you'll need to click the mouse when you are ready to proceed to the next block of questions.

It should be noted that the 45-minute break time is the minimum break time for the day. You can gain extra break time (but not time for the question blocks) by skipping the tutorial or by finishing a block in less than the time allotted.

For security reasons, digital watches will not be allowed. This means that only analog watches will be permitted. You should therefore get used to timing yourself with an analog watch so that you know exactly how much time you have left. Some analog watches come with a bevel that helps keep track of 60-minute periods. This may be useful for keeping track of break time.

Since digital watches are not allowed, get used to keeping track of break time with an analog watch.

Question Types

- Almost all questions are case-based. Some are two to three sentences in length, while others are two to three paragraphs long and contain laboratory data. Very often, a substantial amount of extraneous information is given, making for dense, slow reading. Also, it is common for a clinical scenario to be given followed by a question that could be answered without your having actually read the case. Unfortunately, it is your job to determine which information is superfluous and which is pertinent to the case at hand.

Almost all questions are case-based.

- Questions often describe clinical findings instead of naming eponyms (i.e., they cite "audible hip click" instead of "positive Ortolani's sign"), so it is important to know what each sign and "keyword" actually represents (e.g., "double-bubble sign").
- Subject areas vary randomly from question to question, although groups of matching questions often have a unifying theme.

Most questions have a single best answer, and there have been no negatively phrased questions on recent exams. Some questions are matching sets that call for multiple responses—the number to select is specified at the end of each question. The questions usually describe clinical situations which require that you identify a diagnosis, the underlying pathophysiology of the disease being described, the next appropriate step in management, interpretation of laboratory findings, potential for prevention, or overall prognosis. The part of the vignette that actually asks the question—the stem—is usually at the end of the scenario. From student experience, there are a few stems that are consistently addressed throughout the exam:

- What is the most likely diagnosis? (40%)
- Which of the following is the most appropriate initial step in management? (20%)
- Which of the following is the most appropriate next step in management? (20%)
- Which of the following is the most likely cause of . . . ? (5%)
- Which of the following is the most likely pathogen . . . ? (3%)
- Which of the following would most likely prevent . . . ? (2%)
- Other (10%)

Scoring and Failure Rates

Except for an initial delay, CBT scores should be mailed within two weeks. Like the Step 1 score report, it includes your pass/fail status, two numeric scores, and a performance profile by discipline and disease process (Figs. 6A and 6B). The first score is a three-digit scaled score based on a predefined proficiency standard as set by the September 1991 group of examinees. Over the past few exams, the mean and standard deviation for first-time test takers from US and Canadian medical schools were 207 and 23, respectively, with most scores falling between 140 and 260. In 1998, a score of 170 was required to pass. The second score scale, the two-digit score, defines 75 as the minimum passing score (equivalent to a score of 170 on the first scale). A score of 82 is equivalent to a score of 200 on the first scale.

United States
Medical
Licensing
Examination
™

UNITED STATES MEDICAL LICENSING EXAMINATION™

USMLE Step 2 is administered to students and graduates of U.S. and Canadian medical schools by the
NATIONAL BOARD OF MEDICAL EXAMINERS® (NBME®)
3750 Market Street, Philadelphia, Pennsylvania 19104-3190.
Telephone: (215) 590-9700

STEP 2 SCORE REPORT

Schmoe, Joe T	USMLE ID: 1-234-567-8
Anytown, CA 12345	Test Date: August 1998

The USMLE is a single examination program for all applicants for medical licensure in the United States; it has replaced the Federation Licensing Examination (FLEX) and the certifying examinations of the National Board of Medical Examiners (NBME Parts I, II and III). The program consists of three Steps designed to assess an examinee's understanding of and ability to apply concepts and principles that are important in health and disease and that constitute the basis of safe and effective patient care. **Step 2** is designed to assess whether an examinee possesses the medical knowledge and understanding of clinical science considered essential for the provision of patient care under supervision, including emphasis on health promotion and disease prevention. The inclusion of Step 2 in the USMLE sequence ensures that attention is devoted to principles of clinical science that undergird the safe and competent practice of medicine. Results of the examination are reported to medical licensing authorities in the United States and its territories for use in granting an initial license to practice medicine. The two numeric scores shown below are equivalent; each state or territory may use either score in making licensing decisions. These scores represent your results for the administration of Step 2 on the test date shown above.

PASS	This result is based on the minimum passing score set by USMLE for Step 2. Individual licensing authorities may accept the USMLE-recommended pass/fail result or may establish a different passing score for their own jurisdictions.
200	This score is determined by your overall performance on Step 2. For recent administrations, the mean and standard deviation for first-time examinees from U.S. and Canadian medical schools are approximately 208 and 23, respectively, with most scores falling between 140 and 260. A score of 170 is set by USMLE to pass Step 2. The standard error of measurement (SEM)‡ for this scale is approximately six points.
82	This score is also determined by your overall performance on the examination. A score of 82 on this scale is equivalent to a score of 200 on the scale described above. A score of 75 on this scale, which is equivalent to a score of 170 on the scale described above, is set by USMLE to pass Step 2. The SEM‡ for this scale is one point.

‡Your score is influenced both by your general understanding of clinical science and the specific set of items selected for this Step 2 examination. The standard error of measurement (SEM) provides an estimate of the range within which your scores might be expected to vary by chance if you were tested repeatedly using similar tests.

267PU007

NOTE: Original score report has copy-resistant watermark.

FIGURE 6A. Sample Score Report—Front Page

The overall pass rate for first-time NBME-registered examinees has ranged between 90% and 93% over the past few years. The pass rate for a specific group may be higher, reaching as high as 99% for first-time allopathic test takers. However, the overall pass rate for ECFMG-registered examinees declined in 1996–1997 (43%) when compared to 1995–1996 (47%) (see Table 1).

The preceding information is based on students' experience with the August 1997 and the March 1998 administrations of the USMLE Step 2, CBT field trials, and information published by the NBME. The format and scoring of the examination are subject to change, especially with the introduction of CBT in 1999. Please consult the latest NBME publications, the USMLE website at http://www.usmle.org, and your medical school for the most current and accurate information about the examination.

INFORMATION PROVIDED FOR EXAMINEE USE ONLY
The Performance Profile below is provided solely for the benefit of the examinee.
These profiles are developed as assessment tools for examinees only and will not be reported or verified to any third party.

USMLE STEP 2 PERFORMANCE PROFILES

PHYSICIAN TASK PROFILE	Lower Performance	Borderline Performance	Higher Performance
Preventive Medicine & Health Maintenance			xxxxxxxxxxx*
Understanding Mechanisms of Disease			xxxx*
Diagnosis			xxxxxx*
Principles of Management			xxxxxxxxxx*

NORMAL CONDITIONS & DISEASE CATEGORY PROFILE

	Lower Performance	Borderline Performance	Higher Performance
Normal Growth & Development; Principles of Care			xxxxxxxxxxxxxxxx*
Immunologic Disorders			xxxxxxxxxxxxxx*
Diseases of Blood & Blood Forming Organs			xxxxxxxxxxxx*
Mental Disorders			xxxxxxxxxxxx*
Diseases of the Nervous System & Special Senses			xxxxxxxxxxx*
Cardiovascular Disorders			xxxxxxxxxxxxxxxx
Diseases of the Respiratory System			xxxxxxxxxxxxx*
Nutritional & Digestive Disorders			xxxxxxxxxxx*
Gynecologic Disorders			xxxxxxxxxxxxx*
Renal, Urinary & Male Reproductive Systems			xxxxxxxxxxx*
Disorders of Pregnancy, Childbirth & Puerperium			xxxxxxxxxxxxxxxxxxx
Musculoskeletal, Skin & Connective Tissue Diseases			xxxxxxxxxx*
Endocrine & Metabolic Disorders			xxxxxxxxxxxxx*

DISCIPLINE PROFILE

	Lower Performance	Borderline Performance	Higher Performance
Medicine			xxx*
Obstetrics & Gynecology			xxxxxxxxxxx*
Pediatrics			xxxxxxxx*
Psychiatry			xxxxxxxxxxxx*
Surgery			xx*

The above Performance Profile is provided to aid in self-assessment. The shaded area defines a borderline level of performance for each content area; borderline performance is comparable to a HIGH FAIL / LOW PASS on the total test.

Performance bands indicate areas of relative strength and weakness. Some performance bands are wider than others. The width of a performance band reflects the precision of measurement: narrower bands indicate greater precision. An asterisk indicates that your performance band extends beyond the displayed portion of the scale. Small differences in the location of bands should not be over interpreted. If two bands overlap, the performance in the associated areas should not be interpreted as significantly different.

This profile should not be compared to those from other Step 2 administrations.

Additional information concerning the topics covered in each content area can be found in the *USMLE Step 2 General Instructions, Content Description, and Sample Items.*

007PU267

FIGURE 6B. Sample Score Report—Back Page

USMLE Publications

The USMLE provides a number of publications that can be helpful—if not invaluable—as you begin your test preparation process. Many students overlook these publications. They are as follows:

- *USMLE Bulletin of Information on Computer-Based Testing.* This publication provides you with nuts-and-bolts details about the exam.
- *Step 2 Computer-Based Content and Sample Test Questions.* This is a hard copy of test questions and test content also found on the CD-ROM.
- *USMLE Information on Computer-Based Step 1 and Step 2 CD-ROM.* This CD-ROM provides much of the same information described above, including a video tour of an STC and sample test items. Make sure to spend time thoroughly reviewing the sample test items. In

TABLE 1. Passing Rates for 1997 USMLE Step 2

	March 1997		August 1997		Total 1997	
	No. Tested	Passing (%)	No. Tested	Passing (%)	No. Tested	Passing (%)
NBME-Registered Allopathic						
First-Time Takers	6,413	94	10,673	95	17,086	95
Repeaters	879	61	748	64	1,627	62
NBME Total	**7,292**	**90**	**11,421**	**93**	**18,713**	**92**
ECFMG*-Registered Examinees						
First-Time Takers	7,892	50	8,013	58	15,906	54
Repeaters	6,094	32	6,199	41	12,293	37
ECFMG Total	**13,986**	**42**	**14,212**	**50**	**28,198**	**46**

* Educational Commission for Foreign Medical Graduates.

addition to allowing you to become familiar with the CBT format, the sample items provide the only questions direct from the test makers. Consider taking one block of questions from the sample test a few days before the actual exam. Allowing yourself one minute per question will approximate the pacing of the "real thing."

Consider saving a block of questions from the sample test to take a few days before the exam.

If I Freak Out and Leave, What Happens to My Score?

The 15-minute tutorial portion of the CBT exam is not considered part of the actual exam. Therefore, if you leave during or after the tutorial and before you actually begin the exam, there will be no record of your exam sitting.

Once you proceed to the first block of questions, you will be marked as having opened the exam. However, no score will be reported if you do not complete the exam. In fact, if you leave at any time from the start of the test to the last block, no score will be reported. However, the fact that you started but did not complete the exam will appear on your USMLE score transcript.

The exam ends when all blocks are completed or time has expired. As you leave the testing center, you will receive a written test-completion notice to document your completion of the exam.

In order to receive an official score, you must finish the entire exam. This means that you must start and either finish or run out of time for each block of the exam. Again, if you do not complete all the blocks, your exam will be documented as an incomplete attempt, and no score will be reported.

Adaptive Testing: The Next Generation

In the near future, the NBME plans to implement computer-adaptive sequential testing (CAST) in order to customize "the difficulty of the [USMLE] to the proficiency of each examinee across various stages of the examination." Essentially, this means that an "adaptive" exam will eventually use your performance on a block of questions to determine the difficulty of the block that follows. This will supposedly allow the exam to accurately assess your proficiency using fewer questions. Unlike most standardized exams you've seen, this means that all questions will not be created equal (i.e., they will not be worth the same).

When the NBME field-tested a CAST version of Step 1, its exam algorithm (Fig. 7) selected an easy, moderate, or difficult block of 60 new items based on the examinee's answers to the previous block. Highly proficient examinees tended to get progressively harder test materials, whereas less proficient examinees tended to get progressively easier test materials.

Under CAST, the difficulty of the items is directly factored into each examinee's final score. The NBME claims that "this process of customizing the test difficulty to each examinee's proficiency increases the overall accuracy of the scores and any related pass/fail decisions." The NBME adds, however, that although some examinees may receive more difficult blocks of questions, " . . . the score you achieve will not be affected by the difficulty of the question blocks selected for you." The NBME states that "every examinee will be tested on equivalent content."

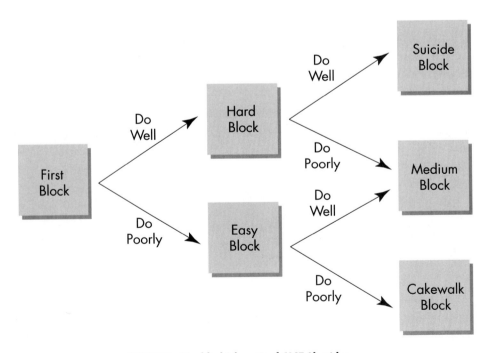

FIGURE 7. Simplified Schematic of CAST Algorithm

Will the new computerized USMLE be an "adaptive" exam? Not now, but eventually it will be. As of January 1999, NBME officials stated that the new computerized boards format would initially not be adaptive. This means that the new format for 1999 will simply be a computerized version of what was previously a written exam. After a period of testing, the NBME plans to change the exam to a CAST format, but no date has yet been set (probably sometime in the year 2000).

The Sylvan Learning Centers

Until now, Sylvan Learning Centers were known primarily for their focus on improving reading, writing, and arithmetic skills among children. In recent years, however, SLCs have expanded their scope to include the administration of graduate-level exams such as the Graduate Records Exam, the Graduate Management Admissions Test, and the National Board of Podiatric Medical Examiners (NBPME) tests. Sylvan administers testing programs for educational institutions, professional associations, corporations, and others through more than 500 test centers in over 80 countries globally.

The division responsible for the administration of the USMLE Step 2 is known as Sylvan Prometric. Sylvan Prometric represents a worldwide distribution network for computer-based testing services for academic admissions and professional licensure/certification.

Sylvan Technology Centers are centers that will be specially equipped with the computer hardware to deliver the CBT format. According to the NBME, these centers provide the "resources necessary for secure administration of USMLE, including video and audio monitoring and recording, and use of digital cameras to record the identity of individuals registered to take the examinations."

Up-to-date examination information may be obtained from the Sylvan website, http://www.educate.com, or from their toll-free number, 1-800-EDU-CATE (800-338-2283).

DEFINING YOUR GOAL

Arguably the first and most important thing to do in your Step 2 preparation is to define how well you want to do on the USMLE Step 2 exam. Your goals will ultimately determine the extent of preparation that will be necessary. The amount of time spent in preparation for this exam varies widely among med-

Less Competitive	More Competitive	Most Competitive
Pediatrics	Emergency Medicine	Dermatology
Family Practice	OB/GYN	ENT
Internal Medicine	Radiology	Orthopedics
Anesthesiology	General Surgery	Ophthalmology
Psychiatry		

FIGURE 8. Competitive Specialties

ical students, ranging anywhere from several months to two days (as in the jokingly stated adage "two weeks for Step 1, two days for Step 2, and a number-2 pencil for Step 3") to no preparation at all. Possible goals include:

- **"Simply passing."** This goal may be sufficient for the majority of US medical students. This may apply to you if you are entering a less competitive specialty.

- **Beating the mean.** Beating the mean (207 for recent exam administrations) signifies an ability to integrate your clinical and factual knowledge to an extent which is superior to that of your peers. Others redefine this goal as achieving a score one standard deviation above the mean (230). This is also the so-called "magic number" that many students have aimed for on the USMLE Step 1, as it supposedly represents the score that one must receive in order to be strongly considered by the more competitive residency programs (Fig. 8). Highly competitive residency programs may use your Step 1 and Step 2 (if available) scores as a screening tool or as selection criteria (Fig. 9). IMGs should aim to beat the mean, as USMLE scores are likely to be a selection factor even for less competitive US residency programs. For additional discussion of the residency application process and the USMLE Step 2, please refer to *First Aid for the Match* (ISBN 0838525962).

- **Acing the exam.** Perhaps you are one of those individuals for whom nothing less than the best will do—and for whom excelling on standardized exams is a source of pride and satisfaction. For you, the USMLE Step 2 will represent the culmination of several years of exams as well as a final opportunity as a medical student to excel at what you do best. An exceptional score on the USMLE Step 2 might also represent a way to "make up" for a less-than-satisfactory score on Step 1, especially if taken in the fall, so that it can be seen by residency programs and used to strengthen your application.

- **Evaluating your clinical knowledge.** This is a commendable goal that can be used as an addendum to any of the other goals mentioned in this section.

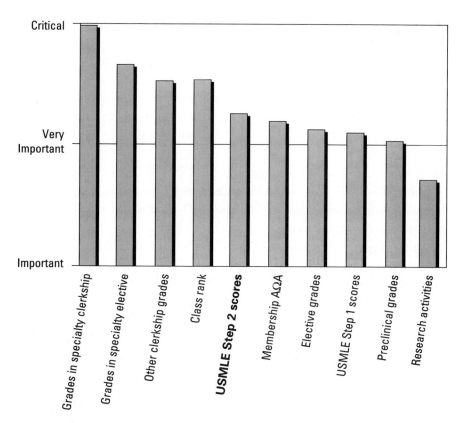

FIGURE 9. Academic Factors Important to Residency Directors

In many ways, this should be the ultimate rationale for taking the exam, since it is technically the reason the exam was designed in the first place. Specifically, the case-based nature of the USMLE Step 2 differs significantly from the more fact-based Step 1 exam in that it more thoroughly examines your ability to recognize classic clinical presentations, deal with acute emergent situations, and go through the step-by-step thought processes involved in the treatment of particular diseases. In short, this exam will allow you to assess your ability to apply your vast collection of medical facts to the situations you are likely to encounter during your residency.

- **Preparing for internship.** Making the transition to internship can be challenging. Studying for the USMLE Step 2 is an excellent way to review and consolidate all of the information that has slowly but surely been fading from memory during your third year. Use the Step 2 preparation as an opportunity to gear up for internship, especially if you are taking the exam in the spring.

When to Take the Exam

With CBT, you now have a wide variety of options regarding when to take Step 2. Here are a few factors to consider:

Step 2 is an opportunity to consolidate your clinical knowledge and prepare for internship.

17

- The nature of your objectives as defined above.
- The specialty in which you are applying. Some competitive residency programs may request your Step 2 scores. Ask your advisor or residency director at your school if this applies to you. If you already have a strong application, then taking Step 2 in the fall could potentially hurt you if you do poorly. However, if you need to shore up your application in a strong field, consider taking the exam (and truly preparing for it) in the fall.
- At many medical schools, passing the USMLE Step 2 is a prerequisite for graduation. This would be another reason to take the exam in the fall or winter. Should you fail, the CBT will allow you to retake the exam 60 days after your last exam date.
- **Proximity to clerkships.** Many students feel that the core clerkship material is fresher in their minds early in the fourth year, making a good argument for taking Step 2 earlier in the fall. Many students organize their rotation schedules such that they have numerous electives and a relatively "light" clinical load during their fourth year. Such students often discover that much of the clinical information they learned on their core rotations has faded. But don't forget that preparation for the USMLE Step 2 is also an excellent tool for review before internship.
- **The extent to which you seek a stress-free fourth year.** If you think it's very likely that you'll pass, you may want to take the exam later so that you don't have to worry about the possibility that your score will affect your match possibilities. On the other hand, taking the USMLE Step 2 exam early gets it out of the way allowing for a stress-free fourth year without the specter of an exam looming on the horizon.
- **The nature of your schedule.** Some students like to plan the test around a clerkship or vacation month in which they have some free time—or at least not when they are on their toughest fourth-year clerkship. It would be counterproductive to take the exam at the same time that you have scheduled a sub-internship in your planned specialty, since you will want to concentrate on performing well on the rotation for a good evaluation and, possibly, a letter of recommendation.

STUDY RESOURCES

Quality and Cost Considerations

Although there is an ever-increasing number of USMLE Step 2 review books and software on the market, the quality of the material is highly variable (see Section III, Database of Review Resources). Some common problems are as follows:

- Certain review books are too detailed to be reviewed in a reasonable amount of time or cover subtopics not emphasized on the exam (e.g., a 400-page anesthesiology book).
- Many sample question books were originally written years ago and have not been updated to reflect trends on the revised USMLE Step 2.
- Many sample question books use poorly written questions or contain factual errors in the explanations.
- Explanations for sample questions range from nonexistent to overly detailed.
- Software for boards review is of highly variable quality, may be difficult to install, and may be fraught with bugs.

Clinical Review Books

Most review books are the products of considerable effort by experienced educators. There are many such books, so you must choose which ones to buy on the basis of their relative merits. Although recommendations from other medical students are useful, many students simply recommend whatever books they used without having compared them to other books on the same subject. In a similar fashion, some students blindly advocate one publisher's series without considering the broad range of quality encountered within most series. Weigh different opinions against each other, read the reviews and ratings in Section III of this guide, and examine the books closely in the bookstore. You are investing not only money but also your limited study time. Do not worry about finding the "perfect" book, as many subjects simply do not have one. The best review book for you reflects the way you like to learn.

There are two types of review books: books that are stand-alone titles and books that are part of a series. Books in a series generally have the same style, and you must decide if that style is helpful for you. However, a given style is not optimal for every subject.

Find out which books are up to date. Some new editions represent major improvements, whereas others contain only cursory changes. You should take into consideration how a book reflects the format of the USMLE Step 2. Some may not have been updated adequately to reflect the changing question style and format of the current USMLE Step 2.

Texts and Notes

Unless you are planning an all-out offensive against Step 2 (and actually have the time), avoid standard texts in preparing for it. Many textbooks are too detailed for high-yield boards review. Even popular handbooks like the *Washington Manual* can be a chore to read, as they were designed for directed reading and reference rather than for cover-to-cover perusal. When using

If a given review book is not working for you, stop using it no matter how highly rated it may be.

texts or notes, engage in active learning by making tables, diagrams, new mnemonics, and conceptual associations whenever possible. If you already have your own mnemonics, then do not bother trying to memorize those of someone else. Supplement incomplete or unclear material with reference to other appropriate textbooks. Keep a good medical dictionary on hand to sort out definitions.

Commercial Courses

Commercial preparation courses can be helpful for some students, but they are expensive and require significant time commitment. They are often effective in organizing study material for students who feel overwhelmed by the sheer volume of material involved in preparing for Step 2. Note, however, that multiweek courses may be quite intense and may thus leave limited time for independent study. Note also that some commercial courses are designed for first-time test takers while others focus on students who are repeating the examination. Still other courses focus on IMGs, who must take all three Steps in a limited amount of time. See page 384 for contact information on several commercial review courses.

Practice Tests

Taking practice tests provides valuable information about strengths and weaknesses in your fund of knowledge and test-taking skills. Some students use practice examinations simply as a means of breaking up the monotony of studying and adding variety to their study schedule. Other students study almost entirely from practice tests. Students report that many practice tests have questions that are, on average, shorter and less clinically oriented than the current USMLE Step 2. Step 2 questions demand fast reading skills and application of clinical facts in a problem-solving format. Approach sample examinations critically, and do not waste time with low-quality questions until you have exhausted better sources.

Use practice tests to identify concepts and areas of weakness, not just facts that you missed.

After taking a practice test, try to identify concepts and areas of weakness, not just the facts that you missed. Use the experience to motivate your study and prioritize what areas need the most work.

Use quality practice examinations to improve your test-taking skills. This is especially important to help familiarize yourself with the style of the USMLE Step 2. Analyze your ability to pace yourself so that you have enough time to complete each block comfortably. Practice examinations are also a good means of training yourself to concentrate for long periods of time under appropriate time pressure. Analyze the pattern of your responses to questions to determine if you have made systematic errors in answering questions. Common mistakes are reading too much into the question, second-guessing your initial impression, and misinterpreting the question.

TEST-TAKING STRATEGIES

By now, you are probably familiar with USMLE exams and most likely have worked out some of your own strategies. However, the clinical vignette style of USMLE Step 2 may be unfamiliar to you. Using student experience from recent Step 2 exams, here are a few strategies that may be helpful.

Planning

If you are unfortunate enough to be on a difficult rotation at the time of the USMLE Step 2, you will need to plan ahead and start studying earlier. A demanding call schedule may leave you chronically tired. Ask your resident early if you can take a couple of call nights off in order to catch up on some rest just before the exam. Regardless of what rotation you are on, make sure to give your resident and the attending advance warning of exam dates. This will allow them to make adjustments in the call schedule for you, as well as to arrange for coverage of your patients if you are on a sub-internship.

Things to Bring with You to the Exam

Don't forget your scheduling permit and a photo ID that includes your signature. You will **not** be admitted to the exam if you fail to bring your permit, and Sylvan will charge a $90.00 rescheduling fee. A watch is useful to help you pace yourself, although digital timers are not allowed. It may also be nice to have some snacks on hand for a little "sugar rush." They will need to be stored in a locker until you take a break. It might also be a good idea to bring your lunch because break time is limited. Also consider bringing fluids, but not too much; you don't want to waste valuable time running to the bathroom. Should you need earplugs, they will be provided at the STC. Finally, consider layering clothing to deal with temperature variations at the testing center.

Pacing

You have 60 minutes per block in which to complete 50 questions. The test is quite fast-paced. Many scenarios are lengthy and time-consuming to read. Many students report feeling pressed for time before they find a rhythm, so keep close track of time using the clock in the corner of the screen and possibly your analog watch. With CBT, examinees report that the most efficient use of time is to answer questions in order. You may, however, return to any problematic question within the same block.

Pacing is key with lengthy clinical vignettes.

Difficult Questions

Do not waste valuable time on difficult or impossible questions.

The cruel reality of the USMLE Step 2 exam is that no matter how much you study, there will still be questions you won't be able to answer. Plan for these. If you recognize that a question is not solvable in a reasonable period of time, do not waste time on it. Move on after making an educated guess; you will not be penalized for wrong answers. Remember, each USMLE exam contains 10–20% experimental questions that will not count toward your score. Don't let tough questions throw you.

Images

Many of the questions can be answered without the picture.

Don't be afraid of questions that include imaging, which may arise with topics such as radiology, dermatology, and ophthalmology. Most questions will be basic and will include common diagnoses. A quick review, however, can be helpful. Use the high-yield glossy section of this book and consider using short glossy segments of textbooks such as the one found in Harrison's. Try reading the clinical scenario, question, and answers prior to studying the x-ray or picture. If all else fails, pick the most common diagnosis. It is helpful to know the normal radiographic appearance of hands, feet, chest, and pelvis in order to recognize gross abnormalities that may be given on the exam.

Finding the "Meat" of the Question

Many of the clinical vignettes on Step 2 are painfully long and contain a significant amount of superfluous information. If you think you may be pressed for time, consider reading the stem of the question first and skimming the answers prior to reading the vignette. Sometimes, after reading the stem and answers, you might be able to seek out key pieces of information in the vignette to help you answer the question. A word of caution, however: Do not overlook details in tricky or tough questions. If you have time, it might indeed be worthwhile to read each vignette carefully to avoid making errors. Try the "meat of the question" technique on the sample items. It may not be useful for everyone.

Other Tidbits

Other helpful hints include the following:

- Note the age and race of the patient in each clinical scenario. In most questions, ethnicity is not given. When it is given, the ethnicity of the patient is often relevant. For example, African-American heritage contributes to the epidemiology, pathophysiology, prognosis, outcome, and even treatment of some diseases. Know these well (see high-yield facts), especially for more common diagnoses.
- Some of the questions that many students felt were the most difficult involved choosing the "most important initial step" or the "next step in

management" of a disease. It can be difficult to prioritize treatment options, so pay close attention to management strategies as you study. Students who took the fall 1998 Step 2 exam noted that treatment and management issues are often more important than differentials.

- Be able to recognize key factors that distinguish major diagnoses.
- Consider completing an emergency medicine rotation prior to taking Step 2. Questions about acute patient management (e.g., trauma) in an emergency setting are common.

TESTING AGENCIES

National Board of Medical Examiners (NBME)
Department of Licensing Examination Services
3750 Market Street
Philadelphia, PA 19104-3190
(215) 590-9700
http://www.nbme.org

Educational Commission for Foreign Medical Graduates (ECFMG)
3624 Market Street, Fourth Floor
Philadelphia, PA 19104-2685
(215) 386-5900 or (202) 293-9320
Fax: (215) 386-9196
http://www.ecfmg.org

Federation of State Medical Boards (FSMB)
400 Fuller Wiser Road, Suite 300
Euless, TX 76039-3855
(817) 571-2949
Fax: (817) 868-4099
http://www.fsmb.org

USMLE Secretariat
3750 Market Street
Philadelphia, PA 19104-3190
(215) 590-9600
http://www.usmle.org

NOTES

First Aid for the International Medical Graduate

International Medical Graduate (IMG) is the term now used to describe any student or graduate of a non-US or non-Canadian medical school, regardless of whether he or she is a US citizen. The old term "Foreign Medical Graduate" (FMG) was replaced because it was misleading when applied to US citizens attending medical schools outside the United States.

THE IMG'S STEPS TO LICENSURE IN THE UNITED STATES

In order to become licensed to practice in the United States, an IMG must go through the following steps (not necessarily in this order). You must complete these steps even if you are already a practicing physician and have completed a residency program in your own country:

- Complete the basic sciences program of your medical school (equivalent to the first two years of US medical school).
- Take the USMLE Step 1. You can do this while still in school or after graduating, but in either case your medical school must certify that you have completed the basic sciences part of your school's curriculum.
- Complete the clinical clerkship program of your medical school (equivalent to the third and fourth years of US medical school).
- Take the USMLE Step 2. If you are still in medical school, your school must certify that you are within one year of graduating if you are to be allowed to take Step 2.
- Take the Educational Commission for Foreign Medical Graduates (ECFMG) English test (or an equivalent to the Test of English as a Foreign Language recognized by the ECFMG).
- Graduate with your medical degree.
- Once you have passed Step 1, Step 2, and the English test, you must obtain an ECFMG certificate. You can get this from ECFMG (see below) after you have sent them a copy of your degree, which they will verify with your medical school. This can take eight weeks or more. You must have an ECFMG certificate if you wish to obtain a position in an accredited residency program; some programs do not allow you to apply unless you already have this certificate.
- Applicants who have not met all of the requirements for ECFMG certification on or before June 30, 1998, will be required to pass the Clinical Skills Assessment exam (see below) in order to obtain an ECFMG certificate.
- Apply for residency positions in your field of interest, either directly or through the National Residency Matching Program ("the Match"). You do not need to have an ECFMG certificate, to have graduated, or to have passed any USMLE step or the English test in order to apply for residencies, either directly or through the Match—but you do need to have passed all the examinations necessary for ECFMG certification (i.e., Step 1, Step 2, and the English test) by a certain deadline in order to be entered into the Match itself. If you have not passed all these exams, you will be automatically withdrawn from the Match.

- If you are not already a US citizen or green-card holder (permanent resident), you must obtain a visa that will allow you to enter and work in the United States.

- Some states require that IMGs obtain an educational/training/limited medical license that allows them to practice as a resident in the state in which their residency program is located. Your residency program may assist you with this application. Note that medical licensing is the prerogative of each individual state, not of the federal government, and that states vary with respect to their laws about licensing (although all 50 states recognize the USMLE).

- Take USMLE Step 3 during your residency, and then obtain a permanent medical license. Note that as an IMG you will not be able to take Step 3 and obtain an independent license until you have completed one, two, or three years of residency, depending on which state you live in (except in the states that allow IMGs to take Step 3 before starting residency—a fact important to IMGs seeking the H1B visa). However, even if you live in a state that requires two or three years of residency as a prerequisite to taking Step 3, you can still take Step 3 and then obtain a license in another state. Once you have a license in any state, you are permitted to practice in federal institutions such as VA hospitals and Indian Health Service facilities throughout the country. This can open the door to "moonlighting" opportunities. For details on individual state rules, write to the licensing board in the state in question or contact the Federation of State Medical Boards (FSMB; see below).

- Complete your residency and then take the appropriate specialty board exams in order to become board certified (e.g., in internal medicine or surgery). If you already have a specialty certification in your home country (e.g., in surgery or cardiology), some specialty boards may grant you six months' or one year's credit toward your total residency time.

Timing of the USMLE

For an IMG, the timing of a complete application is critical. It is extremely important that you send in your application early if you are to garner the maximum number of interview calls. A rough guide would be to complete all exam requirements by June of the year in which you wish to apply. This would translate into sending both your score sheets and your ECFMG certificate, which is imperative for an interview call, by this date.

Many IMGs also benefit from taking the USMLE Step 1 before Step 2 because a sizable portion of the Step 2 exam tests fundamental concepts of basic sciences. It should be added, however, that it is up to each candidate to arrive at his or her own time frame and to avoid procrastinating about taking this crucial test.

USMLE STEP 1 AND THE IMG

The USMLE Step 1 is administered by the ECFMG worldwide. The USMLE Step 1 is often the first—and, for most IMGs, the most challenging—hurdle to overcome. The USMLE is a standardized licensing system that gives IMGs a level playing field; that is to say, it is the same exam series taken by US graduates, even though it is administered by the ECFMG rather than by the National Board of Medical Examiners (NBME). This means that pass marks for IMGs for both Step 1 and Step 2 are determined by a standardized statistical process. In general, to pass Step 1, you will probably have to score higher than the bottom 8–10% of US and Canadian graduates in Step 1. In 1996, however, only 55% of ECFMG candidates passed Step 1 on their first attempt, compared with 93% of US and Canadian medical students and graduates.

Developing good test-taking strategies is especially critical for the IMG.

Of note, 1994–1995 data showed that USFMGs (US citizens attending non-US medical schools) performed 0.4 SD lower than IMGs (non-US citizens attending non-US medical schools).

As an IMG, you must do as well as you can on Step 1. Few if any students feel totally prepared to take Step 1, but IMGs in particular require serious study and preparation in order to reach their full potential on this exam. A poor score on Step 1 is a distinct disadvantage when applying for most residencies. Remember that if you pass Step 1, you cannot retake it to try to improve your score. Good Step 1 scores will lend credibility to your residency application.

Of interest is the fact that students from non-US medical schools perform worst in behavioral science and biochemistry (1.9 and 1.5 SDs below US students) and comparatively better in gross anatomy and pathology (0.7 and 0.9 SDs below US students). Although they are derived from 1994–1995, these data may help you focus your studying efforts.

A good Step 1 score is key to a strong IMG application.

Do commercial review courses help improve your scores? Reports vary, and such courses can be expensive. Many IMGs decide to try the USMLE on their own first and then consider a review course only if they fail. But many states require that you pass the USMLE within three attempts, so you do not have many chances. (For more information on review courses, see p. 384.)

28

In the past, the Step 2 examination had a reputation for being much easier than Step 1, but this no longer seems to be the case for IMGs or US medical students. In August 1996, 54% of ECFMG candidates passed Step 2 on their first attempt, compared with 95% of US and Canadian candidates. Also note that because this is a clinical sciences exam, cultural and geographic considerations play a greater role than is the case with Step 1. For example, if your medical education gave you a lot of exposure to malaria, brucellosis, and malnutrition but little to alcohol withdrawal, child abuse, and cholesterol screening, you must do some work to familiarize yourself with topics that are more heavily emphasized in US medicine. You must also have a basic understanding of the legal and social aspects of US medicine, because you will be asked questions about communicating with and advising patients.

Native English-speaking IMGs are also required to take the language test.

The English Language Test

All IMGs (including U.S. citizens) must take an English test, irrespective of their citizenship and native language. Although taking this exam may strike the native English speaker as absurd, the test is generally considered to be fair and appropriate. It does not involve any use of medical knowledge or medical terminology. In the first part, candidates listen to tape recordings of typical English conversations and are asked questions that assess their language comprehension. In the second part, written sentences with missing words are presented, and candidates are asked to choose an appropriate replacement that is both grammatically correct and meaningful. This test is strictly pass-fail—there is no numerical grade—and is generally not difficult for those who feel comfortable conversing in English.

There is a big difference between textbook learning of a language and actually being immersed in the culture that goes with it.

Clinical Skills Assessment

The ECFMG introduced the Clinical Skills Assessment (CSA) in 1998 in an effort to level the disparities that existed among the more than 1400 medical schools worldwide in terms of both curricula used and educational standards applied. The goal of the CSA was to ensure that IMGs could gather and interpret histories, perform physical examinations, and communicate in the English language at a level comparable to that of US graduates.

The CSA center simulates clinical encounters that would commonly occur in clinics, doctors' offices, and emergency departments. The test is standardized, which means that "standardized patients" (SPs)—i.e., actors who have been extensively trained to simulate various clinical problems—are trained to give the same responses to all candidates participating in the assessment. For quality assurance purposes, a videotape monitors all clinical encounters. Eleven cases are presented that are mixed in terms of age, sex, ethnicity, organ system, and discipline. The five main areas emphasized are:

- Eye, ear, nose, throat, and musculoskeletal system
- General symptoms
- Cardiopulmonary system
- GI and GU systems
- Neuropsychiatry

Candidates are scored on only 10 of the 11 patient encounters. The non-scored encounter is added for research purposes, with results applied to future administrations of the CSA.

Test Administration. Before entering each room, candidates are given an opportunity to review preliminary information on each SP. This information, which is posted on the door of each room, includes the following:

- Patient characteristics (name, age, sex)
- Chief complaint and vitals (temperature, respiratory rate, pulse, BP)

After entering each room, candidates are given 15 minutes (with a warning bell sounded at 10 minutes) to perform the clinical encounter, which should include introducing themselves to SPs, obtaining an appropriate history, performing a focused clinical exam, formulating a differential diagnosis, and planning a diagnostic workup. Candidates are expected to answer any questions SPs might pose as well as to discuss the diagnoses being considered and to advise SPs with respect to their follow-up plans. After candidates leave the room, they have 10 minutes to write a patient note (PN).

"Do's and Don'ts." A number of ground rules can be used to guide the clinical encounter. These include the following:

- Candidates are not permitted to perform rectal, pelvic/genital, or female breast exams. If a candidate feels that such examinations are warranted, he or she may suggest that they be conducted as part of the diagnostic workup.
- Candidates are not allowed to reenter a room once they have left it. It is therefore necessary to obtain all the information needed before ending the clinical encounter.
- Time is limited, so it is advisable to "home in" on relevant problems and to conduct a focused clinical exam. For example, if a 40-year-old diabetic and smoker presents with chest pain, candidates should rule out problems of cardiopulmonary, gastrointestinal, and musculoskeletal origin in efforts to narrow the examination down to these systems. A CNS exam should therefore be the last one on the candidate's list in this particular example.

Scoring of the CSA. Your score will be based on the clinical encounter as a whole and on your overall communication skills.

- **Integrated Clinical Encounter (ICE) score.** Your skills with respect to the clinical encounter will be evaluated as follows:

1. Although SPs will not evaluate your performance, they will document your ability to gather data pertinent to the clinical encounter. Specifically, SPs will document on checklists whether or not you successfully obtained relevant information or correctly performed the physical exam. Your final data gathering (DG) score will represent an average of your performance with all 10 SPs.

2. Health care professionals will rate your PN score according to predefined criteria, with your final PN score representing the average of your individual PN scores over all 10 clinical encounters. Your ICE score will then represent the sum of your DG and PN scores.

$$ICE = DG + PN$$

- **Communication (COM) score.** In addition to assessing your data-gathering skills, SPs will evaluate your interpersonal skills (IPS) and your proficiency in spoken English. Your IPS will be assessed on the following four criteria: rapport, interviewing skills, personal manner, and counseling. Your overall COM score will then represent the average of the sum of your IPS scores and your spoken English proficiency rating.

The grade you receive on the CSA will be either a "pass" or a "fail." To receive a "pass" grade, you will need to independently clear the standards set by experts on both the ICE and COM clinical encounter. CSA scores, like those of all ECFMG tests, are mailed in six to eight weeks.

Do You Need to Take the CSA? Well in advance of the CSA (i.e., months beforehand), you should take steps to ascertain whether you need to take this test. Candidates will be required to pass the CSA if they have not met all of the requirements for ECFMG certification on or before June 30, 1998. Those who are ECFMG certified or who have met all criteria for ECFMG certification before June 30, 1998, and who are applying for residency positions may be asked to take the CSA. The criteria for selecting candidates for residency spots vary according to individual programs, but historically programs have tended to select those candidates who have met the requirements that are current at the time of the selection process.

Applying for CSA. Applicants seeking to take the CSA must complete the four-part application form (Form 706O) in full and mail to the ECFMG along with a $1200 registration fee. By calling (215) 790-1982 (Monday through Friday, 8 AM to midnight EST), you can have an operator help you schedule your test date. It is advisable to have several preferred dates in mind (all within one year of your notification of registration). The operator will formally schedule you on a mutually acceptable day, and your admissions permit will then be mailed to you. Alternatively, you can schedule your CSA date through the Internet at http://www.ecfmg.org. There is no application deadline, since the CSA is administered throughout the year (except on major US holidays).

After the ECFMG receives your fee and application form and determines that you are eligible to take the CSA, you must schedule your test date within four months and take the CSA within one year of the date indicated on your notification of registration.

Test Site Location. The CSA is only administered at the following address:

ECFMG
3624 Market Street
CSA Center, 3rd Floor
Philadelphia, PA 19104-2685

If you are living outside the US, you will need to apply for a visa that will allow your lawful entry into the US in order to take the CSA. A B2 visa may be issued by a consulate. Documents that are recommended to facilitate this process include:

- The CSA admission permit
- Your medical diploma
- Transcripts from your medical school
- Your USMLE score sheets
- A sponsor letter or affidavit of support stating that you (if you are sponsoring yourself) or your sponsor will bear the expenses of your trip and that you have sufficient funds to meet that expense
- An alien status affidavit

Preparing for the CSA. You can prepare for the CSA by addressing common outpatient clinical issues. To improve doctor–patient communication skills, you can try "acting out" dialog with friends or relatives. Since time will be a major factor, do not forget to time the encounter as if it were a real test by giving yourself 15 minutes for data gathering and 10 minutes for the patient note. The following volumes may also be of use to you in your preparation for the CSA:

- *Manual of Family Practice*, Robert Taylor (Little, Brown)
- *Family Practice Review: Problem-Oriented Approach*, R. Swanson (Mosby)

RESIDENCIES AND THE IMG

It is becoming harder for IMGs to obtain United States residencies given the rising concerns about an oversupply of physicians in the United States. Official bodies such as the Council on Graduate Medical Education (COGME) have recommended that the total number of residency slots be reduced from the current 144% of the number of US graduates to 110%. Furthermore, changes introduced in the 1996 immigration law are likely to make it much harder for noncitizens or legal residents of the US to remain in the country after completing a residency.

In the 1997 residency Match, US-citizen IMG applications rose from 735 in 1995 to 1467 in 1997, but the percentage of such IMGs accepted dropped from 49.8% to 43.5%; for non-US-citizen IMGs, applications rose from 5675 in 1995 to 8090 in 1997, while the percentage accepted fell dramatically from 50.5% to 34.5%. These percentages are likely to drop further in the future, especially as some large hospitals that traditionally hire many IMGs (such as those in New York) cut back sharply on their residency slots.

VISA OPTIONS FOR THE IMG

As an IMG, you need a visa to work or train in the US unless you are a US citizen or a permanent resident (i.e., hold a green card). Two types of visas will enable you to accept a residency appointment in the US: J1 and H1B. Sponsoring residency programs (SRPs) prefer a J1 visa, since they need only issue a form (IAP 66) directly to an IMG, whereas in the case of an H1B visa, they have to go through considerable paperwork.

The J1 Visa. Also known as the Exchange Visitor Program, the J1 visa was started to give IMGs the chance to use their training experience in the United States to improve conditions in their home countries. As mentioned above, the INS authorizes most SRPs to issue Form IAP 66 in the same manner that I20s are issued to other international students in the US.

To enable an SRP to issue an IAP 66, you must obtain a certificate from the ECFMG indicating that you are eligible to participate in a residency program in the US. You must ask also the Ministry of Health in your country to issue a statement indicating that there is a need in your country for individuals with the medical skills you would acquire by joining a US residency program. This statement must bear the seal of your country's government and must be signed by a duly designated government official. The Health Ministry in your country should then send this statement to the ECFMG (or they may allow you to mail it directly to the ECFMG).

How does one know that the government in a given country will issue such a statement? In many countries, the Ministry of Health maintains a list of medical specialties in which there is a need for further training abroad. You can also consult seniors in your medical school or officials in the Ministry of Health in advance about these medical specialties. A word of caution, however: If you are applying for a residency in internal medicine and internists are not in short supply in your country, you may have to indicate an intention to pursue a subspecialty after completing your residency training.

The text of the statement should read as follows:

> Name of applicant for visa: _____. There currently exists in (your country) a need for qualified medical practitioners in the specialty of _____. (Name of applicant for visa) has filed a written assurance with the government of this country that he/she will return to (your country) upon completion of training in the United States and intends to enter the practice of medicine in the specialty for which training is being sought.
>
> Stamp (or seal and signature) of issuing official of named country.
> Dated_____

To facilitate the issuing of such a statement by the Ministry of Health in your country, you should submit a certified copy of the agreement or contract from your SRP in the US. The agreement or contract must be signed by you and the residency program official responsible for the training.

With a completed Form IAP 66, you should go to the nearest US consulate. As with other nonimmigrant visas, you must still show that you have a genuine nonimmigrant intent to return to your home country.

When you enter the US, bring your Form IAP 66 along with your visa. You are usually admitted to the US for the length of the J1 program, designated as "D/S," or duration of status. The duration of your program is indicated on the IAP 66.

Duration of Participation. The duration of a resident's participation in a program of graduate medical education or training is limited to the time normally required to complete such a program. If you would like to get an idea of the training time involved for the various medical subspecialties, you may consult the *Directory of Medical Specialties*, published by Marquis Who's Who for the American Board of Medical Specialties. The authority charged with determining the duration of time required by an individual IMG is the United States Information Agency (USIA). This may change, however, because the USIA is likely to be merged into the State Department.

The maximum amount of time for participation in a training program is ordinarily limited to seven years unless the IMG involved has demonstrated to the satisfaction of the USIA director that his or her home country has an exceptional need for further training. The USIA director may grant an extension of stay in the event that an IMG needs to repeat a year of clinical medical training or needs time for training or education to enable him or her to take an exam required for board certification.

Requirements After Entry into the US. Each year, all IMGs participating in a residency program on a J1 visa must provide the Attorney General of the United States with an affidavit (Form I-644) attesting that they are in good standing in the program of graduate medical education or training in which they are participating and that they will return to their home upon completion of their education or training.

Restrictions Under the J1 Visa. Not later than two years after the date of entry into the United States, an IMG participating in a residency program on a J1 visa is allowed one opportunity to change his or her designated program of graduate medical education or training if his or her director approves that change.

The J1 visa includes a condition called the "two-year foreign residence requirement." The relevant section of the Immigration and Nationality Act states:

> "Any exchange visitor physician coming to the United States on or after January 10, 1977, for the purpose of receiving graduate medical education or training is automatically subject to the two-year home-country physical presence requirement of section 212(e) of the Immigration and Nationality Act."

The law thus requires that a J1 visa holder, upon completion of the training program, leave the US for a period of at least two years. Currently there is pressure from the American Medical Association to extend this period to five years.

As an IMG on a J1 visa, you are ordinarily not allowed to change from J1 to other types of visas or (in most cases) to change from J1 to permanent residence while in the US until you have fulfilled the "foreign residence requirement." The purpose of the foreign residence requirement is to ensure that you as an IMG use the training obtained in the US for the benefit of your country. The US government may, however, waive the two-year foreign residence requirement under the following circumstances:

- If you can demonstrate a "well-founded fear of persecution" if forced to return to your country;
- If you can prove that returning to your country would result in "exceptional hardship" to you or to members of your immediate family who are US citizens or permanent residents; or
- If you are sponsored by an " interested governmental agency."

Applying for a J1 Visa Waiver. IMGs who have sought a waiver based on the last alternative have found it beneficial to approach the following potentially "interested government agencies":

- **The Department of Health and Human Services (HHS).** HHS's considerations for a waiver have been as follows: (1) the program or activity in which the IMG is engaged is "of high priority and of national or international significance in an area of interest" to HHS (merely providing medical services in a medically underserved area would not be sufficient); (2) the IMG must be an "integral" part of the program or activity "so that the loss of his/her services would necessitate discontinuance of the program or a major phase of it"; and (3) the IMG "must possess outstanding qualifications, training, and experience well beyond the usually expected accomplishments at the graduate, postgraduate, and residency levels and must clearly demonstrate the capability to make original and significant contributions to the program." In practice, HHS is more likely to recommend waivers for IMGs engaged in research than for those who treat patients. HHS waiver applications should be mailed to Joyce E. Jones, Executive Secretary, Exchange Visitor Review Board, Room 627-H, Hubert H. Humphrey Building, Department of Health and Human Services, 200 Independence Avenue, S.W., Washington, D.C. 20201.

- **The Veterans Administration (VA).** With over 170 health care facilities located in various parts of the US, the VA is a major employer of physicians in this country. In addition, many VA hospitals are affiliated with university medical centers. Unlike HHS, the VA will sponsor IMGs involved not only in research but also in patient care (regardless of specialty) and in teaching. The waiver applicant may engage in teaching and research in conjunction with clinical duties. Not unlike the HHS, however, the VA's latest guidelines (issued on June 22, 1994) provide that it will act as an "interested government agency" only when the loss of the IMG's services would necessitate the discontinuance of a program or a major phase of it and when recruitment efforts have failed to locate a US physician to fill a position.

  The procedure for obtaining a VA sponsorship for a J1 waiver is as follows: (1) the IMG should deal directly with the Human Resources Department at the local VA facility; and (2) the facility must request that the VA's chief medical director sponsor the IMG for a waiver. The waiver request should include the following documentation: (1) a letter from the director of the local facility describing the program, the IMG's immigration status, the health care needs of the facility, and the facility's recruitment efforts; (2) recruitment efforts, including copies of all job advertisements run within the preceding year; and (3) copies of the IMG's licenses, test results, board certifications, IAP 66 forms, etc.

The VA contact person in Washington, D.C., Brian McVeigh, should be contacted by the local medical facility rather than by IMGs or their attorneys.

- **The Appalachian Regional Commission (ARC).** The ARC is composed of more than a dozen states on the East Coast and in the South, including Alabama, Georgia, Kentucky, Maryland, Mississippi, New York, North Carolina, Ohio, Pennsylvania, South Carolina, Tennessee, Virginia, and West Virginia. Since 1992, the ARC has sponsored approximately 200 primary care IMGs annually in counties within its jurisdiction that have been designated as health professional shortage areas (HPSAs) by HHS.

In accordance with its February 1994 revision of its J1 waiver policies, the ARC requires that waiver requests be submitted initially to the ARC contact person in the state of intended employment. If the state concurs, a letter from the state's governor recommending the waiver must be addressed to Jesse J. White, Jr., the federal co-chairman of the ARC. The waiver request should include the following: (1) a letter from the facility to Mr. White stating the proposed dates of employment, the IMG's medical specialty, the address of the practice location, an assertion that the IMG will practice primary care for at least 40 hours per week in the HPSA, and details as to why the facility needs the services of the IMG; (2) a J1 Visa Data Sheet; (3) the ARC federal co-chairman's J1 Visa Waiver Policy and the J1 Visa Waiver Policy Affidavit and Agreement with the notarized signature of the IMG; (4) a contract of at least two years' duration; (5) evidence of the IMG's qualifications, including a resume, medical diplomas and licenses, and IAP 66 forms; and (6) evidence of recruitment efforts within the preceding six months. Copies of advertisements, copies of resumes received, and reasons for rejection must also be included. The ARC will not sponsor IMGs who have been out of status for six months or longer.

Requests for ARC waivers are processed in Washington, D.C. by Laura Dean Greathouse, ARC, 1666 Connecticut Avenue, N.W., Washington, D.C. 20235. ARC is usually able to forward a letter confirming that a waiver has been recommended to the USIA to the requesting facility or attorney within 30 days of the request.

- **The US Department of Agriculture (USDA).** The USDA sponsors physicians who practice in the following areas: family medicine, general surgery, pediatrics, obstetrics and gynecology, emergency medicine, internal medicine, and general psychiatry. The USDA will not sponsor a physician to practice in an area located within the jurisdiction of the ARC.

In order for an area to be deemed "rural," the county in which the health care facility is located would have had to have a population of under 20,000 according to the last census. Also, the facility must be located in an HPSA. The IMG must sign a contract with a health care facility for a minimum period of three years. No IMG whose immigration status has lapsed for six months or more will be considered for sponsorship by USDA.

Since August 1994, USDA has required that each request for a waiver be supported by a letter of concurrence ("no objection") from the Department of Health in the state of intended employment. A few states (e.g., Georgia, Mississippi, New York, and Ohio) require that the USDA waiver request and accompanying documentation be submitted directly to them. If they concur with the request, they forward the entire packet together with a no-objection letter to USDA.

USDA waiver requests should be mailed to Linda Seckel, Program Manager, J1 Visa Residency Waiver Program, Bldg. 005, Room 320, BARC-West, 10300 Baltimore Blvd., Beltsville, MD 20705-2350. The current processing time is approximately four months.

- **State Departments of Public Health.** There is no application form for a state-sponsored J1 waiver. However, USIA regulations specify that an application must include the following documents: (1) a letter from the State Department of Public Health identifying the physician and specifying that it would be in the public interest to grant him a J1 waiver; (2) an employment contract that is valid for a minimum of three years and that states the name and address of the facility for which the physician will be employed and the geographic areas in which he will practice medicine; (3) evidence that these geographic areas are located within HPSAs; (4) a statement by the physician agreeing to the contractual requirements; (5) copies of all IAP 66 forms; and (6) a completed USIA Data Sheet. In addition, each application is numbered sequentially, since the number of physicians who may be granted waivers in a particular state is limited to 20 per year. Individual states may choose to participate or not to participate in this program. Participating states include Alabama, Alaska, Arkansas, Arizona, Delaware, Florida, Georgia, Illinois, Indiana, Iowa, Kentucky, Maine, Massachusetts, Michigan, Minnesota, Mississippi, Missouri, Nebraska, Nevada, New Hampshire, New Mexico, New York, North Carolina, North Dakota, Ohio, Oklahoma, Pennsylvania, Rhode Island, South Carolina, Vermont, and Washington. Undecided states include California, Connecticut, New Jersey, Virginia and Wyoming. Nonparticipating states include Hawaii, Idaho, Kansas, Louisiana, Montana, Oregon, South Dakota, Tennessee, Texas, and Utah.

- **The H1B Visa.** Since 1991, the law has allowed medical residency programs to sponsor foreign-born medical residents for H1B visas. There are no restrictions to changing the H1B visa to any other kind of visa, including permanent resident status (green card), through employer sponsorship or through close relatives who are US citizens or permanent residents. There was an overall ceiling of 65,000 H1B visas for professionals in all categories until mid-1998, when the number was raised to 95,000. It is advisable for SRPs to apply for H1B visas as soon as possible in the official year (beginning October 1) when the new quota officially opens up.

H1B visas are intended for "professionals" in a "specialty occupation." This means that an IMG intending to pursue a residency program in the US with an H1B visa needs to pass all three steps of the USMLE before becoming eligible for the H1B. The ECFMG administers Steps 1 and 2. Step 3 is conducted by the individual states. You will need to contact the FSMB or the medical board of the state where you intend to take the Step 3 for details.

Basic eligibility requirements for USMLE Step 3 are as follows:

- Obtain the MD degree (or its equivalent) or a DO degree by the application deadline.
- Pass both USMLE Step 1 and Step 2 (or the equivalents). Applicants must receive notice of a passing score by the application deadline.
- Graduates of foreign medical schools should be ECFMG certified or successfully complete a "fifth pathway" program (at a date no later than the application deadline).
- Apply to the following states, which do not have postgraduate training as an eligibility requirement:

  1. **California**
     Medical Board of California
     1426 Howe Ave., Suite 54
     Sacramento, CA 95825-3236
     www.medbd.ca.gov
     Phone: (916) 263-2389; Fax: (916) 263-2387
     Licensure inquiries: (916) 263-2499; (916) 263-2344

  2. **Connecticut**
     Connecticut Department of Public Health
     PO Box 340308
     Hartford, CT 06134-0308
     Phone: (860) 509-7579; Fax: (860) 509-8457
     Step 3 inquiries: FSMB at (817) 571-2949

3. **Louisiana**
   Louisiana State Board of Medical Examiners
   PO Box 30250
   New Orleans, LA 70190-0250
   Phone: (504) 524-6763; Fax: (504) 568-8893

4. **Maryland**
   Maryland Board of Physician Quality Assurance
   PO Box 2571
   Baltimore, MD 21215-0095
   Phone: (410) 764-4777; Fax: (410) 764-2478
   Step 3 inquiries: (800) 877-3926

5. **Nebraska***
   Nebraska Department of Health
   PO Box 94986
   Lincoln, NE 68509-4986
   www.hhs.state.ne.us
   Phone: (402) 471-2118; Fax: (402) 471-3577
   Step 3 inquiries: FSMB at (817) 571-2949

6. **Nevada**
   Nevada State Board of Medical Examiners
   P.O. Box 7238
   Reno, NV 89510
   (702) 688-2559; Fax: (702) 688-2321
   Step 3 inquiries: FSMB at (817) 571-2949

7. **New York**
   New York State Board of Medicine
   Cultural Education Center, Room 3023
   Empire State Plaza
   Albany, NY 12230
   Phone: (518) 474-3841; Fax: (518) 473-6995

8. **Rhode Island**
   Rhode Island Board of Medical Licensure and Discipline
   Department of Health
   Cannon Building, Room 205
   Three Capitol Hill
   Providence, RI 02908-5097
   Phone: (401) 277-3855; Fax: (401) 277-2158
   Step 3 inquiries: FSMB at (817) 571-2949

*Nebraska requires that IMGs obtain a "valid indefinitely" ECFMG certificate.

9. **South Dakota**
   South Dakota State Board of Medical and Osteopathic Examiners
   1323 S. Minnesota Ave.
   Sioux Falls, SD 57105
   Phone: (605) 334-8343; Fax: (605) 336-0270
   Step 3 inquiries: FSMB at (817) 571-2949

10. **Tennessee**
    Tennessee Board of Medical Examiners
    425 5th Avenue North
    1st Floor, Cordell Hull Building
    Nashville, TN 37247-1010
    Phone (615) 532-4384; Fax: (615) 532-5369
    Step 3 inquiries: FSMB at (817) 571-2949

11. **Utah**
    Utah Department of Commerce
    Division of Occupational & Professional Licensure
    PO Box 146741
    Salt Lake City, UT 84114-6741
    Phone: (801) 530-6628; Fax: (801) 530-6511

12. **West Virginia**
    West Virginia Board of Medicine
    101 Dee Dr.
    Charleston, WV 25311
    Phone (304) 558-2921; Fax: (304) 723-2877

H1B Application. An application for an H1B visa is not filed by the intending immigrating professional but by his or her employment sponsor—in your case, by the SRP in the US. If an SRP is willing to do so, you will be told about it at the time of your interview for the residency program.

Before filing an H1B application with the INS, an SRP must file an application with the US Labor Department affirming that the SRP will pay at least the normal salary for your job that a US professional would earn. After receiving approval from the Labor Department, your SRP should be ready to file the H1B application with the INS. The SRP's supporting letter is the most important part of the H1B application package; it must describe the job duties involved to make it clear that the physician is needed in a "specialty occupation" (resident) under the prevalent legal definition of that term.

Most SRPs prefer to issue an IAP 66 for a J1 visa to filing papers for an H1B visa because of the burden of paperwork and the attorney costs involved in securing approval of an H1B visa application. Even so, a sizable number of SRPs are willing to go through the trouble, particularly if an IMG is an excellent candidate or if the SRP concerned finds it difficult to fill all the available residency slots (rarer with continuing cuts in residency spots). If an SRP is unwilling to do so because of attorney costs, it is advisable for you to suggest that you would be willing to bear the burden of such costs. The entire process of getting an H1B visa can take anywhere from 10 to 20 weeks.

Although an H1B visa can be stamped by any US consulate abroad, it is advisable to get it done at the US consulate where you first applied for a visitor visa to travel to the US for interviews.

Summary. Despite some significant obstacles, a number of viable methods are available to IMGs who seek to pursue a residency program or eventually practice medicine in the US.

There is no doubt that the best alternative for IMGs is to obtain H1B visas to pursue their medical residencies. However, in cases where an IMG joins a residency program with a J1 visa, there are some possibilities of obtaining waivers of the two-year foreign residency requirement, particularly for those who are willing to make a commitment to perform primary care medicine in medically underserved areas.

RESOURCES FOR THE IMG

- ECFMG
  3624 Market Street, Fourth Floor
  Philadelphia, PA 19104-2685
  (215) 386-5900 or (202) 293-9320
  Fax: (215) 386-9196
  http://www.ecfmg.org

  This number is answered only between 9:00 AM and 12:30 PM and between 1:30 PM and 5:00 PM Monday through Friday EST. The ECFMG often takes a long time to answer the phone and is frequently busy at peak times of the year, and there is then a long voice-mail message, so it is better to write or fax early than to rely on a last-minute phone call. Do not contact the NBME, as all IMG exam affairs are conducted by the ECFMG. The ECFMG also publishes the *Handbook for Foreign Medical Graduates and Information Booklet* on ECFMG certification and the USMLE program, which gives details of dates and locations of forthcoming USMLE, CSA, and English tests for IMGs together with application forms. It is free of charge and is also available from the public affairs offices of US embassies and consulates worldwide, as well as from Overseas Educational Advisory Centers. Single copies of the handbook may also be ordered by calling (215) 386-5900, preferably on weekends or between 6 PM and 6 AM Philadelphia time, or by faxing to (215) 387-9963. Requests for multiple copies must be made by fax or mail on organizational letterhead. The full text of the booklet is also available on the ECFMG's website at http://www.ecfmg.org/content.htm#Top.

- Federation of State Medical Boards
  400 Fuller Wiser Road, Suite 300
  Euless, TX 76039-3855
  (817) 868-4000
  Fax: (817) 868-4099

The FSMB publishes Exchange, Section I, which gives detailed information on examination and licensing requirements in all US jurisdictions. The 1996–1997 edition costs $25. (Texas residents must add 7.75% state sales tax.) To obtain publications, write to Federation Publications at the above address. All orders must be prepaid by a personal check drawn on a US bank, a cashier's check, or a money order payable to the Federation. Foreign orders must be accompanied by an international money order or the equivalent, payable in US dollars through a US bank or a US affiliate of a foreign bank. For Step 3 inquiries, the telephone number is (817) 868-4000, and the fax number is (817) 868-4099.

- Some of the Step 1 commercial review courses listed in Section III are conducted outside the United States. Write or call the course providers for details.
- The ECFMG has a home page on http://www.ecfmg.org with the complete *ECFMG Information Booklet* available online. Late announcements (e.g., dates of mailing out score reports) are also made on this site.
- The FSMB has a home page at http://www.fsmb.org
- The Internet newsgroups misc.education.medical and bit.listsery.medforum can be valuable forums through which to exchange information on licensing exams, residency applications, and so on.
- Some immigration information for IMGs is available from the various sites of Siskind, Susser, Haas & Chang, a firm of attorneys specializing in immigration law, on the following websites, which include a searchable index and a free e-mail subscription to immigration law bulletins:
  http://www.telalink.net/~gsiskind/bulletin.html
  http://www.visalaw.com/~gsiskind/95feb/2feb95.html
  http://www.telalink.net/~gsiskind/95feb/2feb95.html
  http://www.americanlaw.com/q&a28.html
- Another source of immigration information can be found on the website of the law offices of Carl Shusterman, a Los Angeles lawyer specializing in medical immigration law:
  http://websites/earthlink.net/~visalaw
- International Medical Placement Ltd., a US company specializing in recruiting foreign physicians to work in the United States, has a site at http://www.cyberdeas.com/imp. This site includes ordering information for several publications by FMSG, Inc., including USMLE Study Guides and residency matching information, as well as details on USMLE lecture courses offered by the author of these publications, Dr. Stanley Zaslau. The site also has information on seminars held by the company in foreign countries for physicians who are thinking of moving to the United States.

43

- *The International Medical Graduates' Guide to U.S. Medicine: Negotiating the Maze* by Louise B. Ball (199 pages; ISBN 1883620163) can be obtained from:
Galen Press
PO Box 64400
Tucson, AZ 85728-4400
(800) 442-5369 (United States and Canada) or (520) 577-8363
Fax: (520) 520-6459

This book has a lot of detailed information and is particularly strong on the intricacies of immigration law as it applies to foreign-citizen IMGs who wish to practice in the United States—although this is a rapidly changing field, and some of the information is probably out of date already. Also note that much of the book's contents may be relevant only to some IMGs, as many chapters are geared toward specific problems or situations (e.g., how to sponsor a relative, how a small American town may try to sponsor a foreign physician, how a US faculty member can sponsor a foreign clinical research fellow), and there is considerable repetition across chapters.

Bottom line: Great for foreign citizens who need help in understanding how to "negotiate the maze" of medical immigration regulations, but not necessarily high yield for many other IMGs.

Preclinical Primer

Anatomy
Behavioral Science
Biochemistry
Microbiology
Pathology
Pharmacology
Physiology

The second edition of *First Aid for the USMLE Step 2* introduces a basic sciences review for Step 2. A significant portion of material tested on Step 2 includes clinically relevant basic science facts normally tested on Step 1. The Preclinical Primer is a collection of highly clinical basic science facts taken directly from *First Aid for the USMLE Step 1*. The facts are organized according to the seven traditional basic medical science disciplines (anatomy, behavioral science, biochemistry, microbiology, pathology, pharmacology, and physiology). Individual facts are generally presented in a three-column format, with the **Title** of the fact in the first column, the **Description** of the fact in the second column, and the **Mnemonic** or **Special Note** in the third column. Each fact was selected for its **clinical relevance** to Step 2. Think of it as our greatest Step 1 "hits" collection. Most of this material will be very familiar to you, so it should be a nice stroll down memory lane.

| **Meckel's diverticulum** 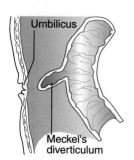 | Persistence of the vitelline duct or yolk stalk. May contain ectopic acid–secreting gastric mucosa and/or pancreatic tissue. Most common congenital anomaly of the GI tract. Can cause bleeding or obstruction near the terminal ileum. Contrast with omphalomesenteric cyst = cystic dilatation of vitelline duct. | The five 2's: 2 inches long. 2 feet from the ileocecal valve. 2% of population. Commonly presents in first 2 years of life. May have 2 types of epithelia. |

Amniotic fluid abnormalities

| Polyhydramnios | > 1.5–2 L of amniotic fluid; associated with esophageal/duodenal atresia, anencephaly. |
| Oligohydramnios | < 0.5 L of amniotic fluid; associated with bilateral renal agenesis or posterior urethral valves (in males). |

| **Unhappy triad/ knee injury** 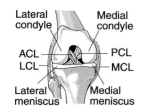 | This common football injury (caused by clipping from the lateral side) consists of damage to medial collateral ligament (MCL), medial meniscus, and anterior cruciate ligament (ACL). PCL = posterior cruciate ligament. LCL = lateral collateral ligament. | Positive anterior drawer sign indicates tearing of the anterior cruciate ligament. "Anterior" and "posterior" in ACL and PCL refer to sites of **tibial** attachment. |

| **Chorea** | Sudden, jerky, purposeless movements. Characteristic of basal ganglia lesion (e.g., Huntington's disease). | *Chorea* = dancing (Greek). Think choral dancing or choreography. |

| **Athetosis** | Slow, writhing movements, especially of fingers. Characteristic of basal ganglia lesion. | *Athetos* = not fixed (Greek). Think snakelike. |

| **Hemiballismus** | Sudden, wild flailing of one arm. Characteristic of contralateral subthalamic nucleus lesion. | Half ballistic (as in throwing a baseball). |

| **Tremors: cerebellar versus basal** | Cerebellar tremor = intention tremor. Basal ganglion tremor = resting tremor. | Basal = at rest (**Park**inson's disease) when **Park**ed. |

Brain lesions

Area of lesion	Consequence	
Broca's area	Motor (expressive) aphasia	**BRO**ca's is **BRO**ken speech.
Wernicke's area	Sensory (fluent) aphasia	Wernicke's is **W**ordy but
Amygdala (bilateral)	Klüver–Bucy syndrome (hyperorality, hypersexuality, disinhibited behavior)	makes no sense.
Frontal lobe	Frontal release signs (e.g., personality changes and deficits in concentration, orientation, judgment)	
Right parietal lobe	Spacial neglect syndrome (agnosia of the contralateral side of the world)	
Reticular activating system	Coma	
Mamillary bodies (bilateral)	Wernicke–Korsakoff's encephalopathy (confabulations, anterograde amnesia).	

Internuclear ophthalmoplegia	Lesion in the medial longitudinal fasciculus (MLF). Results in medial rectus palsy on attempted lateral gaze. Nystagmus in abducting eye. Convergence is normal. MLF syndrome is seen in many patients with multiple sclerosis.	MLF = **M**S
Lower motor neuron (LMN) signs	LMN injury signs: atrophy, flaccid paralysis, absent deep tendon reflexes. Fasciculations may be present.	**Lower** MN ≈ everything **lower**ed (less muscle mass, **decreased** muscle tone, **decreased** reflexes, **down**going toes).
Upper motor neuron (UMN) signs	UMN injury signs: little atrophy, spastic paralysis (clonus), hyperactive deep tendon reflexes, possible positive Babinski.	**Upper** MN ≈ everything **up** (tone, DTRs, toes).

Reportable diseases	Only some infectious diseases are reportable, including AIDS (but not HIV positivity), chickenpox, gonorrhea, hepatitis A and B, measles, mumps, rubella, salmonella, shigella, syphilis, tuberculosis.

Exceptions to confidentiality

1. Potential harm to third parties is serious
2. Likelihood of harm is high
3. No alternative means exist to warn or to protect those at risk
4. Third party can take steps to prevent harm

Examples include:
1. Infectious diseases—physicians may have a duty to warn public officials and identifiable people at risk
2. The Tarasoff decision—law requiring physician to protect potential victim from harm; may involve breach of confidentiality
3. Child and/or elder abuse
4. Impaired automobile drivers
5. Suicidal/homicidal patient
6. Domestic violence

Developmental milestones

	Approximate age	Milestone
Infant	3 mo	Holds head up, social smile, Moro reflex disappears
	4–5 mo	Rolls front to back, sits when propped
	7–9 mo	Stranger anxiety, sits alone, orients to voice
	12–14 mo	Upgoing Babinski disappears
	15 mo	Walking, few words, separation anxiety
Toddler	12–24 mo	Object permanence
	18–24 mo	Rapprochement
	24–48 mo	Parallel play
	24–36 mo	Core gender identity
Preschool	30–36 mo	Toilet training
	3 y	Group play, rides tricycle, copies line or circle drawing
	4 y	Cooperative play, simple drawings (stick figure), hops on one foot
School age	6–11 y	Development of conscience (superego), same-sex friends, identification with same-sex parent
Adolescence (puberty)	11 y (girls) 13 y (boys)	Abstract reasoning (formal operations), formation of personality

Grief

Normal bereavement characterized by shock, denial, guilt and somatic symptoms. Typically lasts 6 mo–1 yr.

Pathologic grief includes excessively intense or prolonged grief, or grief that is delayed, inhibited or denied.

HIGH-YIELD FACTS

Preclinical Primer

Sleep apnea	Central sleep apnea: no respiratory effort. Obstructive sleep apnea: respiratory effort against airway obstruction. Person stops breathing for at least 10 sec during sleep. Associated with obesity, loud snoring, systemic/pulmonary hypertension, arrhythmias, and possibly sudden death. Individuals may become chronically tired.
Somatoform disorders	Both illness production and motivation are unconscious drives. Several types: 1. Conversion—symptoms suggest motor or sensory neurologic or physical disorder but tests and physical exam are negative 2. Somatoform pain disorder—conversion disorder with pain as presenting complaint 3. Hypochondriasis—misinterpretation of normal physical findings, leading to preoccupation with and fear of having a serious illness in spite of medical reassurance 4. Somatization—variety of complaints in multiple organ systems 5. Body dysmorphic disorder—patient convinced that part of own anatomy is malformed 6. Pseudocyesis—false belief of being pregnant associated with objective signs of pregnancy

BIOCHEMISTRY

Galactosemia	Absence of galactose-1-phosphate uridyltransferase. Autosomal recessive. Damage is caused by accumulation of toxic substances (including galactitol) rather than absence of an essential compound. Symptoms: cataracts, hepatosplenomegaly, mental retardation. Treatment: exclude galactose and lactose (galactose + glucose) from diet.
Lactase deficiency	Age-dependent and/or hereditary lactose intolerance (blacks, Asians). Symptoms: bloating, cramps, osmotic diarrhea. Treatment: avoid milk or add lactase pills to diet.
Phenylketonuria	Normally, phenylalanine is converted into tyrosine (nonessential aa). In PKU, there is ↓ phenylalanine hydroxylase or ↓ tetrahydrobiopterin cofactor. Tyrosine becomes essential and phenylalanine builds up, leading to excess phenylketones. Findings: mental retardation, fair skin, eczema, musty body odor. Treatment: ↓ phenylalanine (contained in Nutrasweet) and ↑ tyrosine in diet.	Screened for at birth. Phenylketones = phenylacetate, phenyllactate, and phenylpyruvate in urine.

Hyperbilirubinemia

From conjugated (direct; glucuronidated) and/or unconjugated (indirect) bilirubin.

Causes: massive hemolysis, block in subsequent catabolism of heme, displacement from binding sites on albumin, decreased excretion (e.g., liver damage or bile duct obstruction). Bilirubin is yellow, causing jaundice.

UNconjugated is **IN**direct and **IN**soluble.
Conjugated bilirubin is excreted in the urine.

Ketone bodies

In liver: fatty acid and amino acids → acetoacetate + β-hydroxybutyrate (to be used in muscle and brain). Ketone bodies found in prolonged starvation and diabetic ketoacidosis. Excreted in urine. Made from HMG-CoA. Ketone bodies are metabolized by the brain to 2 molecules of acetyl CoA.

Breath smells like acetone (fruity odor). Urine test for ketones does not detect β-hydroxybutyrate (favored by high redox state).

Vitamins

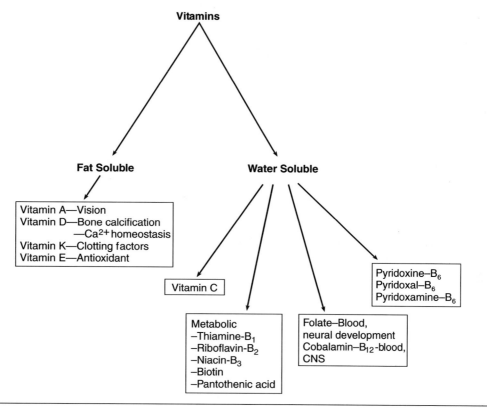

Vitamin A (retinol)

Deficiency	Night blindness and dry skin.	Retinol is vitamin A, so think Retin-A (used topically for wrinkles and acne).
Function	Constituent of visual pigments (retinal).	
Excess	Arthralgias, fatigue, headaches, skin changes, sore throat, alopecia.	

Vitamin B$_1$ (thiamine)

Deficiency	Beriberi and Wernicke–Korsakoff syndrome. Seen in alcoholism and malnutrition.	Beriberi: characterized by polyneuritis, cardiac pathology, and edema. Spell beriberi as Ber1Ber1.
Function	In thiamine pyrophosphate, a cofactor for oxidative decarboxylation of α-keto acids (pyruvate, α-ketoglutarate) and a cofactor for transketolase.	Wet beriberi may lead to high output cardiac failure.

Vitamin B$_2$ (riboflavin)

Deficiency	Angular stomatitis, Cheilosis, Corneal vascularization.	The 2 C's
Function	Cofactor in oxidation and reduction (e.g., $FADH_2$).	FAD and FMN are derived from riboFlavin (B$_2$ = 2 ATP).

Vitamin B$_3$ (niacin)

Deficiency	Pellagra can be caused by Hartnup disease, malignant carcinoid syndrome and INH.	Pellagra's symptoms are the 3 D's: Diarrhea, Dermatitis, Dementia (also beefy glossitis).
Function	Constituent of NAD^+, $NADP^+$ (used in redox reactions). Derived from tryptophan.	NAD derived from Niacin (B$_3$ = 3 ATP).

Vitamin B$_5$ (pantothenate)

Deficiency	Dermatitis, enteritis, alopecia, adrenal insufficiency.	
Function	Constituent of CoA, part of fatty acid synthase. Cofactor for acyl transfers.	Pantothen-A is in Co-A.

Vitamin B$_6$ (pyridoxine)

Deficiency	Convulsions, hyperirritability (deficiency inducible by INH).
Function	Converted to pyridoxal phosphate, a cofactor used in transamination (e.g., ALT and AST), decarboxylation, and trans-sulfuration.

Biotin

Deficiency	Dermatitis, enteritis. Caused by antibiotic use, ingestion of raw eggs.	
Function	Cofactor for carboxylations (pyruvate carboxylase, acetyl-CoA carboxylase, propionyl-CoA carboxylase) but not decarboxylations.	"Buy-a-tin of CO_2" for carboxylations.

Folic acid

Deficiency
- Most common vitamin deficiency in US.
- Macrocytic, megaloblastic anemia (often no neurologic symptoms), sprue.

Function
- Coenzyme for one-carbon transfer; involved in methylation reactions.
- Important for the synthesis of nitrogenous bases in DNA and RNA.

Folate from Foliage.
Eat green leaves (because folic acid is not stored very long). Supplemental folic acid in early pregnancy reduces neural tube defects.
PABA is the folic acid precursor in bacteria. Sulfa drugs and dapsone are PABA analogs.

Vitamin B$_{12}$ (cobalamin)

Deficiency
- Macrocytic, megaloblastic anemia; neurologic symptoms (optic neuropathy, subacute combined degeneration, paresthesia); glossitis.

Function
- Cofactor for homocysteine methylation and methyl-malonyl-CoA handling.
- Stored primarily in the liver.
- Synthesized only by microorganisms.

Found only in animal products.
Vit. B$_{12}$ deficiency is usually caused by malabsorption (sprue, enteritis, *Diphyllobothrium latum*), lack of intrinsic factor (pernicious anemia), or absence of terminal ileum (Crohn's disease).
Use Schilling test to detect deficiency.

Vitamin C (ascorbic acid)

Deficiency
- Scurvy.

Function
- Necessary for hydroxylation of proline and lysine in collagen synthesis.
- Scurvy findings: swollen gums, bruising, anemia, poor wound healing.

Vitamin C Cross-links Collagen. British sailors carried limes to prevent scurvy (origin of the word "limey").

Vitamin D

- D$_2$ = ergocalciferol, consumed in milk.
- D$_3$ = cholecalciferol, formed in sun-exposed skin.
- 25-OH D$_3$ = storage form.
- 1,25 (OH)$_2$ D$_3$ = active form.

Deficiency
- Rickets in children (bending bones), osteomalacia in adults (soft bones), and hypocalcemic tetany.

Function
- Increases intestinal absorption of calcium and phosphate.

Excess
- Hypercalcemia, loss of appetite, stupor. Seen in sarcoidosis, a disease where the epithelioid macrophages convert vit. D into its active form.

Remember that drinking milk (fortified with vitamin D) is good for bones.

Vitamin E

Deficiency
- Increased fragility of erythrocytes.

Function
- Antioxidant (protects erythrocytes from hemolysis).

Vitamin E is for Erythrocytes.

Vitamin K

Deficiency	Neonatal hemorrhage with ↑ PT, ↑ aPTT, but normal bleeding time.	K for Koagulation. Note that the vitamin K–dependent clotting factors are II, VII, IX, X, and protein C and S. Warfarin is a vitamin K antagonist.
Function	Catalyzes γ-carboxylation of glutamic acid residues on various proteins concerned with blood clotting. Synthesized by intestinal flora. Therefore, vit. K deficiency can occur after the prolonged use of broad-spectrum antibiotics.	

MICROBIOLOGY

Clostridia (with exotoxins)	All gram-positive, spore-forming, anaerobic bacilli. *Clostridium tetani* produces an exotoxin causing tetanus. C. *botulinum* produces a preformed, heat-labile toxin that inhibits ACh release, causing botulism. C. *perfringens* produces α toxin, a hemolytic lecithinase that causes myonecrosis or gas gangrene. C. *difficile* produces a cytotoxin, an exotoxin that kills enterocytes, causing pseudomembranous colitis. Often secondary to antibiotic use, especially clindamycin or ampicillin.	**Tet**anus is **tet**anic paralysis (blocks glycine, an inhibitory neurotransmitter). **Bot**ulinum is from bad **bot**tles of food (causes a flaccid paralysis). **Perf**ringens **perf**orates a gangrenous leg. **Diffi**cile causes **di**arrhea. Treat with metronidazole.
Bugs causing food poisoning	*Vibrio parahaemolyticus* and *Vibrio vulnificus* in contaminated seafood. *Bacillus cereus* in reheated rice. *Staphylococcus aureus* in meats, mayonnaise, custard. *Clostridium perfringens* in reheated meat dishes.	**V**omit **B**ig **S**melly **C**hunks. *Staphylococcus aureus* food poisoning starts quickly, ends quickly. "Food poisoning from reheated rice? Be serious!" (B. cereus)
Pseudomonas aeruginosa	*PSEU*domonas causes wound and burn infections, Pneumonia (especially in cystic fibrosis), Sepsis (black lesions on skin), External otitis (swimmer's ear), UTI, and hot tub folliculitis. Aerobic gram-negative rod. Non–lactose fermenting, oxidase positive. Produces pyocyanin (blue-green) pigment. Water source. Produces endotoxin (fever, shock) and exotoxin A (inactivates EF-2). Treat with aminoglycoside plus extended-spectrum penicillin (e.g., piperacillin, ticarcillin).	**AER**uginosa—**AER**obic. Think water connection and blue-green pigment.

Helicobacter pylori Causes gastritis and up to 90% of duodenal ulcers. Risk factor for peptic ulcer and gastric carcinoma. Gram-negative rod. Urease positive (e.g., urease breath test). Creates alkaline environment. Treat with triple therapy: bismuth (Pepto-Bismol), metronidazole, and either tetracycline or amoxicillin.

Pylori—think pylorus of stomach. *Proteus* and *H. pylori* are both urease positive (cleave urea to ammonia).

Zoonotic bacteria

Species	Disease	Transmission and source
Borrelia burgdorferi	Lyme disease	Tick bite; *Ixodes* ticks that live on deer and mice
Brucella spp.	Brucellosis/ Undulant fever	Dairy products, contact with animals
Francisella tularensis	Tularemia	Tick bite; rabbits, deer
Yersinia pestis	Plague	Flea bite; rodents, especially prairie dogs
Pasteurella multocida	Cellulitis	Animal bite; cats, dogs

Bugs **F**rom **Y**our **P**et **U**ngulates and **U**npasteurized dairy products give you **U**ndulant fever.

1° and 2° tuberculosis

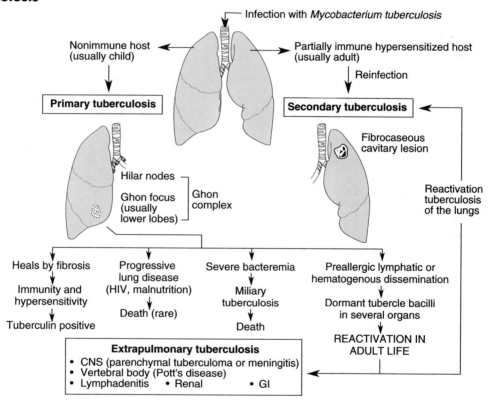

VDRL false positives

VDRL detects nonspecific Ab that reacts with beef cardiolipin. Used for diagnosis of syphilis, but many biologic false positives, including viral infection (mononucleosis, hepatitis), some drugs, rheumatic fever, rheumatoid arthritis, SLE, and leprosy.

HIGH-YIELD FACTS

Preclinical Primer

Normal flora: dominant

Skin–*S. epidermidis*
Nose–*S. aureus*
Oropharynx–Viridans streptococci
Dental plaque–*S. mutans*
Colon–*B. fragilis* > *E. coli*
Vagina–*Lactobacillus, E. coli,* group B strep

Neonates delivered by cesarean section have no flora but are rapidly colonized after birth.

Common causes of pneumonia

Children (6 wk–18 y) →	Adults (18–40 y) →	Adults (40–65 y) →	Elderly
Viruses (RSV)	**Mycoplasma**	*S. pneumoniae*	**S. pneumoniae**
Mycoplasma	*C. pneumoniae*	*H. influenzae*	Anaerobes
Chlamydia pneumoniae	*S. pneumoniae*	Anaerobes	*H. influenzae*
S. pneumoniae		Viruses	Gram-negative rods
		Mycoplasma	**Viruses**

Special groups

Nosocomial (hospital acquired)	*Staphylococcus,* gram-negative rods
Immunocompromised	*Staphylococcus,* gram-negative rods, **fungi,** viruses, ***Pneumocystis carinii*—with HIV**
Aspiration	Anaerobes
Alcoholic/IV drug user	*S. pneumoniae, Klebsiella, Staphylococcus*
Postviral	*Staphylococcus, H. influenzae*
Neonate	Group B streptococci, *E. coli*
Atypical	*Mycoplasma, Legionella, Chlamydia*

Causes of meningitis

Newborn (0–6 mo) →	Children (6 mo–6 y) →	6 y–60 y →	60 y +
Group B streptococci	***H. influenzae* B**	**N. meningitidis**	**S. pneumoniae**
E. coli	*S. pneumoniae*	Enteroviruses	Gram-negative rods
Listeria	*N. meningitidis*	*S. pneumoniae*	*Listeria*
	Enteroviruses	HSV	

In HIV—*Cryptococcus,* CMV, toxoplasmosis (brain abscess), JC virus (PML)
Note: Incidence of *H. influenzae* meningitis has ↓ greatly with introduction of *H. influenzae* vaccine in last 10–15 years.

Urinary tract infections

Ambulatory: *E. coli* (50–80%), *Klebsiella* (8–10%).
Staphylococcus saprophyticus (10–30%) is the second most common cause of UTI in young ambulatory women.
Hospital: *E. coli, Proteus, Klebsiella, Serratia, Pseudomonas.*
Epidemiology: women to men = 30 to 1 (short urethra colonized by fecal flora).

UTIs mostly caused by ascending infections. In males: babies with congenital defects; elderly with enlarged prostates.
UTI: dysuria, frequency, urgency, suprapubic pain.
Pyelonephritis: fever, chills and flank pain.

Nosocomial infections	By risk factor:	The two most common causes
	Newborn nursery: CMV, RSV	of nosocomial infections are
	Urinary catheterization: *E. coli, Proteus mirabilis*	*E. coli* (UTI) and *S. aureus*
		(wound infection).
	Respiratory therapy equipment: *P. aeruginosa*	Presume *Pseudomonas*
	Work in renal dialysis unit: HBV	*air-uginosa* when **air** or
	Hyperalimentation: *Candida albicans*	burns are involved.
	Water aerosols: *Legionella*	*Legionella* when water source
		is involved.

Bug hints (if all else fails)	Pus, empyema, abscess: *S. aureus*	
	Pediatric infection: *H. influenzae* (including epiglottitis)	
	Pneumonia in CF, burn infection: *P. aeruginosa*	
	Branching rods in oral infection: *Actinomyces israelii*	
	Traumatic open wound: *C. perfringens*	
	Surgical wound: *S. aureus*	
	Dog or cat bite: *Pasteurella multocida*	
	Currant jelly sputum: *Klebsiella*	

Mumps virus	A paramyxovirus with one serotype.	**M**umps gives you **b**umps
	Symptoms: aseptic **M**eningitis, **O**rchitis (inflammation of testes), and **P**arotitis. Can cause sterility (especially after puberty).	(parotitis). **MOP**

Measles virus	A paramyxovirus that causes measles. Koplik spots (bluish-gray spots on buccal mucosa) are diagnostic. SSPE, encephalitis (1 in 2000), or giant cell pneumonia (rarely, in immunosuppressed) are possible sequelae.	3 C's of measles: **C**ough **C**oryza **C**onjunctivitis Also look for **K**oplik spots.

Mononucleosis	Caused by EBV, a herpesvirus. Characterized by fever, hepatosplenomegaly, pharyngitis, and lymphadenopathy (especially posterior auricular nodes). Peak incidence 15–20 y old. Positive heterophil Ab test. Abnormal circulating cytotoxic T cells (atypical lymphocytes).	Most common during peak kissing years ("kissing disease").

Immune deficiencies

Bruton's agammaglobulinemia	**B**-cell deficiency. X-linked recessive defect in a tyrosine-kinase gene associated with low levels of all classes of immunoglobulins. Associated with recurrent bacterial infections after 6 months of age, when levels of maternal IgG antibody decline.
Thymic aplasia (DiGeorge's syndrome)	**T**-cell deficiency. Thymus and parathyroids fail to develop owing to failure of development of the 3rd and 4th pharyngeal pouches. Presents with **T**etany owing to hypocalcemia. Congenital defects of heart and great vessels. Recurrent viral, fungal, and protozoal infections.
Chronic mucocutaneous candidiasis	T-cell dysfunction specifically against *Candida albicans*.
Severe combined immunodeficiency (SCID)	B- and T-cell deficiency. Defect in early stem-cell differentiation. Presents with recurrent viral, bacterial, fungal, and protozoal infections. May have multiple causes (e.g., failure to synthesize class II MHC antigens, defective IL-2 receptors, or adenosine deaminase deficiency).
Wiskott–Aldrich syndrome	B- and T-cell deficiency. Defect in the ability to mount an IgM response to capsular poly-saccharides of bacteria. Associated with elevated IgA levels, normal IgE levels, and low IgM levels. Triad of symptoms includes recurrent pyogenic infections, eczema, and thrombocytopenia.
Ataxia–telangiectasia	B- and T-cell deficiency, with associated IgA deficiency. Presents with cerebellar problems (ataxia) and spider angiomas (telangiectasia).
Selective immunoglobulin deficiency	Deficiency in a specific class of immunoglobulins. Possibly due to a defect in isotype switching. Selective IgA deficiency is the most common selective immunoglobulin deficiency.
Chronic granulomatous disease	Phagocyte deficiency. Defect in phagocytosis of neutrophils owing to lack of NADPH oxidase activity or similar enzymes. Presents with marked susceptibility to opportunistic infections with bacteria, especially *S. aureus* and *E. coli,* and *Aspergillus.*
Chédiak–Higashi disease	Autosomal recessive defect in phagocytosis that results from microtubular and lysosomal defects of phagocytic cells. Presents with recurrent pyogenic infections by staphylococci and streptococci.
Job's syndrome	Neutrophils fail to respond to chemotactic stimuli. Associated with high levels of IgE. Presents with recurrent cold staphylococcal abscesses.

Autosomal trisomies

Down's syndrome (trisomy 21), 1:700	Most common chromosomal disorder and cause of congenital mental retardation. Findings: mental retardation, flat facial profile, prominent epicanthal folds, simian crease, duodenal atresia, congenital heart disease (most common malformation is endocardial cushion defect), Alzheimer's disease in affected individuals > 35 years old, associated with an increased risk of ALL. Ninety-five percent of cases are due to meiotic nondisjunction of homologous chromosomes, 4% of cases are due to Robertsonian translocation, and 1% of cases are due to Down mosaicism. Associated with advanced maternal age (from 1:1500 in women under 20 to 1:25 in women over 45).	Drinking age (21)
Edwards' syndrome (trisomy 18), 1:8000	Findings: severe mental retardation, rocker bottom feet, low-set ears, micrognathia, congenital heart disease, clenched hands (flexion of fingers), prominent occiput. Death usually occurs within 1 year of birth.	Election age (18)
Patau's syndrome (trisomy 13), 1:6000	Findings: severe mental retardation, microphthalmia, microcephaly, cleft lip/palate, abnormal forebrain structures, polydactyly, congenital heart disease. Death usually occurs within 1 year of birth.	Puberty (13)

Genetic gender disorders

Klinefelter's syndrome [male] (XXY), 1:850	Testicular atrophy, eunuchoid body shape, tall, long extremities, gynecomastia, female hair distribution. Presence of inactivated X chromosome (Barr body).	One of the most common causes of hypogonadism in males.
Turner's syndrome [female] (XO), 1:3000	Short stature, ovarian dysgenesis, webbing of neck, coarctation of the aorta, most common cause of primary amenorrhea. No Barr body.	"Hugs & kisses" (XO) from Tina Turner (female).
Double Y males [male] (XYY), 1:1000	Phenotypically normal, very tall, severe acne, antisocial behavior (seen in 1–2% of XYY males).	Observed with increased frequency among inmates of penal institutions.

HIGH-YIELD FACTS

Preclinical Primer

Autosomal dominant diseases

Adult polycystic kidney disease	Bilateral massive enlargement of kidneys due to multiple large cysts. Patients present with pain, hematuria, hypertension, progressive renal failure. Ninety percent of cases are due to mutation in APKD1 (chromosome 16). Associated with polycystic liver disease, **berry aneurysms,** mitral valve prolapse. Juvenile form is recessive.
Familial hypercholesterolemia	Elevated LDL owing to defective or absent LDL receptor. Heterozygotes (1 in 500) have cholesterol ≈ 300 mg/dL. Homozygotes (very rare) have cholesterol ≈ 700+ mg/dL, severe atherosclerotic disease early in life, and tendon xanthomas (classically in the Achilles tendon). Myocardial infarction may develop before age 20.
Marfan's syndrome	Fibrillin gene mutation → connective tissue disorders. Skeletal abnormalities: tall with long extremities, hyperextensive joints, and long, tapering fingers and toes Cardiovascular: cystic medial necrosis of aorta → aortic incompetence and dissecting aortic aneurysms. Floppy mitral valve. Ocular: subluxation of lenses.
Von Recklinghausen's disease (NFT1)	Findings: café-au-lait spots, neural tumors, Lisch nodules (pigmented iris hamartomas). On long arm of chromosome 17; 17 letters in von Recklinghausen.
Von Hippel–Lindau disease	Findings: hemangioblastomas of retina/cerebellum/medulla; about half of affected individuals develop multiple bilateral renal cell carcinomas and other tumors. Associated with deletion of VHL gene (tumor suppressor) on chromosome 3 (3p).
Huntington's disease	Findings: depression, progressive dementia, choreiform movements, caudate atrophy and decreased levels of GABA and acetylcholine in the brain. Symptoms manifest in affected individuals between the ages of 20 and 50. Gene located on chromosome 4; triplet repeat disorder.
Familial **A**denomatous **P**olyposis	Colon becomes covered with adenomatous polyps after puberty. Features: deletion on chromosome **F**ive; **A**utosomal dominant inheritance; **P**ositively will get colon cancer (100% without resection).
Hereditary spherocytosis	Spheroid erythrocytes; hemolytic anemia; increased MCHC. Splenectomy is curative.

Teratogens

Most susceptible in 3rd–8th week of pregnancy.

Examples	Effects
ACE inhibitors	Renal damage
Cocaine	Abnormal fetal development and fetal addiction
DES	Vaginal clear cell adenocarcinoma
Iodide	Congenital goiter or hypothyroidism
13-cis-retinoic acid	Extremely high risk for birth defects
Thalidomide	Limb defects
Warfarin, x-rays	Multiple anomalies

Fetal infections can also cause congenital malformations.

Conditions associated with neoplasms	Condition	Neoplasm
	1. **Down's** syndrome	1. **Acute Lymphoblastic** Leukemia. "We will **ALL** go **DOWN** together."
	2. Xeroderma pigmentosum	2. Squamous cell and basal cell carcinomas of skin
	3. Chronic atrophic gastritis, pernicious anemia, postsurgical gastric remnants	3. Gastric adenocarcinoma
	4. Tuberous sclerosis (facial angiofibroma, seizures, mental retardation)	4. Astrocytoma and cardiac rhabdomyoma
	5. Actinic keratosis	5. Squamous cell carcinoma of skin
	6. Barrett's esophagus (chronic GI reflux)	6. Esophageal adenocarcinoma
	7. Plummer–Vinson syndrome (atrophic glossitis, esophageal webs, anemia; all due to iron deficiency)	7. Squamous cell carcinoma of esophagus
	8. Cirrhosis (alcoholic, hepatitis B/C)	8. Hepatocellular carcinoma
	9. Ulcerative colitis	9. Colonic adenocarcinoma
	10. Paget's disease of bone	10. Secondary osteosarcoma and fibrosarcoma
	11. Immunodeficiency states	11. Malignant lymphomas
	12. AIDS	12. Aggressive malignant lymphomas and Kaposi's sarcoma
	13. Autoimmune diseases (e.g., Hashimoto's thyroiditis, myasthenia gravis)	13. Malignant thymomas, benign thymomas, thymic hyperplasia
	14. Acanthosis nigricans (hyperpigmentation and epidermal thickening)	14. Visceral malignancy (stomach, lung, breast, uterus)

Tumor markers

PSA, prostatic acid phosphatase	Prostatic carcinoma	Tumor markers should not be used as the primary tool for cancer diagnosis. They may be used to confirm diagnosis, to monitor for tumor recurrence, and to monitor response to therapy.
CEA	Carcinoembryonic antigen. Very nonspecific but produced by ~70% of colorectal and pancreatic cancers; also by gastric and breast carcinomas.	
α-fetoprotein	Normally made by fetus. Hepatocellular carcinomas. Nonseminomatous germ cell tumors of the testis (e.g., yolk sac tumor).	
β-hCG	**H**ydatidiform moles, **C**horiocarcinomas, and **G**estational trophoblastic tumors.	
α₁-antitrypsin	Liver and yolk sac tumors.	
CA-125	Ovarian tumors.	
S-100	Melanoma, neural tumors, astrocytomas.	

Local effects of tumors

Local effect	Cause
Mass	Tissue lump or tumor.
Nonhealing ulcer	Destruction of epithelial surfaces (e.g., stomach, colon, mouth, bronchus).
Hemorrhage	From ulcerated area or eroded vessel.
Pain	Any site with sensory nerve endings. Tumors in brain are initially painless.
Seizures	Tumor mass in brain.
Obstruction	Of bronchus → pneumonia.
	Of biliary tree → jaundice.
	Of left colon → constipation.
Perforation	Of ulcer in viscera → peritonitis, free air.
Bone destruction	Pathologic fracture, collapse of bone.
Inflammation	Of serosal surface → pleural effusion, pericardial effusion, ascites.
Space-occupying lesion	Raised intracranial pressure with brain neoplasms. Anemia due to bone marrow replacement.
Localized loss of sensory or motor function	Compression or destruction of nerve (e.g., recurrent laryngeal nerve by lung or thyroid cancer, with hoarseness).
Edema	Venous or lymphatic obstruction.

Skin cancer

Squamous cell carcinoma	Very common. Associated with excessive exposure to sunlight. Commonly appear on hands and face. Locally invasive but rarely metastasizes.	Actinic keratosis is a precursor to squamous cell carcinoma. Keratin "pearls." Arsenic exposure.
Basal cell carcinoma	Most common in sun-exposed areas of body. Locally invasive but almost never metastasizes. Gross pathology: pearly papules.	Basal cell tumors have "palisading" nuclei.
Melanoma	Common tumor with significant risk of metastasis. Associated with sunlight exposure. Incidence increasing. **Depth** of tumor correlates with risk of metastasis.	Increased risk in fair-skinned persons. Dysplastic nevus is a precursor to melanoma.

Cancer epidemiology

	Male	Female	
Incidence	Prostate (32%)	Breast (32%)	Deaths from lung cancer have plateaued in males, but
	Lung (16%)	Lung (13%)	deaths continue to increase
	Colon and rectum (12%)	Colon and rectum (13%)	in females.
Mortality	Lung (33%)	Lung (23%)	Cancer is the second leading
	Prostate (13%)	Breast (18%)	cause of death in the U.S. (heart disease is first).

Leukemias

General considerations: ↑ number of circulating leukocytes in blood; bone marrow infiltrates of leukemic cells; marrow failure can cause anemia (↓RBCs), infections (↓WBCs), and hemorrhage (↓platelets); leukemic cell infiltrates in liver, spleen, and lymph nodes are common.

ALL—children; lymphoblasts; most responsive to therapy.

AML—Auer rods; myeloblasts; adults.

CLL—lymphadenopathy; hepatosplenomegaly; few symptoms; indolent course; ↑ smudge cells in peripheral blood smear; warm Ab autoimmune hemolytic anemia; very similar to SLL (small lymphocytic leukemia).

CML—most commonly associated with Philadelphia chromosome [t(9;22), *bcr-abl*]; myeloid stem cell proliferation; may accelerate to AML ("blast crisis").

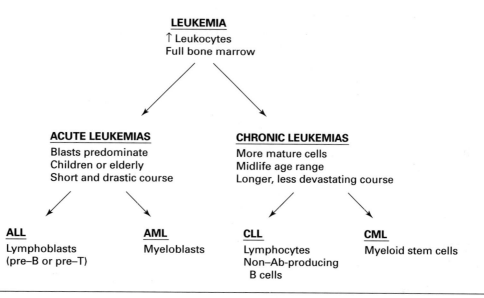

LEUKEMIA
↑ Leukocytes
Full bone marrow

ACUTE LEUKEMIAS
Blasts predominate
Children or elderly
Short and drastic course

CHRONIC LEUKEMIAS
More mature cells
Midlife age range
Longer, less devastating course

ALL
Lymphoblasts
(pre–B or pre–T)

AML
Myeloblasts

CLL
Lymphocytes
Non–Ab-producing
 B cells

CML
Myeloid stem cells

Cirrhosis/ portal hypertension

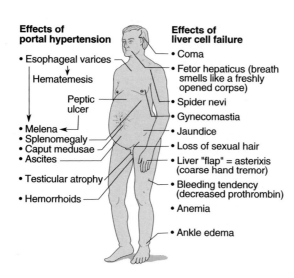

Effects of portal hypertension
- Esophageal varices
  ↓
  Hematemesis
- Peptic ulcer
- Melena ◄
- Splenomegaly
- Caput medusae
- Ascites
- Testicular atrophy
- Hemorrhoids

Effects of liver cell failure
- Coma
- Fetor hepaticus (breath smells like a freshly opened corpse)
- Spider nevi
- Gynecomastia
- Jaundice
- Loss of sexual hair
- Liver "flap" = asterixis (coarse hand tremor)
- Bleeding tendency (decreased prothrombin)
- Anemia
- Ankle edema

Cirrho (Greek) = tawny yellow.
Diffuse fibrosis of liver, destroys normal architecture.
Nodular regeneration.
Micronodular: nodules < 3 mm, uniform size.
Macronodular: nodules > 3 mm, varied size.
Micronodular cirrhosis is due to metabolic insult (e.g., alcohol), whereas macronodular is usually due to significant liver injury leading to hepatic necrosis (e.g., postinfectious or drug-induced hepatitis).
Increased risk of hepatocellular carcinoma.

Lung cancer

Bronchogenic carcinoma	Tumors that arise centrally: 1. Squamous cell carcinoma—clear link to Smoking 2. Small cell carcinoma—clear link to Smoking; associated with ectopic hormone production Tumors that arise peripherally: 1. Adenocarcinoma 2. Bronchioalveolar carcinoma (thought not to be related to smoking) 3. Large cell carcinoma—undifferentiated	Lung cancer is the leading cause of cancer death. Presentation: cough, hemoptysis, bronchial obstruction, wheezing, pneumonic "coin" lesion on x-ray. **SPHERE** of complications: **S**uperior vena caval syndrome **P**ancoast's tumor **H**orner's syndrome **E**ndocrine (paraneoplastic) **R**ecurrent laryngeal symptoms (hoarseness) **E**ffusions (pleural or pericardial)
Carcinoid tumor	Can cause carcinoid syndrome.	
Metastases	Very common. Brain (epilepsy), bone (pathologic fracture), and liver (jaundice, hepatomegaly).	

Wernicke–Korsakoff syndrome

Caused by vitamin B_1 (thiamine) deficiency in alcoholics. Classically may present with triad of psychosis, ophthalmoplegia, and ataxia (Wernicke's encephalopathy). May progress to memory loss, confabulation, confusion (Korsakoff's syndrome; irreversible). Associated with periventricular hemorrhage/necrosis, especially in mamillary bodies.
Treatment: IV vitamin B_1 (thiamine).

Diagnosis of MI

In the first six hours, EKG is the gold standard.
Troponin is used within the first 8 hours.
CK-MB is test of choice in the first 24 hours post-MI.
LDH_1 is test of choice from 2 to 7 days post-MI.
AST is nonspecific and can be found in cardiac, liver, and skeletal muscle cells. EKG changes can include ST elevation (transmural ischemia) and Q waves (transmural infarct).

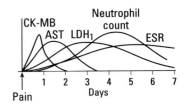

MI complications

1. Cardiac arrhythmia (90%)
2. LV failure and pulmonary edema (60%)
3. Thromboembolism: mural thrombus
4. Cardiogenic shock (large infarct: high risk of mortality)
5. Rupture of ventricular free wall, interventricular septum, papillary muscle (4–10 days post-MI), cardiac tamponade
6. Fibrinous pericarditis: friction rub (3–5 days post-MI)
7. Dressler's syndrome: autoimmune phenomenon resulting in fibrinous pericarditis (several weeks post-MI)

Cardiomyopathies

Dilated (congestive) cardiomyopathy	Most common cardiomyopathy (90% of cases). Etiologies include chronic **A**lcohol abuse, **B**eriberi, postviral myocarditis by **C**oxsackievirus B, chronic **C**ocaine use, **D**oxorubicin toxicity, peripartum cardiomyopathy. Heart dilates and looks like a balloon on chest x-ray.	Systolic dysfunction ensues. **A**lcohol **B**eriberi (wet) **C**oxsackievirus B, **C**ocaine **D**oxorubicin
Hypertrophic cardiomyopathy (formerly IHSS)	Hypertrophy often asymmetric and involving the intraventricular septum. 50% of cases are familial and are inherited as an AD trait. Cause of sudden death in young athletes. Walls of LV are thickened and chamber becomes banana-shaped on echocardiogram.	Diastolic dysfunction ensues.
Restrictive/obliterative cardiomyopathy	Major causes include sarcoidosis, amyloidosis, endocardial fibroelastosis, and endomyocardial fibrosis (Löffler's).	

Valvular heart disease

Aortic stenosis	Crescendo-decrescendo systolic ejection murmur, with LV >> aortic pressure during systole.
Aortic regurgitation	High-pitched "blowing" diastolic murmur. Wide pulse pressure.
Mitral stenosis	Rumbling late diastolic murmurs. LA >> LV pressure during diastole. Opening snap.
Mitral regurgitation	High-pitched "blowing" holosystolic murmur.
Mitral prolapse	Systolic murmur with midsystolic click. Most frequent valvular lesion, especially in young women.

Wegener's granulomatosis

Characterized by focal necrotizing vasculitis and necrotizing granulomas in the lung and upper airway and by necrotizing glomerulonephritis.

Symptoms	Perforation of nasal septum, chronic sinusitis, otitis media, mastoiditis, cough, dyspnea, hemoptysis.
Findings	C-ANCA is a strong marker of disease; CXR may reveal large nodular densities; hematuria and red cell casts.
Treatment	Cyclophosphamide, corticosteroids, and/or methotrexate.

Acidosis/alkalosis

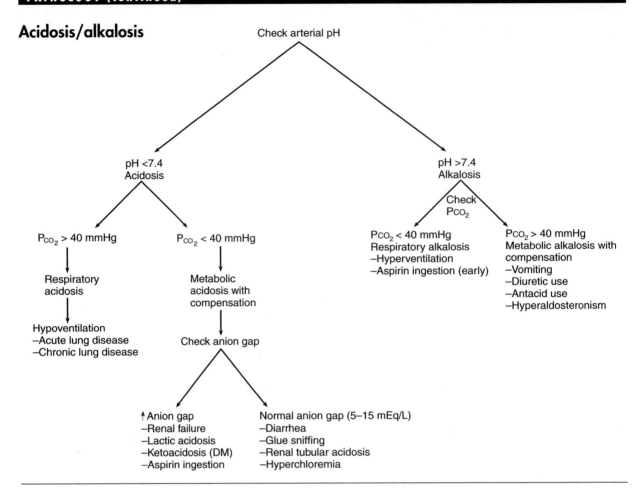

Check arterial pH

pH <7.4
Acidosis

pH >7.4
Alkalosis

$P_{CO_2} > 40$ mmHg

$P_{CO_2} < 40$ mmHg

Check
P_{CO_2}

$P_{CO_2} < 40$ mmHg
Respiratory alkalosis
–Hyperventilation
–Aspirin ingestion (early)

$P_{CO_2} > 40$ mmHg
Metabolic alkalosis with
compensation
–Vomiting
–Diuretic use
–Antacid use
–Hyperaldosteronism

Respiratory
acidosis

Metabolic
acidosis with
compensation

Hypoventilation
–Acute lung disease
–Chronic lung disease

Check anion gap

↑Anion gap
–Renal failure
–Lactic acidosis
–Ketoacidosis (DM)
–Aspirin ingestion

Normal anion gap (5–15 mEq/L)
–Diarrhea
–Glue sniffing
–Renal tubular acidosis
–Hyperchloremia

Ampicillin, amoxicillin

Mechanism	Same as penicillin. Wider spectrum, penicillinase sensitive. Also, combine with clavulanic acid (penicillinase inhibitor) to enhance spectrum. AmOxicillin has greater Oral bioavailability than ampicillin.	
Clinical use	Extended-spectrum penicillin: certain gram-positive bacteria and gram-negative rods (*Haemophilus influenzae*, *Escherichia coli*, *Listeria monocytogenes*, *Proteus mirabilis*, *Salmonella*).	Coverage: ampicillin/ amoxicillin **HELPS**
Toxicity	Hypersensitivity reactions; ampicillin: rash.	

Cephalosporins

Mechanism	β-lactam drugs that inhibit cell wall synthesis but are less susceptible to penicillinases. Bactericidal.	
Clinical use	First generation: gram-positive cocci, *Proteus mirabilis*, *E. coli*, *Klebsiella pneumoniae*.	1st generation: **PEcK**
	Second generation: gram-positive cocci, *Haemophilus influenzae*, *Enterobacter aerogenes*, *Neisseria* species, *Proteus mirabilis*, *E. coli*, *K. pneumoniae*, *Serratia marcescens*.	2nd generation: **HEN PEcKS**
	Third generation: serious gram-negative infections.	
	Cefo**tax**ime and ceftri**ax**one can penetrate the CNS (use for meningitis).	Think of an "**ax** to the head" (CNS).
Toxicity	Hypersensitivity reactions, increased nephrotoxicity of aminoglycosides, disulfiram-like reaction with ethanol (in cephalosporins with a methylthiotetrazole group, e.g., cefamandole).	

Nonsurgical antimicrobial prophylaxis

Meningococcal infection	Rifampin (drug of choice), minocycline
Gonorrhea	Ceftriaxone
Syphilis	Benzathine penicillin G
History of recurrent UTIs	Trimethoprim-sulfamethoxazole (TMP-SMX)
PCP	TMP-SMX (drug of choice), aerosolized pentamidine

Sympathomimetics

Drug	Mechanism/selectivity	Applications
Catecholamines		
Epinephrine	Direct general agonist (α_1, α_2, β_1, β_2)	Anaphylaxis, glaucoma (open angle), asthma, hypotension
Norepinephrine	α_1, α_2, β_1	Hypotension
Isoproterenol	$\beta_1 = \beta_2$	AV block (rare)
Dopamine	$D_1 = D_2 > \beta > \alpha$	Shock ($\uparrow$renal perfusion), heart failure
Dobutamine	$\beta_1 > \beta_2$	Shock, heart failure
Other		
Amphetamine	Indirect general agonist, releases stored catecholamines	Narcolepsy, obesity, attention deficit disorder
Ephedrine	Indirect general agonist, releases stored catecholamines	Nasal congestion, urinary incontinence, hypotension
Phenylephrine	$\alpha_1 > \alpha_2$	Pupil dilator, vasoconstriction, nasal decongestion
Albuterol, terbutaline	$\beta_2 > \beta_1$	Asthma
Cocaine	Indirect general agonist, uptake inhibitor	Causes vasoconstriction and local anesthesia

β-Blockers

Propranolol, metoprolol, atenolol, nadolol, timolol, pindolol, esmolol, labetalol

Application	Effect
Hypertension	$\downarrow$ cardiac output, $\downarrow$ renin secretion
Angina pectoris	$\downarrow$ heart rate and contractility, resulting in decreased oxygen consumption
MI	β-blockers decrease mortality
SVT (propranolol, esmolol)	$\downarrow$ AV conduction velocity
Glaucoma (timolol)	$\downarrow$ secretion of aqueous humor
Toxicity	Impotence, exacerbation of asthma, cardiovascular adverse effects (bradycardia, AV block, CHF), CNS adverse effects (sedation, sleep alterations)
Selectivity	Nonselective ($\beta_1 = \beta_2$): propranolol, timolol, pindolol, nadolol, and labetalol (also blocks α_1 receptors) β_1 selective ($\beta_1 > \beta_2$): metoprolol, atenolol, esmolol (short-acting)

Tricyclic antidepressants

Imipramine, amitriptyline, desipramine, nortriptyline, clomipramine, doxepin

Mechanism — Block reuptake of norepinephrine and serotonin.

Clinical use — Endogenous depression, bedwetting (imipramine), obsessive–compulsive disorder (clomipramine).

Side effects — Sedation, α-blocking effects, atropine-like (anticholinergic) side effects (tachycardia, urinary retention). Tertiary TCAs (amitriptyline) have more anticholinergic effects than secondary TCAs (nortriptyline). Desipramine is the least sedating.

Toxicity — Convulsions, coma, respiratory depression, hyperpyrexia, arrhythmias. Confusion and hallucinations in elderly.

SSRIs

Fluoxetine, sertraline, paroxetine

Mechanism — Serotonin-specific reuptake inhibitors.

Clinical use — Endogenous depression.

Toxicity — Anxiety, insomnia, tremor, anorexia, nausea, and vomiting.

It normally takes 2–3 wks for antidepressants to have an effect.

Inhaled anesthetics

Halothane, enflurane, isoflurane, sevoflurane, methoxyflurane, nitrous oxide

Principle — The lower the solubility, the quicker the anesthetic induction and the quicker the recovery.

Effects — Myocardial depression, respiratory depression, nausea/emesis, ↑ cerebral blood flow.

Toxicity — Hepatotoxicity (halothane), nephrotoxicity (methoxyflurane), proconvulsant (enflurane), malignant hyperthermia (rare).

Anti-anginal therapy

Goal: Reduction of myocardial O_2 consumption (MVO_2) by decreasing one or more of the determinants of MVO_2: end diastolic volume, blood pressure, heart rate, contractility, ejection time.

Component	Nitrates	β blockers	Nitrates + β blockers
End diastolic volume	↓	↑	No effect or ↓
Blood pressure	↓	↓	↓
Contractility	↑ (reflex response)	↓	Little/no effect
Heart rate	↑ (reflex response)	↓	↓
Ejection time	↓	↑	Little/no effect
MVO_2	↓	↓	↓↓

Calcium channel blockers:
 – **N**ifedipine is similar to **N**itrates in effect
 – Verapamil is similar to β blockers in effect

HIGH-YIELD FACTS

Preclinical Primer

Calcium channel blockers	Nifedipine, verapamil, diltiazem	
Mechanism	Block voltage-dependent L-type calcium channels of cardiac and smooth muscle and thereby reduce muscle contractility. 　　Vascular smooth muscle: nifedipine > diltiazem > verapamil. 　　Heart: verapamil > diltiazem > nifedipine.	
Clinical use	Hypertension, angina, arrhythmias.	
Toxicity	Cardiac depression, peripheral edema, flushing, dizziness, and constipation.	

ACE inhibitors	Captopril, enalapril, lisinopril	**Losartan** is a new angiotensin II receptor antagonist. It is **not** an ACE inhibitor and does not cause cough.
Mechanism	Inhibit angiotensin-converting enzyme, reducing levels of angiotensin II and preventing inactivation of bradykinin, a potent vasodilator. Renin release is ↑ due to loss of feedback inhibition.	
Clinical use	Hypertension, congestive heart failure, diabetic renal disease.	
Toxicity	Cough, angioedema, proteinuria, taste changes, hypotension, fetal renal damage, rash.	

K⁺-sparing diuretics	**S**pironolactone, **T**riamterene, **A**miloride	The K⁺ **STA**ys.
Mechanism	Spironolactone is a competitive aldosterone antagonist in the cortical collecting tubule. Triamterene and amiloride act at same site by blocking Na^+ channels in the CCT.	
Clinical use	Hyperaldosteronism, K^+ depletion.	
Toxicity	Hyperkalemia, endocrine effects (gynecomastia, anti-androgen effects).	

Lead poisoning	**L**ead **L**ines on gingivae and on epiphyses of long bones on x-ray. **E**ncephalopathy and **E**rythrocyte basophilic stippling. **A**bdominal colic and sideroblastic **A**nemia. **D**rops: wrist and foot drop. Dimercaprol and EDTA as first line of treatment.	**LEAD** High risk in houses with chipped paint.

70

Asthma drugs

Nonspecific β agonists — Isoproterenol: relaxes bronchial smooth muscle (β_2). Adverse effect is tachycardia (β_1).

β_2 agonists — Albuterol: relaxes bronchial smooth muscle (β_2). Adverse effects are tremor and arrhythmia.

Methylxanthines — Theophylline: mechanism unclear—may cause bronchodilation by inhibiting phosphodiesterase, enzyme involved in degrading cAMP (controversial).

Muscarinic antagonists — Ipratropium: competitive block of muscarinic receptors preventing bronchoconstriction.

Cromolyn — Prevents release of mediators from mast cells. Effective only for the prophylaxis of asthma. Not effective during an active asthmatic attack. Toxicity is very rare.

Corticosteroids — Prevent release of leukotrienes from arachidonic acid by blocking phospholipase A_2. Are drugs of choice in a patient with status asthmaticus (in combination with albuterol).

Antileukotrienes — Zileuton: blocks synthesis by lipoxygenase; zafirlukast: blocks leukotriene receptors.

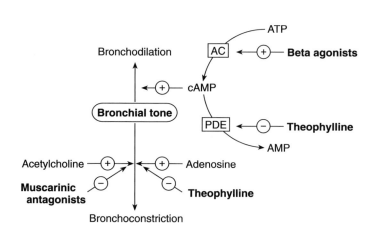

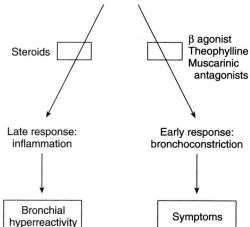

Treatment strategies in asthma

71

Cardiac output variables

Stroke volume affected by **C**ontractility, **A**fterload, and **P**reload.

Contractility (and SV) increased with:
1. Catecholamines ($\uparrow$ activity of Ca^{2+} pump in sarcoplasmic reticulum)
2. $\uparrow$ extracellular calcium
3. $\downarrow$ extracellular sodium
4. Digitalis ($\uparrow$ intracellular Na^+, resulting in $\uparrow Ca^{2+}$)

Contractility (and SV) decreased with:
1. β_1 blockade
2. Heart failure
3. Acidosis
4. Hypoxia/hypercapnea

SV **CAP**

Stroke volume increases in anxiety, exercise, and pregnancy.

Pulse pressure is proportional to stroke volume.

A failing heart has decreased stroke volume.

Myocardial O_2 demand is $\uparrow$ by:
$\uparrow$ afterload ($\propto$ diastolic BP)
$\uparrow$ contractility
$\uparrow$ heart rate
$\uparrow$ heart size ($\uparrow$ wall tension)

Normal pressures

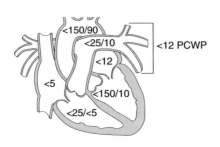

PCWP = pulmonary capillary wedge pressure (in mmHg) is a good approximation of left atrial pressure.

Oxygen dissociation curve

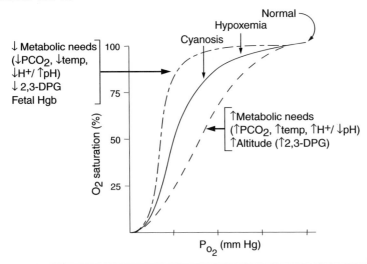

When curve shifts to the right, $\downarrow$ affinity of hemoglobin for O_2 (facilitates unloading of O_2 to tissue).

An $\uparrow$ in all factors (except pH) causes a shift of the curve to the right.

A $\downarrow$ in all factors (except pH) causes a shift of the curve to the left.

72

Bilirubin   Product of heme metabolism, actively taken up by hepatocytes. Conjugated version is water soluble. Jaundice (yellow skin, sclerae) results from elevated bilirubin levels.

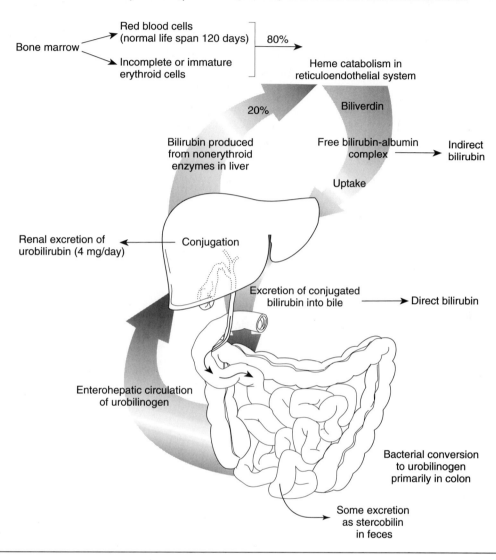

Renal failure   Failure to make urine and excrete nitrogenous wastes. Consequences:

1. Anemia (failure of erythropoietin production)
2. Renal osteodystrophy (failure of active vit. D production)
3. Hyperkalemia, which can lead to cardiac arrhythmias
4. Metabolic acidosis due to ↓ acid secretion and ↓ generation of buffers
5. Uremia (increased BUN, creatinine)
6. Sodium and H_2O excess → CHF and pulmonary edema

Two forms of renal failure: acute renal failure (often due to hypoxia) and chronic renal failure.

Hyperaldosteronism

Primary (Conn's syndrome)	Caused by an aldosterone-secreting tumor, resulting in hypertension, hypokalemia, hypernatremia, metabolic alkalosis, and **low** plasma renin.	Treatment includes spironolactone, a diuretic that works by acting as an aldosterone antagonist.
Secondary	Due to renal artery stenosis, chronic renal failure, CHF, cirrhosis, or nephrotic syndrome. Kidney misperception of low intravascular volume, resulting in an overactive renin-angiotensin system. Therefore, it is associated with **high** plasma renin.	

PTH

Source	Chief cells of parathyroid.	
Function	1. Increases bone resorption of calcium 2. Increases kidney reabsorption of calcium 3. Decreases kidney reabsorption of phosphate 4. Increases 1,25 (OH)$_2$ vit. D (cholecalciferol) production by stimulating kidney 1α-hydroxylase	PTH: increases serum Ca^{2+}, decreases serum PO_4^{3-}, increases urine PO_4^{3-}. PTH stimulates both osteoclasts and osteoblasts.
Regulation	Increase in serum Ca^{2+} decreases secretion.	**PTH** = **P**hosphate **T**rashing **H**ormone

Menstrual cycle

Follicular growth is fastest during second week of proliferative phase.

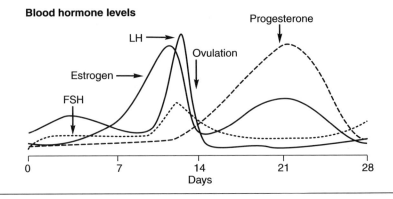

Blood hormone levels

Database of High-Yield Facts

The second edition of *First Aid for the USMLE Step 2* contains a revised and expanded database of clinical science material that student authors and faculty have identified as high yield for boards review. The topics are organized into core clinical specialties and subspecialties. **Mnemonics** and **Key Points** are highlighted in the margins.

New for the second edition are **"reference links"** to the eight clinical titles in the ***Underground Clinical Vignettes* (UCV) series** (S2S Medical Publishing). These annotations link the high-yield fact to a corresponding vignette case which illustrates how that fact may appear in a Step 2 clinical scenario. The sample annotation below refers to cases 23 and 45 from *UCV Internal Medicine, Vol. II.*

UCV *IM2.23, 45*

The Database of High-Yield Topics is not comprehensive. The facts have been condensed to emphasize the most essential material. Remember, as you work with the material, to add your own notes and mnemonics, and recognize that not all memory techniques work for all students.

We encourage medical students and faculty to submit entries and mnemonics so that we may enhance the database for future students. Recommendations of alternate tools for study that may be useful in preparing for Step 2, such as diagrams, charts, and computer-based tutorials, are also welcome (see How to Contribute, page xvii).

UCV REFERENCE LEGEND*	
Abbreviation	**UCV Title**
EM	Bhushan et al. *Underground Clinical Vignettes: Emergency Medicine.* Los Angeles: S2S Medical Publishing, 1999 (ISBN 1890061271).
IM1	Bhushan et al. *Underground Clinical Vignettes: Internal Medicine, Vol. I.* Los Angeles: S2S Medical Publishing, 1999 (ISBN 1890061204).
IM2	Bhushan et al. *Underground Clinical Vignettes: Internal Medicine, Vol. II.* Los Angeles: S2S Medical Publishing, 1999 (ISBN 1890061255).
Neuro	Bhushan et al. *Underground Clinical Vignettes: Neurology.* Los Angeles: S2S Medical Publishing, 1999 (ISBN 1890061263).
OB	Bhushan et al. *Underground Clinical Vignettes: OB/GYN.* Los Angeles: S2S Medical Publishing, 1999 (ISBN 1890061239).
Ped	Bhushan et al. *Underground Clinical Vignettes: Pediatrics.* Los Angeles: S2S Medical Publishing, 1999 (ISBN 1890061212).
Psych	Bhushan et al. *Underground Clinical Vignettes: Psychiatry.* Los Angeles: S2S Medical Publishing, 1999 (ISBN 1890061247).
Surg	Bhushan et al. *Underground Clinical Vignettes: Surgery.* Los Angeles: S2S Medical Publishing, 1999 (ISBN 1890061220).

*Please refer to the back of the book for more information on UCV titles.

Disclaimer

The entries in this section reflect student opinions of what is high yield. Owing to the diverse sources of material, no attempt has been made to trace or reference the origins of entries individually. We have regarded mnemonics as essentially in the public domain. All errors and omissions will be gladly corrected if brought to the attention of the authors, either through the publisher or directly by e-mail.

Cardiovascular

High blood pressure due to an unidentified cause (secondary hypertension is due to a known cause); **accounts for > 95% of all cases of hypertension.** High blood pressure is usually defined as a sustained increase in systolic BP > 140 and/or a diastolic BP > 90, typically based on **two readings separated in time** (Table 2.1–1). Risk factors for primary hypertension include a **family history** of hypertension or heart disease, a **high-sodium diet, obesity,** and **advanced age;** blacks are affected more frequently than whites.

Primary (essential) hypertension is the most common cause of high blood pressure.

History

Asymptomatic until complications develop.

PE

Systolic BP > 140 and/or **diastolic BP > 90,** retinal changes (copper wires, AV nicking; see Figure 2.1–1), and possibly a systolic click and/or loud S2. An S4 may also be auscultated.

Differential

Secondary hypertension (see below), NSAIDs, pregnancy.

Evaluation

Perform tests for secondary causes if the patient's clinical picture is consistent with any type of secondary hypertension (see "Secondary Hypertension") and periodic tests for complications of hypertension (EKG, BUN/creatinine).

Treatment

Begin with diet/lifestyle modification. **Diuretics** (inexpensive and particularly effective in African Americans) and **beta-blockers** (beneficial for patients with CAD) are good first-line agents. Other options are noted in Table 2.1–2.

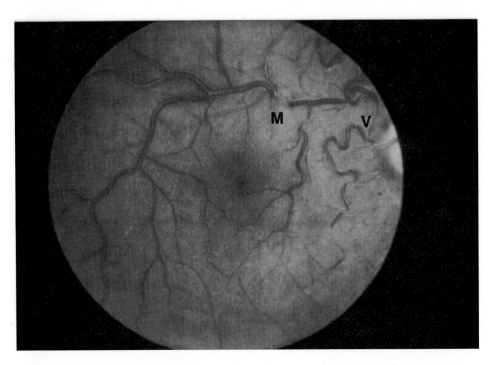

FIGURE 2.1–1.   Hypertensive retinopathy. Note the tortuous retinal veins (V) and venous micro-aneurysms (M). Other findings include hemorrhages, retinal infarcts, detachment of the retina, and disk edema. Please refer to insert for color version of this and other images.

TABLE 2.1–1. Classification and Interpretation of Blood Pressure Measurements.

Category[1]	Systolic Blood Pressure (mmHg)	Diastolic Blood Pressure (mmHg)	Follow-up Recommended
Normal	< 130	< 85	Recheck in two years.
High normal	130–139	85–89	Recheck in one year.[2]
Hypertension			
Stage 1 (mild)	140–159	90–99	Confirm within two months.
Stage 2 (moderate)	160–179	100–109	Evaluate or refer within one month.
Stage 3 (severe)	180–209	110–119	Evaluate or refer within one week.
Stage 4 (very severe)	≥ 210	≥ 120	Evaluate or refer immediately.

[1] When systolic and diastolic pressures fall into different categories, the higher category should be selected to classify the individual's blood pressure.
[2] Consider offering counseling about lifestyle modifications.

TABLE 2.1–2. Selection of Antihypertensive Medications.

	More Effective or Appropriate	Less Effective or Contraindicated
Coexisting conditions		
Prior MI	Beta-blocker, ACE inhibitor	Calcium channel blocker (with reduced ejection fraction)
Angina pectoris	Beta-blocker, calcium channel blocker	Vasodilator (without concomitant beta-blocker)
CHF	Diuretic, ACE inhibitor	Calcium channel blocker, beta-blocker[1]
Diabetes mellitus	ACE inhibitor	Beta-blocker (if hypoglycemia occurs), diuretic (if glucose is high in type II diabetes)
Peripheral vascular disease		Beta-blocker (if there is rest pain or severe claudication)
Bronchospasm		Beta-blocker
BPH	Alpha-blocker	
Migraine	Beta-blocker	
Arthritis		ACE inhibitor (if on chronic NSAID regimen)
Gout		Diuretic
Osteoporosis	Thiazide diuretic ↑Ca	
Pregnancy (current or potential)	Beta-blocker (considerable experience with labetalol; atenolol associated with low birth weight), calcium channel blocker, methyldopa, hydralazine	ACE inhibitor
Demographic factors		
Older patients	Diuretic (especially for isolated systolic hypertension)	ACE inhibitor
Blacks	Calcium channel blocker, diuretic	ACE inhibitor, beta-blocker
Young whites	Beta-blocker, ACE inhibitor	

[1] Growing evidence supports a role for beta-blockers in some patients with CHF, but these drugs may cause acute deterioration and require careful monitoring.

The best way to prevent stroke is to control hypertension.

Complications

CAD, kidney disease, **cerebrovascular disease,** aortic aneurysm, aortic dissection, LVH, CHF.

SECONDARY HYPERTENSION
UCV *IM1.15*

High blood pressure that is due to an **identifiable** organic cause. Surgically correctable causes of hypertension, which account for < 5% of cases of hypertension, include coarctation of the aorta, pheochromocytoma, Conn's syndrome, Cushing's syndrome, renal artery stenosis, and unilateral renal parenchymal disease.

- **Renal disease:** Any primary renal disease can lead to high blood pressure. **ACE inhibitors** will treat the hypertension and slow the progression of renal disease.

- **Renal artery stenosis:** This is especially common in patients < 25 years old as well as in patients > 50 years old with recent-onset hypertension. Etiologies include **fibromuscular dysplasia** (usually seen in **younger** patients) and **atherosclerosis** (more common in older patients). Diagnosis can be made by arteriography as well as by renal vein renin ratio (RVRR), and screening is possible with the captopril provocation test or nuclear perfusion scan. Treat with **angioplasty** and **stenting** if possible; also consider ACE inhibitors as adjunctive or temporary therapy in unilateral disease **(in bilateral disease, ACE inhibitors can accelerate kidney failure).** Surgery is a secondary option if angioplasty is not effective or feasible. *IM2.34*

- **Oral contraceptive use:** Common in women > 35 years old, obese women, and those with long-standing OCP use. Discontinue the OCP (it can take time to see an effect).

- **Pheochromocytoma:** Classically associated with **episodic** hypertension, diaphoresis, and headache but can present less obviously. Patients are **often misdiagnosed** with anxiety disorder. Look for this in patients who are **young** or otherwise atypical, who have severe and/or **paroxysmal symptoms,** or who have a history of endocrine tumors (MEN IIA and IIB syndromes). Pheochromocytoma is diagnosed by **elevated** 24-hour **urinary catecholamines** and/or **VMA** (vanillylmandelic acid) or by the clonidine suppression test. Imaging studies (CT, MRI) or scintigraphy (MIBG scan) can also be used for diagnosis. Treatment consists of **surgical resection** (pretreat with alpha- and beta-blockers).

- **Primary hyperaldosteronism:** Due to excess aldosterone (Conn's syndrome) or glucocorticoid production (Cushing's syndrome), usually from an **adrenal adenoma,** although the lesion can be malignant. Screen for hyperaldosteronism by looking for **hypokalemia,** elevated urinary potassium, and **elevated plasma/urine aldosterone.** Screen for Cushing's syndrome by physical exam (e.g., **central obesity,** hirsutism, "buffalo hump," **striae**) and by testing for **glucose intolerance;** think of iatrogenesis if the patient is on chronic steroid therapy.

Causes of secondary hypertension—

CHAPS
Cushing's syndrome
Hyperaldosteronism
Aortic coarctation
Pheochromocytoma
Stenosis of renal arteries

PHEochromocytoma:

Palpitations
Headache and
  Hypertension
Episodic diaphoresis

A **BP > 200/120 with symptoms** (headache, chest pain, syncope) but **no signs** of impending **end-organ damage**. A **hypertensive emergency** consists of a BP > 200/120 with **signs of end-organ damage.** Signs can include acute renal failure or **hematuria, altered mental status** or other evidence of neurologic disease, intracranial hemorrhage, ophthalmologic findings suggesting retinal damage (**papilledema,** vascular changes), unstable angina/MI, or pulmonary edema. "Malignant hypertension" is defined as progressive **renal failure** and/or **encephalopathy** plus papilledema.

Evaluation

Cardiovascular, neurologic, ophthalmologic, and abdominal exams (see Figure 2.1–2). Obtain head and/or abdominal CT, UA, BUN/creatinine, CBC, and electrolytes to assess the extent of end-organ damage.

Treatment

- **Hypertensive urgency:** BP can be brought down relatively **slowly,** usually with **oral agents** such as beta-blockers, clonidine, and ACE inhibitors. Avoid short-acting calcium channel blockers. If oral therapy is not sufficient, try IV agents (see below).
- **Hypertensive emergency:** IV agents to reduce BP by approximately

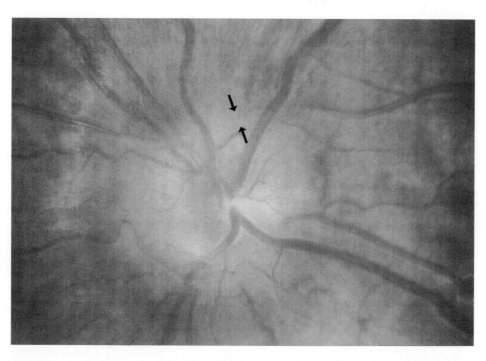

FIGURE 2.1–2. Papilledema. Look for blurred disk margins due to edema of the optic disk (arrows).

HIGH-YIELD FACTS

Cardiovascular

25% **within one hour,** often with **nitroprusside** (very potent; use carefully), nitroglycerin, labetalol, nicardipine, and/or hydralazine. Add a **diuretic** if there is evidence of pulmonary edema/fluid overload.

Exercise or pharmacologic testing aimed at **increasing cardiac workload** to assess myocardial perfusion, cardiac ischemia, and the risk of subsequent MI. Cardiac stress testing should be performed on patients with suspected or known CAD, patients who present with chest pain for the first time, and those with progressively worsening symptoms. If patients can achieve a peak heart rate that is 85% of predicted for age/sex and have an interpretable **EKG** (e.g., no LBBB), an exercise stress test is preferred, often with **nuclear imaging** to look for myocardial **perfusion defects.** If a patient cannot achieve sufficient physical activity (e.g., disabled or older patients), a **pharmacologic** stress test such as an adenosine or Persantine thallium scan or a dobutamine echocardiogram is commonly performed.

Signs of active ischemia during stress testing include angina, ST-segment changes on EKG, or decreased BP. A premature rise in heart rate to > 90% of the patient's predicted heart rate (predicted heart rate = 220 – age) is indicative of **cardiac deconditioning** secondary to a sedentary lifestyle. Patients whose stress tests reveal reversible myocardial ischemia should have **coronary catheterization** if they are appropriate candidates for PTCA or CABG. Exercise stress testing is fairly sensitive but not perfect, so a negative test does not rule out disease, especially if the patient has classic symptoms of CAD.

RHEUMATIC FEVER/RHEUMATIC HEART DISEASE   UCV *IM1.14, Ped.32*

A sequela of **pharyngeal streptococcal infection.** Rheumatic fever is a systemic immune process that may result in rheumatic heart disease.

History/PE

- **Acute rheumatic fever: Major criteria** include migratory polyarthritis, carditis (pericarditis, myocarditis), erythema marginatum, subcutaneous nodules, and chorea (Sydenham's). **Minor criteria** include fever, polyarthralgias, increased ESR, history of rheumatic fever, antecedent strep infection, and prolonged PR interval. Two major criteria or one major and two minor criteria are required for diagnosis.
- **Rheumatic heart disease:** Valvular abnormalities secondary to rheumatic fever; most often **mitral stenosis** *(IM1.10)*, but can be mitral + aortic or mitral + aortic + tricuspid.

Differential

RA, SLE, endocarditis, osteomyelitis, Lyme disease, sickle cell disease.

Pharyngitis gives you rheumatic "phever."

Rheumatic fever, major criteria—

PECCS
Polyarthritis (MIGRATORY)
Erythema marginatum
Carditis
Chorea
Subcutaneous nodules

84

Evaluation

Elevated ESR and **positive ASO** antibody titers are seen. For rheumatic heart disease, perform echocardiography to assess valvular function.

Treatment

Bed rest, **salicylates, penicillin** or erythromycin; steroids if other treatments are not successful. The complications of this disease are the primary reason to treat streptococcal pharyngeal infections. Administer **antimicrobial prophylaxis** against bacterial endocarditis for **medical/dental** procedures in patients with rheumatic heart disease with amoxicillin (erythromycin if the patient is allergic to penicillin).

Treat streptococcal pharyngeal infections to prevent rheumatic heart disease.

ENDOCARDITIS
UCV *IM1.8, IM2.9, 29*

Inflammation of a heart valve, usually secondary to bacterial or other infectious causes. Risk factors include a history of rheumatic heart disease or **valvular heart disease** (including MVP), **IV drug use,** immunosuppression, and the presence of a **prosthetic heart valve.** Subacute bacterial endocarditis is most commonly caused by (viridans streptococci) while acute bacterial endocarditis is most commonly caused by more virulent organisms such as *Staphylococcus aureus* (especially in IV drug users), *Streptococcus pneumoniae,* and *Streptococcus pyogenes.*

History

Patients present with **high fever** that may last for weeks together with cough, shortness of breath, and/or **systemic symptoms** (weakness, fatigue, malaise). In a patient with a history of **valvular disease** or **IV drug use,** fever alone should raise suspicion of this diagnosis. Endocarditis is an intravascular infection that can seed other organs, so look for signs of lung, joint, and neurologic disease.

Endocarditis is a common cause of FUO.

PE

Murmur (often regurgitant), **fever,** and/or joint tenderness. Small, tender nodules on finger and toe pads **(Osler's nodes),** small, peripheral hemorrhages **(Janeway lesions),** subungual petechiae **(splinter hemorrhages),** and retinal hemorrhages **(Roth's spots)** may also be found. Endocarditis is usually left-sided (mitral, aortic) unless patients have a history of IV drug use, in which case it is more commonly right-sided.

ENDOCARDITIS
MJ FOR SENATE

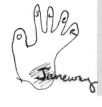

MURMUR
FEVER
OSLER'S (NODULES ON FING PADS)
SPLINTER (SUBUNGUAL PETECHIAE)
ROTH'S (RETINAL HEMORR)
JANEWAY (PERIPH HEMORR)
ON PALM, NON TEND

Differential

Osteomyelitis, abscess, pneumonia, rheumatic fever, joint infection, prostatitis in males, STDs in females, and other causes of FUO.

Evaluation

Obtain at least **three sets of blood cultures** separated in time and location; multiple positive blood cultures revealing the same pathogen are considered strong evidence of bacterial endocarditis. Echocardiography can be used to look for vegetations, but a negative echo does not rule out the diagnosis. CXR may reveal **septic emboli** in right-sided endocarditis. Elevated ESR is common.

Treatment

- Treat empirically with **long-term antibiotic therapy,** usually for 28 days, with therapy initially given to cover gram-positive bugs and then tailored to specific organisms found on culture. Newer regimens with 14-day treatments include 14 days of an antistaphylococcal penicillin (e.g., nafcillin), with an aminoglycoside (e.g., gentamicin) added for the first five days for "augmentation."
- Always monitor for recurrence or relapse; treat relapses with longer courses of antibiotics.
- Give **antibiotic prophylaxis** (i.e., amoxicillin or erythromycin) **before dental work,** as patients now have valvular disease.
- Perform **valve replacement** in cases of worsening valvular function, systemic embolization, abscess formation, or development of conduction disturbances.

AORTIC ANEURYSM   UCV EM.3.14

An aneurysmal dilatation of the aorta, most commonly secondary to **atherosclerosis.** Most aortic aneurysms are abdominal, and > 90% originate below the renal arteries. Risk factors include **hypertension,** other vascular disease (atherosclerosis), family history, and tobacco use; **males** are affected more frequently than females, and risk increases with age.

History

Usually **asymptomatic** and discovered on physical exam or on a radiologic study. However, a ruptured aneurysm can cause hypotension as well as severe, tearing abdominal pain radiating to the back. Many individuals with rupture die before they arrive at the hospital.

PE

Pulsatile abdominal mass, abdominal bruits, hypotension (if ruptured), and evidence of lower extremity arterial insufficiency.

Differential

Pancreatitis/pseudocyst, neoplasms (pancreatic, colonic, other), orthopedic causes of back pain, appendicitis, gallbladder disease.

Evaluation

Abdominal ultrasound for diagnosis or to follow an aneurysm over time, although CT determines the precise anatomy and may be helpful as an adjunct.

Treatment

- In asymptomatic patients, **monitoring** is appropriate for lesions < 5 cm. **If the lesion is > 5 cm or is enlarging rapidly, surgical repair** is indicated.
- Emergent surgery is indicated for symptomatic or ruptured aneurysms.

AORTIC DISSECTION UCV FM.3

The spread of blood into an **intimal tear** in the wall of the aorta, causing a **second lumen** to form. **Type A** dissections involve the ascending aorta; **type B** are distal to the left subclavian artery. Risk factors include **hypertension, trauma, coarctation of the aorta, syphilis, Ehlers–Danlos syndrome, and Marfan's syndrome.**

TYPE A – ASCENDING

TYPE B – BEYOND SUBCLAVIAN

History

Patients present with acute-onset, severe **"tearing" or "ripping" anterior chest pain;** pain can radiate to the back and abdomen as it progresses. Syncope, decreased pulses, and shock may develop as the condition worsens.

Patients classically present with sudden onset of tearing chest pain radiating to the back and with asymmetric upper extremity blood pressures.

PE

Asymmetric or decreased peripheral pulses. Patients may be hypertensive with asymmetric upper extremity BPs and a diastolic murmur secondary to aortic regurgitation.

Differential

MI, pulmonary embolus, angina, thoracic aortic aneurysm, esophageal rupture.

Evaluation

CXR often demonstrates a **widened superior mediastinum.** Diagnosis can be made via **CT with IV contrast,** transesophageal echocardiography, or **angiog-**

raphy (the gold standard). An intimal flap or pseudolumen may be seen. Workup should also include EKG (look for LVH and ischemic changes).

Treatment

- Stabilize the patient by treating high or low blood pressure. Treat high blood pressure with **IV nitrates and beta-blockers.** Pressure may bottom out with nitrates (e.g., sublingual nitroglycerin), so exercise caution.
- Type A dissections require **emergent surgery.** Consider medical management in patients with type B dissections who are poor surgical candidates.

ANGINA PECTORIS

Episodes of chest pain due to **ischemic** cardiac disease (inadequate oxygen delivery to myocardium). Risk factors include age, hypercholesterolemia, diabetes, hypertension, family history, previous angina/MI, tobacco, cocaine, and amphetamine use. Males are affected more frequently than females.

History

The classic triad involves **substernal chest pain** or pressure that is **precipitated by exertion** and **relieved by rest or nitrates.** Angina can radiate to the arms, jaw, and neck and can be associated with diaphoresis, nausea/emesis, or lightheadedness. Anginal symptoms can vary significantly among patients.

PE

Diaphoresis, elevated BP, tachycardia, and apical systolic murmur/gallop may be appreciated during an anginal episode.

GERD and esophageal spasm may also improve with nitroglycerin.

Differential

MI, costochondritis, herpes zoster neuropathy, GERD (may also improve with nitrates), PUD, cholecystitis, pericarditis, aortic dissection, pulmonary embolus, pneumothorax, pneumonia, and pleurisy.

Evaluation

EKG may show transient **ST-segment depression** (or elevation). Check **cardiac enzymes.** Risk-stratify by performing an **exercise stress test** or coronary **catheterization.**

Treatment

- Patients with suspected MI (according to clinical findings) must be admitted and monitored by EKG/telemetry until acute MI is ruled out by serial cardiac enzymes.
- Treat acute symptoms with sublingual **nitroglycerin, aspirin,** and **beta-blockers.** Start heparin drip in patients with EKG changes, multiple attacks, or unstable angina.
- If pain subsides, patients should be given nitrates (for further attacks), beta-blockers, and aspirin. Discuss **risk factor** (e.g., smoking, cholesterol, hypertension) **reduction.** Consider stress test.
- If pain increases in frequency, is unrelieved with nitroglycerin, or occurs at rest **(unstable angina),** proceed to **heparinization, angiography,** and possible **revascularization** (PTCA vs. CABG). Candidates for potential revascularization have symptoms of myocardial ischemia refractory to medical management, a positive stress test despite maximal medical regimen, or recurrent or persistent chest pain. Criteria for CABG include left main stenosis > 50%, three-vessel disease with reduced ejection fraction, and diabetic CAD.

MYOCARDIAL INFARCTION (MI) UCV *EM.1, IM1.11*

An **occlusion or spasm** of coronary vessels causing myocardial ischemia and tissue death, MI is often secondary to acute thrombus formation on a **ruptured atherosclerotic plaque.** Risk factors include age, hypertension, hypercholesterolemia, family history of early CAD, diabetes mellitus, and tobacco use. **Males** are affected more than females, and **postmenopausal females** are affected more than premenopausal females.

> **Risk factors for CAD—**
>
> **CAD HDL**
> **C**igarettes
> **A**ge and sex
> **D**iabetes mellitus
> **H**ypertension
> **D**eath from MI in family
> **L**DL high and **L**ow HDL

History

Patients present with **acute-onset chest pain,** often described as a **pressure or tightness,** that can **radiate to the left arm** or neck. **Diaphoresis,** shortness of breath, lightheadedness, and **nausea**/vomiting may also be seen. Be alert to atypical presentations. MI may cause syncope. Elderly, diabetic, and postoperative patients are particularly likely to have "silent" MIs.

PE

Tachycardia, **new mitral regurgitation** (ruptured papillary muscle), low blood pressure (cardiogenic shock), and crackles **(pulmonary edema).**

Differential

Angina, pulmonary embolism, aortic dissection, pneumothorax, pericarditis, GERD, costochondritis, herpes zoster, esophageal spasm, peptic ulcer, pneumonia, cholecystitis.

Evaluation

Evaluation should include **EKG** and **cardiac enzymes** (CK with CK-MB fraction, LDH, troponin I, troponin T). Diagnosis is based on a rise in cardiac enzymes and/or EKG changes (ST-segment elevation/depression or new LBBB; Figures 2.1–3 and 2.1–4) with an appropriate clinical presentation. MI is also associated with **arrhythmias,** including atrial fibrillation, supraventricular tachycardia, and ventricular arrhythmias. CXR may show signs of CHF.

Treatment

"Time is myocardium."

- **Acute management:** Give **oxygen, aspirin, beta-blockers** (hold in the presence of bradycardia, hypotension, or pulmonary edema), **nitroglycerin** (can cause hypotension), and **morphine** (for pain). Consider **thrombolysis** with TPA, urokinase, or streptokinase or revascularization with **angioplasty.** If hypotensive, start IV fluids and stop nitroglycerin. Patients with suspected MI require hospital admission to a cardiac-monitored bed to watch for continuing ischemia and cardiac arrhythmias, especially in the first 24 hours post-MI.
- **Inpatient:** Treat with **aspirin, heparin, beta-blockers,** and **ACE inhibitors;** perform **stress test** and/or echo after five days to assess future risk. In the event of a positive stress test, perform **catheterization** to assess vessel patency. Consider PTCA or CABG for significant occlusions.
- **Long term:** Give **aspirin, beta-blockers, lipid-lowering agents,** and **ACE inhibitors** if tolerated (especially in patients with pulmonary edema); **modify risk factors** by lowering cholesterol and BP, changing diet, and increasing exercise.

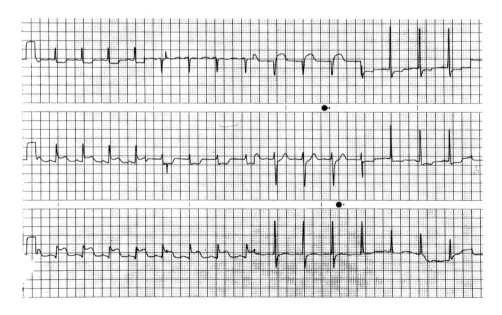

FIGURE 2.1–3. Inferior wall myocardial infarction. In this patient with acute chest pain, the EKG demonstrated acute ST elevation in leads II, III, and aVF with reciprocal ST depression and T-wave flattening in leads I, aVL, and V$_4$ to V$_6$.

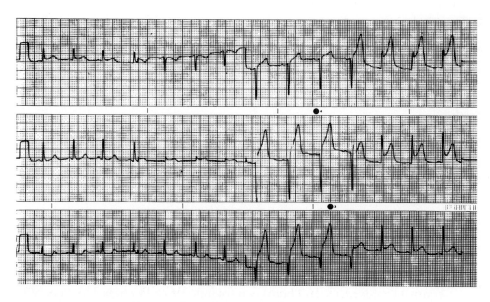

FIGURE 2.1–4. Anterior wall myocardial infarction. The patient presented with acute chest pain. EKG showed ST elevation in leads aVL and V₁ to V₆ and hyperacute T waves.

Complications

Complications following acute MI include reinfarction, LV wall rupture, pericarditis, **Dressler's syndrome,** papillary muscle rupture (with mitral regurgitation), aneurysmal dilatation of the left ventricle, and mural thrombi. **Lethal arrhythmia** is the most common cause of death following acute MI. More than 5 PVCs/min indicates a poor prognosis.

DRESSLER'S
PERICARDITIS
p̄ MI

ATRIAL FIBRILLATION

A supraventricular arrhythmia that causes an irregularly irregular rhythm. Risk factors include mitral or aortic valve abnormalities, cardiomyopathy, hypertension, ASD, hyperthyroidism, alcohol use/withdrawal, old age, pericarditis, pulmonary embolism, and chest surgery/trauma.

History

Atrial fibrillation is often **asymptomatic** but may present with shortness of breath, **palpitations,** chest pain, or syncope.

PE

Irregularly irregular pulse.

Causes of atrial fibrillation—

PIRATES
Pulmonary disease
Ischemia
Rheumatic heart disease
Anemia or atrial myxoma
Thyrotoxicosis
Ethanol
Sepsis

Differential

Multifocal atrial tachycardia, atrial flutter (Figure 2.1–6), tachycardia with variable AV block, ventricular tachycardia.

Evaluation

EKG shows an irregularly irregular rhythm with **absent P waves** and a ventricular rate of 80–200 bpm (Figure 2.1–5). Determine if there is an underlying cardiac or systemic cause.

Treatment

- **Acute:** The goal of treatment is **rate control** and hemodynamic stabilization; restoration of **sinus rhythm** is secondary. Drug therapy for rate control (reduce to < 100 bpm) can include IV or PO **beta-blockers, diltiazem,** and **digoxin.** Once rate is controlled, consider cardioversion. If atrial fibrillation has been present < 48 hours, perform chemical cardioversion (e.g., quinidine, procainamide, amiodarone, and sotalol) or electrical cardioversion. If atrial fibrillation has been present for > 48 hours or its duration is unknown, **anticoagulate** the patient with warfarin and electrically cardiovert in 3–4 weeks or obtain a **transesophageal echocardiogram** to rule out left atrial thrombi before cardioversion. If these measures are not effective or if the patient becomes unstable (e.g., shows signs of increasing chest pain, decreasing mental status, or hypotension), attempt **synchronized cardioversion.** Anticoagulate for four weeks post-cardioversion.
- **Chronic: Rate control** with beta- or calcium channel blockers; **anticoagulate** with aspirin and/or warfarin for stroke prevention.

Complications

Cerebrovascular disease with the formation of mural thrombi that may embolize in cerebral vessels, causing TIAs and/or CVAs.

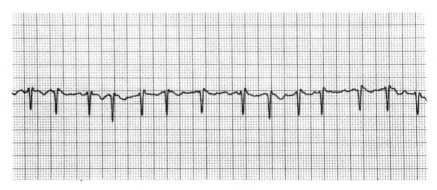

FIGURE 2.1–5. Atrial fibrillation. Note the absence of P waves and irregularly irregular ventricular rhythm.

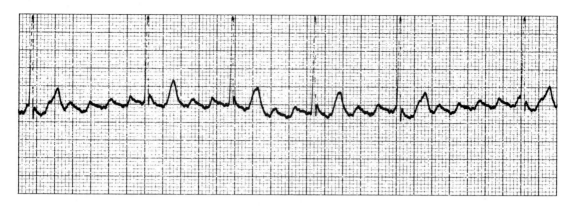

FIGURE 2.1–6. Atrial flutter. The "sawtooth" baseline of rapid but organized atrial activity (usually between 220 and 360 beats per minute) is characteristic.

CONGESTIVE HEART FAILURE (CHF)   **UCV** *IM1.4*

Symptomatic impaired cardiac function. Risk factors include CAD, a family history of hypertrophic cardiomyopathy, hypertension, vascular heart disease, alcohol abuse, and myocarditis.

History

Patients present with **dyspnea on exertion** (or at rest if severe), fatigue, lower extremity edema, **orthopnea, paroxysmal nocturnal dyspnea, nocturia,** and/or abdominal fullness.

PE

Physical exam may reveal sinus tachycardia and a laterally displaced PMI. Patients with right-sided failure may have elevated CVP **(jugular venous distention),** hepatomegaly, **hepatojugular reflex,** and bipedal **edema;** those with left-sided failure may have bilateral **basilar crackles** and **S3** and/or **S4** gallop.

Differential

MI, angina, pericarditis, nephrotic syndrome/renal failure, cirrhosis.

Evaluation

Workup should include EKG, CXR (look for **cardiomegaly, cephalization of pulmonary vessels,** pleural effusions, vascular indistinctness, and prominent hila), and **echocardiogram.** Diagnosis is based on the clinical picture and an echocardiogram showing impaired cardiac function (hypertrophic or dilated cardiomyopathy may be observed). Rule out MI in acute exacerbations. If amyloid or viral myocarditis is suspected (e.g., in cases of previous viral prodrome, young age), a myocardial biopsy may be performed.

Causes of recurrent CHF—

FAILURE
Forgot medication
Arrhythmia/**A**nemia
Ischemia/**I**nfarct/
  Infection
Lifestyle (Na+ and
  fluid intake)
Upregulation (increased CO in
  pregnancy, hyperthyroidism)
Renal failure → fluid
  overload
Embolus (pulmonary)

Treatment

- **Correct treatable causes** such as thyroid disease and valvular disease.
- **Acute:** If the patient has worsening dyspnea and other symptoms, diurese aggressively with a **loop diuretic** (such as furosemide) and a non-loop agent. Use **ACE inhibitors** in all patients who can tolerate them. Patients may require hospital admission and may also require intubation. Dobutamine for inotropy (aka "dobutamine holiday") and nitroprusside for afterload reduction may be helpful.
- **Chronic:** Use **ACE inhibitors**/AII blockers (which have been shown to decrease mortality), **diuretics** (furosemide), and **digoxin.** Treat arrhythmias as they arise; limit dietary sodium and fluid intake. Use beta-blockers if tolerated. Consider **warfarin** for severe dilated cardiomyopathy, atrial fibrillation, or previous embolic episodes.

PERICARDITIS   UC▮V *IM1.13*

Inflammation of the pericardial sac, often with an effusion. Causes include viral infection, TB infection, SLE, uremia, drugs, and neoplasms; pericarditis may also occur after MI, open heart surgery, or radiotherapy.

History

Patients may present with **pleuritic chest pain,** dyspnea, cough, and **fever.** Pain is often **positional** in nature, i.e., it worsens when the patient is supine and is relieved when the patient leans forward or with shallow breathing.

PE

Pericardial **friction rub** on auscultation (best heard with the patient leaning forward). In tamponade, **elevated CVP** and/or **pulsus paradoxus** (a fall in systolic BP > 10 mmHg on inspiration) may be seen.

Differential

Cardiac tamponade, heart failure, MI/angina, pneumonia, pneumothorax.

Evaluation

Obtain CXR, echocardiogram, and tests to rule out systemic causes. **Low-voltage, diffuse ST-segment elevation** or PR-segment depression on EKG (Figure 2.1–7) suggests the diagnosis. A pericardial effusion on echocardiography supports the diagnosis.

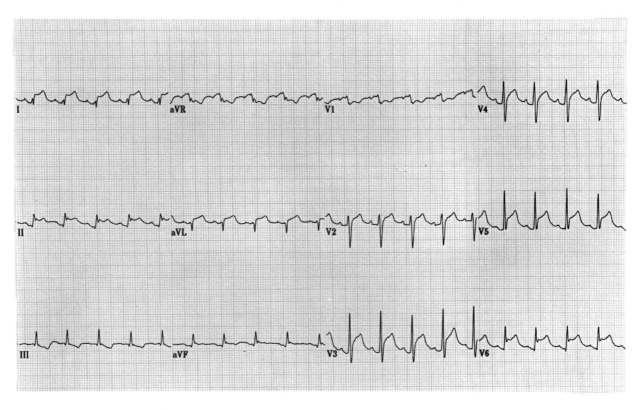

FIGURE 2.1–7. Pericarditis. There is characteristic ST elevation in all leads and PR depression in the precordial leads.

Treatment

- Treat underlying cause, e.g., **steroids**/immunosuppressants for SLE and aspirin/**NSAIDs** for viral pericarditis.
- Small effusions can be followed.
- If tamponade or a large effusion is present, **pericardiocentesis** is indicated with continuous drainage if necessary.

CARDIAC TAMPONADE

UCV EM.2

Fluid in the pericardial sac resulting in compromised ventricular filling and decreased cardiac output. Cardiac tamponade is more closely related to the rate of fluid formation than to the size of the effusion. Risk factors include known pericarditis and trauma (commonly stab wounds medial to the left nipple).

History

Patients present with severe **chest pain, tachycardia,** and **tachypnea** that can rapidly lead to shock and death.

Tamponade should be suspected in any hemodynamically unstable patient who does not respond to initial resuscitative measures.

PE

Physical exam may reveal Beck's triad of **hypotension, distant heart sounds,** and **distended neck veins** (elevated CVP), as well as a narrow pulse pressure, tachypnea, tachycardia, pulsus paradoxus, **Kussmaul's sign** (elevated CVP on inspiration), and a **rapidly worsening clinical picture.**

Differential

Severe MI, tension pneumothorax.

Evaluation

Obtain an immediate **echocardiogram** if time permits. CXR may demonstrate an enlarged, globular heart. EKG may show decreased amplitude.

Treatment

Treat with urgent **pericardiocentesis** (the aspirate will be **nonclotting** blood); a pericardial window may be required. **Volume expansion** with aggressive IV fluids is also helpful.

Dermatology

A delayed (type IV—cell-mediated) hypersensitivity reaction in the form of a skin rash that develops from contact with a substance to which the patient has **previously been sensitized.** Common offending agents include **poison ivy, poison oak, nickel,** perfumes, **soaps** and detergents, and **cosmetics.**

History

Patients most commonly complain of **pruritus** and **rash.** Rarely they may present with edema, fever, lymphadenopathy, and generalized malaise.

PE

Erythematous, weepy, crusted patches, plaques, or **papulovesicles** grouped in **linear arrays** or **geometric shapes** with sharp angles and straight borders (Figure 2.2–1). Characteristic locations are where makeup, clothing, perfume, jewelry, and plants come into contact with the skin.

Differential

Impetigo, herpes simplex, herpes zoster, seborrheic dermatitis, eczema.

Evaluation

Diagnosis is based on **clinical impression** and, if necessary, on skin patch testing.

Treatment

- **Mild cases: Cool compresses** or oatmeal preparation; apply **topical steroids** 3–4 times a day to reduce pruritus.
- **Severe cases: Systemic corticosteroids** may be required; use **antihistamines** for relief of itching.

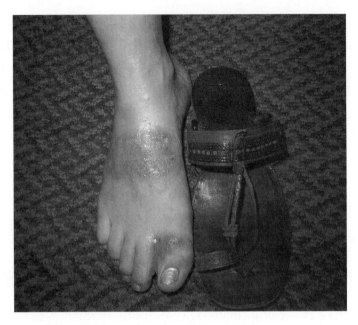

FIGURE 2.2–1. Contact dermatitis. Erythematous papules, vesicles, and serous weeping localized to areas of contact with the offending agent are characteristic.

UCV *IM2.7*

Chronic, superficial inflammatory disorder commonly involving the face; thought to be a reaction to *Pityrosporum* yeast. The rash is most common during the **neonatal** and **postpubertal** periods.

History

Patients present with mild to moderate **pruritus.**

PE

Yellowish, greasy, and **erythematous scaling patches and plaques** of the **scalp, ears,** and **face.** In severe cases, the rash may extend to the chest, back, and intertriginous areas. Scaling of the scalp (**"cradle cap"**) may be present.

Differential

Fungal infection, allergic contact dermatitis, psoriasis, immune deficiencies (e.g., histiocytosis X).

Evaluation

Diagnosis is based on **clinical suspicion.** KOH preparation can rule out **fungal infection.** A biopsy is rarely necessary except in atypical presentations.

Treatment

- **Therapy for the face, body, and intertriginous areas:** 1% hydrocortisone or stronger BID depending on the thickness of the affected skin. In some cases a 2% ketoconazole cream can be used as a substitute for, or in conjunction with, topical steroids. Mild tar cream can be used as an adjunct to topical steroids.
- **Therapy for the scalp: Medicated shampoos** with selenium sulfide, tar, or zinc pyrithione (Selsun or Head and Shoulders) 2–3 times a week. In more severe cases, topical steroids may be used.

PSORIASIS　　　　　　　　　　　　　　　　　　**UCV** *IM2.6*

An idiopathic inflammatory disorder that results in **epidermal hyperproliferation.**

History

Pruritus may be present. Pain, tenderness, and joint stiffness may occur with **psoriatic arthritis** (characterized by involvement of the DIP joints). **Generalized toxicity,** fever, and malaise may occur with the generalized pustular form.

PE

Dark **red plaques with silvery-white scales** and **sharp margins** (Figure 2.2–2). Lesions are classically found over **areas of extension.** Characteristic nail findings include **nail pitting,** "oil spots," and **onycholysis** (lifting of the nail plate).

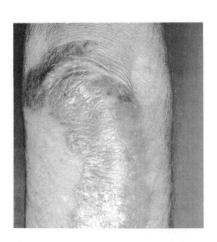
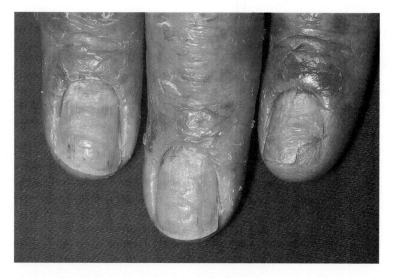

FIGURE 2.2–2. Psoriasis. (A) Skin changes. The classic sharply demarcated dark red plaques with silvery scales are commonly located on extensor surfaces (e.g., elbows, knees). (B) Nail changes. Note the pitting, onycholysis, and "oil spots".

Differential

SLE (possibly without systemic symptoms), syphilis, allergic contact dermatitis, fungal infections, seborrheic dermatitis, cutaneous T-cell lymphoma, eczema.

Evaluation

Diagnosis is based on the **gross appearance** and pattern of distribution of the lesions. **Skin biopsy** shows a thickened epidermis with an absent granular cell layer and preservation of the nuclei within the hyperkeratotic stratum corneum. Neutrophils in the stratum corneum are classic. Blood tests may show elevated uric acid levels, increased ESR, and mild anemia.

Treatment

- **Mild to moderate disease: Topical steroids,** intralesional corticosteroid therapy, tars, anthralin, salicylic acid, tretinoin, 5-FU, topical antifungal agents, systemic antibiotics.
- **Severe or generalized psoriasis: Phototherapy,** PUVA, methotrexate, etretinate.

PITYRIASIS ROSEA

A mild, idiopathic, self-limited cutaneous eruption seen primarily in children.

History

Patients present with mild to moderate pruritus.

PE

A herald patch is pathognomonic for pityriasis rosea.

A diffuse eruption of round to **oval erythematous papules** and plaques covered with a fine "cigarette paper" white scale, with the distribution of the rash on the trunk following skin lines in a **Christmas-tree pattern** (Figure 2.2–3). A **herald patch**—a solitary patch 2–6 cm in diameter that precedes the rest of the rash—is pathognomonic.

Differential

Secondary syphilis, psoriasis, cutaneous T-cell lymphoma (parapsoriasis).

Evaluation

A **skin biopsy** is required if the lesions do not resolve in two months. A serologic test is indicated to rule out secondary syphilis.

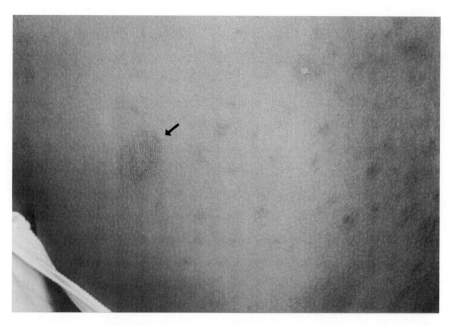

FIGURE 2.2–3. Pityriasis rosea. The round to oval erythematous plaques are often covered with a fine white scale ("cigarette paper") and are often found on the trunk and proximal extremities. The plaques are often preceded by a larger herald patch (arrow).

Treatment

The lesions are **self-limited.** A mild topical steroid or talc may be used for relief of pruritus. Natural sunlight or daily UVB treatments may hasten healing.

HERPES SIMPLEX UCV IM2.3

A painful, **recurrent** vesicular eruption of the mucocutaneous surfaces due to herpes simplex virus infection. The **oral-labial** form of HSV is usually due to herpes simplex type 1. The **genital** form is usually due to herpes simplex type 2.

History

Primary eruptions are more severe and longer-lasting than recurrent eruptions. **Primary** outbreaks may be accompanied by **lymphadenopathy, fever,** discomfort, **malaise,** and edema of the involved tissue. **Recurrent** infections are limited to the mucocutaneous area innervated by the **involved nerve.** Onset is preceded by **tingling,** burning, or frank pain.

PE

Physical exam reveals **grouped vesicles on an erythematous base** (Figure 2.2–4A).

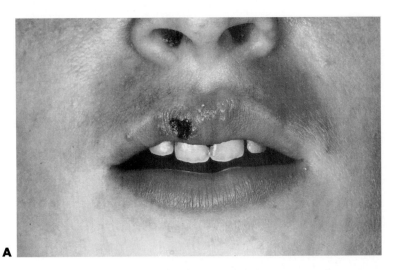

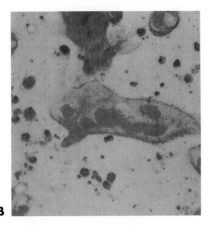

FIGURE 2.2–4. Herpes simplex. (A) Primary infection. Grouped vesicles on an erythematous base on the patient's lips and oral mucosa may progress to pustules before resolving. (B) Tzanck smear. The multinucleated giant cells from vesicular fluid provide a presumptive diagnosis of HSV infection. The Tzanck smear cannot distinguish between HSV and VZV infection.

Differential

Aphthous stomatitis, pemphigus vulgaris, Behçet's disease, syphilis, chancroid, trauma.

Evaluation

Multinucleated giant cells and acantholytic cells on **Tzanck smear** yield a **presumptive** diagnosis (Figure 2.2–4B). However, herpes zoster has the same appearance on the Tzanck, so definitive diagnosis requires culture or direct fluorescent antibody testing.

Treatment

Acyclovir ointment is somewhat effective in reducing the duration of viral shedding but not in preventing recurrence. The mainstay of therapy is oral or IV acyclovir (use IV acyclovir for severe cases or immune-compromised patients), which reduces both the frequency and the severity of recurrences. Daily acyclovir suppressive therapy may be used in patients with > 6 outbreaks per year.

VARICELLA

UCV Ped.34

Infection by the varicella-zoster virus (a member of the herpesvirus family), also known as **chickenpox.** Transmission is via **respiratory droplet contamination** or contact with **skin lesions.** Varicella has an incubation period of 10–20 days. Contagion begins **24 hours** before the eruption appears and continues until crusting has occurred.

History

A **prodrome** of malaise, fever, headache, and myalgia commonly occurs 24 hours before the onset of the rash. **Pruritic lesions appear in crops** over a period of 3–4 days.

PE

Lesions start as pink to red macules and then progress to grouped central vesicles, giving the classic appearance of a **"dewdrop on a rose petal,"** finally crusting over. Lesions are commonly found on the **trunk, face,** and **scalp.**

Differential

Disseminated herpes zoster, exanthem due to coxsackievirus.

Evaluation

Diagnosis is based on **clinical examination** and history and, if necessary, can be confirmed by culture or direct fluorescent antibody testing.

Treatment

The disease is **self-limited** in healthy children. For healthy adults with uncomplicated primary varicella, **oral acyclovir** is the appropriate therapy. For adults with severe disease, immune-compromised patients, and those with primary varicella pneumonia, **IV acyclovir** may be required. A **vaccine** is now available for infants, children, and adults (immune-compromised patients and

Administer varicella immune globulin to pregnant women with primary infection.

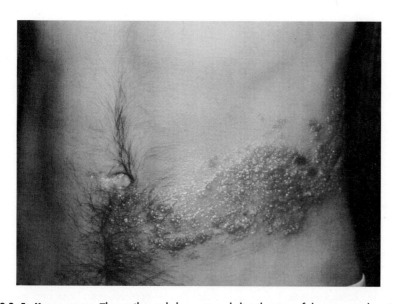

FIGURE 2.2–5. Herpes zoster. The unilateral dermatomal distribution of the grouped vesicles on an erythematous base is characteristic.

adults without previous infection). Recurrent infection can present as **shingles (herpes zoster, Figure 2.2–5)**, which can be quite painful and serious. *IM2.20*

ACTINIC KERATOSIS UCV *IM2.1*

A **premalignant lesion** resulting from **sun exposure** which can lead to squamous cell carcinoma. Actinic keratosis is also known as solar keratosis.

History

Lesions are usually **asymptomatic** unless they are irritated or inflamed.

PE

Physical exam reveals **discrete, rough, scaling patches** and papules 1–5 mm in diameter. Lesions usually have a poorly demarcated erythematous base with an area of rough, **white superficial scaling** and are generally found in sun-exposed areas of the body (Figure 2.2–6).

Differential

Squamous cell carcinoma, eczema.

Evaluation

All actinic keratoses should be biopsied.

Skin biopsy shows areas of **dysplastic squamous epithelium** (hyperkeratosis, with cells of the lower epidermis showing loss of polarity, pleomorphism, and hyperchromatic nuclei) **without invasion.**

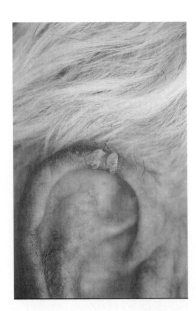

FIGURE 2.2–6. Actinic keratosis. The discrete patch has an erythematous base and rough white scale. Actinic keratosis is a premalignant lesion that may progress to squamous cell carcinoma. It is most commonly found in sun-exposed areas.

Treatment

Treat with **topical 5-FU,** cryosurgery, curettage, and chemical peel. **Prevent with UVA/UVB sunscreens** and by avoiding prolonged and unnecessary sun exposure.

SQUAMOUS CELL CARCINOMA UCV *IM2.8*

Risk factors include **exposure** to sun and ionizing radiation, actinic keratosis, immunosuppression, arsenic, and industrial carcinogens.

History

Lesions are usually slowly evolving and **asymptomatic;** occasionally, bleeding or pain may develop.

PE

Physical examination reveals small, red, **exophytic nodules** with varying degrees of scaling or crusting (Figure 2.2–7). Lesions are commonly found in **sun-exposed areas.** Lesions are usually found on the ears, cheeks, lower lip, and dorsum of the hands.

Differential

Basal cell carcinoma, warts, actinic keratosis.

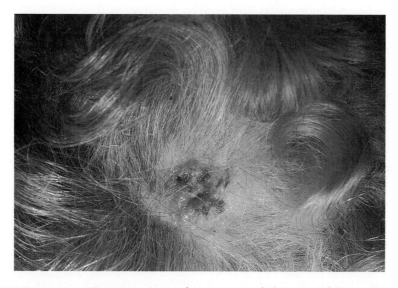

FIGURE 2.2–7. Squamous cell carcinoma. Note the crusting and ulceration of this erythematous plaque. Most lesions are exophytic nodules with erosion or ulceration.

Evaluation

Biopsy shows irregular masses of anaplastic epidermal cells proliferating down to the dermis.

Treatment

Surgical excision is necessary for larger lesions and for those involving the periorbital, periauricular, perilabial, genital, and perigenital areas. **Mohs' micrographic surgery** (serial excisions with fresh-tissue microscopic examination to maximize cosmesis) may be performed for recurrent lesions and on areas of the face that are difficult to reconstruct, as well as for poorly differentiated tumors and those with ill-defined margins. **Radiation** may be necessary in cases where surgery is not a viable option. **Prevent with UVA/UVB sunscreens** and by avoiding prolonged and unnecessary sun exposure.

BASAL CELL CARCINOMA

The **most common type of skin cancer.** Basal cell carcinoma is associated with excessive sun exposure and may take many different forms, including nodular, ulcerative, pigmented, and superficial.

History

Lesions are usually asymptomatic unless secondarily infected or inflamed or in advanced disease.

PE

Pearly-colored papule of variable size. The external surface is frequently covered with fine **telangiectasias** and appears **translucent** (Figure 2.2–8). Lesions may be found anywhere on the body but are most commonly found in sun-exposed areas.

Differential

Squamous cell carcinoma, actinic keratosis, seborrheic keratosis.

Evaluation

Skin biopsy shows characteristic basophilic **palisading cells.**

Treatment

Therapy depends on the size and location of the tumor, the histologic type, the history of prior treatment, the underlying health of the patient, and cos-

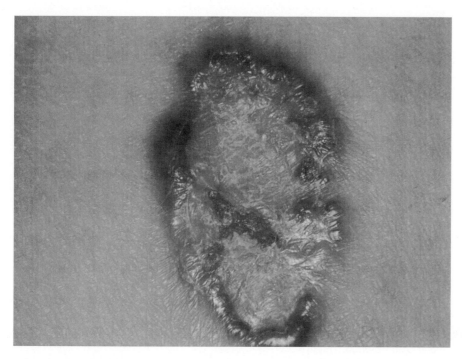

FIGURE 2.2–8. Basal cell carcinoma. Note the pearly, translucent surface (often covered with fine telangectasias), rolled border, and central ulceration.

metic considerations. Options include curettage, surgical excision, Mohs' micrographic surgery, cryosurgery, and radiation. **Prevent with UVA/UVB sunscreens** and by avoiding prolonged and unnecessary sun exposure.

MELANOMA UCV *Surg.4*

An **aggressive** skin malignancy of melanocytic origin. Risk factors include sun exposure, fair skin, a positive family history (e.g., dysplastic nevus syndrome), xeroderma pigmentosa, a large number of nevi, and the presence of dysplastic nevi. Melanoma is the leading cause of death from skin disease.

History

Melanoma is usually **asymptomatic** until late in the disease process. Patients may present with pruritus and mild discomfort. **A pigmented skin lesion that has recently changed in size or appearance should raise concern.** Lesions may be seen on sun-exposed areas as well as on the plantar aspect of the feet.

PE

Lesions are characterized by the **ABCD**s of melanoma (see sidebar) and may occur anywhere on the body (Figure 2.2–9).

ABCDs of melanoma:

Asymmetry
Border irregularity
Color variation
Diameter (large)

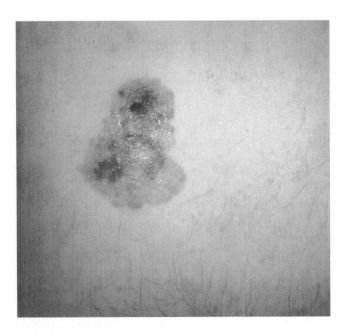

FIGURE 2.2–9. Melanoma. Note the **a**symmetry, **b**order irregularity, **c**olor variation, and large **d**iameter of this plaque.

Differential

Nevi, seborrheic keratosis, freckles, pigmented basal cell carcinoma.

Evaluation

Skin biopsy shows **melanocytes with marked cellular atypia** (vacuolated cytoplasm, hyperchromatic nuclei with prominent nucleoli, and pleomorphism) and melanocytic invasion into the dermis.

Treatment

Surgical excision is the treatment of choice. In cases of metastases, lymph node dissection and **chemotherapy** are necessary. Advanced disease may not respond to therapy. The thickness of the melanoma **(depth of invasion)** is the most important prognostic factor.

ERYTHEMA MULTIFORME

UCV EM.30

An acute, usually self-limited reaction of the skin and mucous membranes characterized by macules, papules, vesicles, and bullae. Erythema multiforme is an immune-mediated disorder that is due to drugs (e.g., penicillin, sulfonamides, phenytoin), infection (especially herpes simplex and *Mycoplasma*), vaccination, or malignancy.

History

The appearance of skin lesions may be preceded by a mild **prodrome** consisting of malaise and myalgias. Lesions may be associated with pain and fever. Mucosal involvement may result in dysphagia and dysuria.

PE

Pink-red to red-blue **macules, papules, gyrate erythematous plaques, target lesions,** and **bullae** are found on physical examination (Figure 2.2–10). Lesions can be found anywhere but are most common on the **extremities, palms, and soles.** Erythema multiforme major (Stevens–Johnson syndrome) may present with systemic toxicity, involvement of the oral mucosa and conjunctiva, and skin denudation.

Differential

Urticaria, viral exanthem, staphylococcal scalded skin syndrome, bullous pemphigoid, pemphigus vulgaris.

Evaluation

Diagnosis is based on a clinical history of **exposure** to agents known to cause erythema multiforme. An elevated eosinophil count or positive serologic tests for hepatitis, infectious mononucleosis, histoplasmosis, or mycoplasma may be seen. Skin biopsy may show perivascular lymphocytes and necrotic keratinocytes.

Treatment

Mild cases resolve on their own. If the condition is drug-induced, **discontinue the inciting agent** immediately. If due to herpes simplex, acyclovir should be given. Severe forms require **corticosteroids** and analgesia for painful eruptions and may also necessitate hospitalization for dehydration due to poor PO intake and/or skin loss in Stevens–Johnson syndrome.

Erythema multiforme is due to drugs, infection, vaccination, or malignancy.

Stevens–Johnson syndrome can be fatal and is commonly treated in a burn unit.

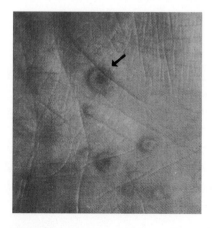

FIGURE 2.2–10. Erythema multiforme. The classic target lesion has a dull red center, pale zone, and darker outer ring (arrow). This acute self-limited reaction may occur with infection, antibiotic use, exposure to radiation or chemicals, or malignancy.

CELLULITIS

A primary skin infection commonly caused by **group A streptococci** or **staphylococci.** Risk factors include diabetes, IV drug use, venous stasis, and immune-compromised states.

History

The area of involvement is **red, swollen,** and either **painful** or burning. Fever and chills may be present.

PE

Red, hot, swollen, tender skin lesions. Tinea pedis with resultant skin fissures is a common portal of bacterial entry (often not apparent on physical exam). Look for signs of compartment syndrome.

Differential

Necrotizing fasciitis, osteomyelitis, abscess, urticaria, allergic contact dermatitis, phlebitis.

Evaluation

A culture of material obtained from the wound may aid in diagnosis. Blood cultures should be obtained when bacteremia is suspected. Otherwise, the diagnosis is based on clinical signs and symptoms.

Treatment

For mild to moderate cases, prescribe **oral antibiotics** (usually cephalexin or dicloxacillin for penicillinase-producing organisms) for 7–10 days. Hospitalization and IV antibiotics (e.g., oxacillin) are necessary if there are any signs of systemic toxicity, comorbid conditions, extremes of age, hand or orbital involvement, or other concerns.

ERYTHEMA NODOSUM   UCV *IM2.4*

Erythema nodosum results from hypersensitivity reactions to drugs, infections, sarcoid, or IBD.

An inflammation of the subcutaneous fat that produces tender erythematous nodules, usually on the **anterior tibial areas,** most commonly in young women. Lesions result from hypersensitivity reactions to drugs or infections (including beta-hemolytic strep, coccidioidomycosis, histoplasmosis, TB, and syphilis), sarcoid, rheumatic fever, or inflammatory bowel disease (IBD).

History

Lesions are usually **painful** and located on the anterior aspects of both legs. Malaise, arthralgias, and fever may precede the rash.

PE

Tender, erythematous pretibial nodules without ulceration (Figure 2.2–11). Lesions rarely occur on the face, arms, or trunk.

Differential

Polyarteritis nodosa, other types of panniculitis.

Evaluation

Skin biopsy provides a definitive diagnosis. Other helpful laboratory findings include an elevated ESR, mild leukocytosis, a high ASO titer, and a false-positive VDRL. CXR, cultures, and a Gram stain of the lesion may also be performed. (Gram stain should be negative, since erythema nodosum is a reactive lesion.)

Treatment

Therapy is supportive and includes elevation of the leg, bed rest, and

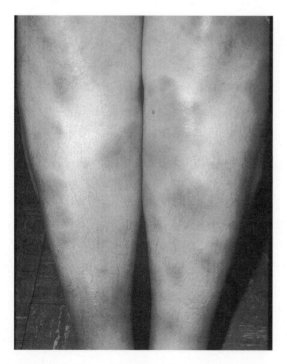

FIGURE 2.2–11. Erythema nodosum. The erythematous plaques and nodules are commonly located on pretibial areas. Lesions are painful and indurated and heal spontaneously without ulceration.

NSAIDs. Potassium iodide may be given as well. Systemic corticosteroids may be necessary for persistent cases. Before steroid therapy is initiated, a thorough evaluation should be performed to confirm the etiology of the lesion.

TINEA VERSICOLOR

A common superficial skin infection caused by the fungus *Malassezia furfur*.

History

Lesions are usually asymptomatic but may cause mild itching.

PE

Physical exam reveals **small, scaling macules** that tend to enlarge and sometimes coalesce. They can be pinkish, lightly pigmented, or **hypopigmented.** The usual sites are the chest and back, but lesions can be found anywhere (Figure 2.2–12).

Differential

Vitiligo, eczema, psoriasis, seborrheic dermatitis.

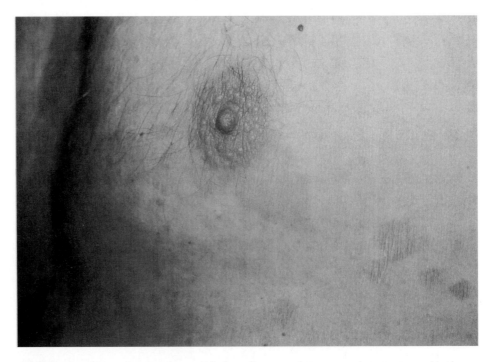

FIGURE 2.2–12. Tinea versicolor. These pinkish scaling macules commonly appear on the chest and back. Lesions may also be lightly pigmented or hypopigmented depending on the patient's skin color and sun exposure.

Evaluation

KOH examination reveals **short, blunt hyphae and small spores** ("spaghetti and meatballs"). Wood's light examination distinguishes pigmented from hypopigmented areas and is helpful in evaluating the extent of the disease.

Treatment

Initial treatment is with a **topical antifungal agent,** with resolution occurring in approximately 2–3 weeks. Selenium sulfide shampoo may be used 1–3 times a week for three weeks; the lotion is applied to the skin for 10 minutes and is then scrubbed off. In light of their serious side effects, systemic antifungals should be used only in the most resistant cases. Oral ketoconazole therapy is used in some cases. Eighty percent of cases recur within two years, since the organism colonizes the skin.

TINEA CORPORIS

Tinea corporis, or ringworm, is a fungal infection on the body.

History

Patients complain primarily of pruritic scaly plaques.

PE

Ring-shaped, erythematous, and **scaling plaques** are seen, often with central clearing and **elevated borders.** The lesions are usually few in number (Figure 2.2–13).

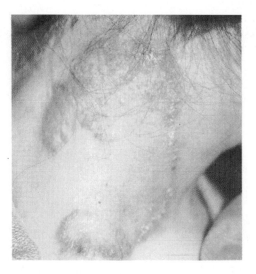

FIGURE 2.2–13. Tinea corporis. Ring-shaped, erythematous, scaling macules with central clearing seen here on the neck are characteristic.

Differential

Pityriasis rosea, psoriasis, SLE, secondary syphilis, nummular eczema.

Evaluation

Diagnosis is based on physical findings and on **hyphae** seen on **KOH preparation.** Culture is confirmatory.

Treatment

Topical antifungal cream should be applied twice a day for four weeks. Griseofulvin may be necessary if the lesions do not respond to topical therapy.

MOLLUSCUM CONTAGIOSUM

A poxvirus infection that is most common in **young children** and is also among the most common cutaneous findings in **AIDS patients.**

History

Lesions are **asymptomatic** unless inflamed or irritated.

PE

Physical exam reveals discrete, **dome-shaped, shiny papules,** frequently with central **umbilication** (Figure 2.2–14). Lesions are usually 2–5 mm in diameter. In children, the lesions are commonly found on the trunk, extremities, and face. In adults they are more frequently found in the perianal and perigenital areas.

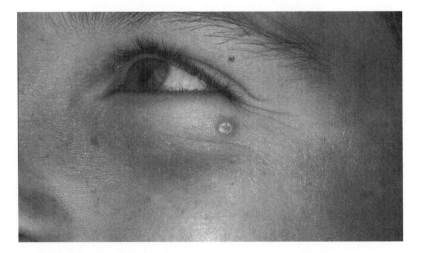

FIGURE 2.2–14. Molluscum contagiosum. The dome-shaped, fleshy, umbilicated papule on the child's eyelid is characteristic.

Differential

Warts, acne, milia.

Evaluation

Expressing and staining the contents confirms the diagnosis. Giemsa or Wright's stain allows for the identification of large inclusion or molluscum bodies. Ask adults about HIV risk factors.

Treatment

Treatment consists of curretting the lesion, liquid nitrogen cryotherapy, or application of **trichloroacetic acid.** Lesions resolve spontaneously over periods of months or years and are often left untreated in children.

CANDIDAL INTERTRIGO

An infection of the skin caused by *Candida albicans.* Predisposing factors include **obesity, diabetes, recent antibiotic therapy,** and a **warm, moist environment.**

History

Pruritus and **pain** are the most common presenting symptoms.

PE

Well-demarcated, beefy-red **erythematous patches** surrounded by satellite pustules. The infection is usually restricted to **intertriginous areas** (Figure 2.2–15). In infants, it often presents as a rash in the **diaper area.**

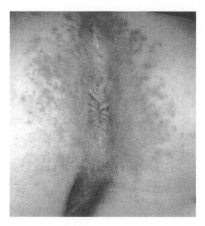

FIGURE 2.2–15. Candidal intertrigo. Erythematous areas surrounded by satellite pustules are restricted to warm, moist intertriginous areas.

Differential

Tinea cruris, irritant intertrigo, psoriasis, eczema, seborrheic dermatitis, erythrasma.

Evaluation

Diagnosis can be confirmed by scraping a satellite lesion, placing it in **KOH,** and observing **pseudohyphae** under a microscope.

Treatment

Reduce moisture and friction through **weight loss** and **body powder.** A **topical antifungal agent** should be used and may be combined with a low-potency topical steroid to alleviate the pruritis associated with the lesions.

IMPETIGO   UCV *Ped.26*

A contagious and autoinoculable infection of the skin caused by **staphylococcal or streptococcal organisms,** impetigo is more common in **children** than in adults. Bullous impetigo is due to coagulase-positive staphylococci that produce exfoliatin, a toxin that leads to vesicle or bulla formation. Nonbullous impetigo is caused by group A streptococci, which produce superficial pustular lesions.

History

Patients often present with **pruritic facial lesions** that develop over a few days.

PE

Classically, **honey-colored crusts** are seen on the lesions, which often involve the face. **Bullous impetigo** begins as small, erythematous macules that develop into thin-walled vesicles or bullae on an erythematous base. **Nonbullous impetigo** is characterized by superficial pustules with surrounding erythema. Common sites of distribution are the **face, neck,** and **extremities** (Figure 2.2–16).

Differential

Ecthyma (thick crust overlying a deep ulcer), allergic contact dermatitis.

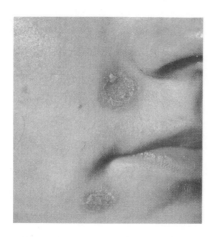

FIGURE 2.2–16. Impetigo. Dried pustules with superficial golden-brown crust are most commonly found around the nose and mouth.

Evaluation

A bacterial culture may help assess sensitivity to the chosen antibiotic therapy.

Treatment

Affected areas should be gently washed with a mild soap. **Systemic antibiotics** should have activity against both staphylococcus and streptococcus, since the distinction may at times be difficult to make. Because of contagion, the patient's towels and washcloths should be segregated from other household members.

Endocrine

DIABETES MELLITUS
UCV IM1.20

A metabolic disease that manifests as hyperglycemia secondary to **insulin deficiency** or to end-organ **insulin resistance.** Diabetes mellitus is classified into two major types:

- **Type I:** Also known as insulin-dependent diabetes mellitus (IDDM), type I diabetes mellitus is most commonly diagnosed in **children,** is characterized by **insulin deficiency,** requires **exogenous insulin,** and is strongly associated with HLA-DR3 and HLA-DR4 serotypes.
- **Type II:** Also known as non-insulin-dependent diabetes mellitus (NIDDM) or adult-onset diabetes mellitus (AODM), type II diabetes mellitus usually occurs in **obese patients > 40** and is due to end-organ **insulin resistance.** NIDDM tends to run in families.

History/PE

Patients present with **polydipsia, polyuria** (including nocturia), **polyphagia, weight loss,** recurrent infections, and blurred vision. Patients with IDDM may present with rapid weight loss and symptoms of ketoacidosis.

Differential

Pancreatic diseases (e.g., chronic pancreatitis, hemochromatosis), hormonal abnormalities (e.g., glucagonoma [IM1.22], Cushing's syndrome), **medication side effects** (e.g., corticosteroids, thiazide diuretics, phenytoin), gestational diabetes.

Evaluation

Criteria include **symptoms** of diabetes (polyuria, polydipsia, unexplained weight loss) plus **random** plasma glucose concentration > **200 mg/dL** OR **fasting** plasma glucose > **126 mg/dL** OR two-hour postprandial glucose > 200 on oral glucose tolerance test (each criterion must be **repeated** on a subsequent day). Elevated hemoglobin A_{1c} (glycosylated hemoglobin) and the presence of urine glucose and urine ketones also support the diagnosis.

Treatment

- **Type I:** Treat with **insulin.**
- **Type II:** Treat initially with **weight loss** and **exercise** and then with **oral hypoglycemics** (e.g., glipizide, glyburide, metformin). Use **insulin for refractory cases.**

Complications

Table 2.3–1 lists complications commonly associated with diabetes.

TABLE 2.3–1. Complications of Diabetes.

Complication	Description
Diabetic ketoacidosis IM1.21	Hyperglycemia-induced crisis that occurs most commonly in **type I diabetics** and that may be precipitated by infections, MI, alcohol, drugs (e.g., corticosteroids, thiazide diuretics), pancreatitis, and noncompliance with insulin therapy. Patients often present with **abdominal pain, vomiting, Kussmaul respirations** (increased tidal volume), and a **fruity, acetone odor.** Patients are severely dehydrated with many electrolyte abnormalities (e.g., hypokalemia, hypophosphatemia, **increased anion gap metabolic acidosis**) and may also develop mental status changes. Treatment includes **insulin** and aggressive **fluid and electrolyte replacement** in addition to treatment of initiating event.
Nonketotic hyperglycemic coma IM1.28	Presents as **profound dehydration,** mental status changes, and an extremely high plasma glucose (> 600 mg/dL); occurs most commonly in **type II diabetics** and is often fatal. Treatment includes **insulin** and **aggressive fluid and electrolyte replacement.**
Retinopathy	Generally does not appear until diabetes has been present for at least **3–5 years.** Risk factors include hyperglycemia, hypertension, and pregnancy. Preventive measures include control of hyperglycemia and hypertension and **laser therapy for neovascularization.**
Diabetic nephropathy	Characterized by glomerular hyperfiltration followed by **microalbuminuria.** Begin therapy with an **ACE inhibitor;** control hyperglycemia; control hypertension.
Neuropathy	Peripheral, symmetric, sensorimotor neuropathy leading to foot trauma and diabetic ulcers. Treat with preventive **foot care, analgesics,** and tricyclic antidepressants.
Macrovascular complications	Cardiovascular, cerebrovascular, peripheral vascular disease. **Cardiovascular disease** is the most common cause of death in diabetic patients. Goal BP is 135/85; lower LDL to < 130. In presence of known CAD, lower LDL to < 100 and triglycerides to < 200 mg/dL.

Graves' disease is the most common etiology of hyperthyroidism. It is most often seen in women 20–40 years of age. Other etiologies include toxic nodular goiter, toxic adenomas, and subacute thyroiditis. Less common etiologies include pituitary TSH hypersecretion, exogenous iodide (Jod–Basedow disease), struma ovarii, and Hashimoto's thyroiditis.

History

Weight loss and increased appetite as well as heat intolerance, nervousness, weakness, increased bowel frequency, and menstrual abnormalities.

PE

Warm, moist skin, goiter, sinus tachycardia or atrial fibrillation, thyroid bruit, fine tremor, and hyperactive reflexes. Exophthalmos and pretibial myxedema are seen in Graves' disease (Figure 2.3–1).

Differential

Anxiety, neurosis, mania, pheochromocytoma, malignancy, chronic alcoholism, primary myopathy, myasthenia gravis.

Evaluation

Suppressed TSH is the most sensitive test for primary hyperthyroidism; also look for elevated T_4, increased free T_4, and elevated free T_4 index. ESR will be elevated in thyroiditis.

TSH receptor antibodies are seen in patients with Graves' disease.

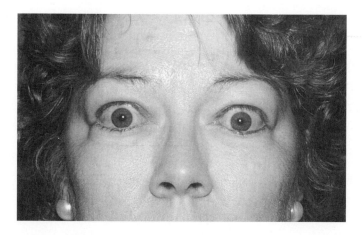

FIGURE 2.3–1. Graves' ophthalmopathy. Proptosis with lid retraction that results from lymphocytic infiltration and edema of the extraocular muscles may progress to fibrosis with limited eye movement and blindness from optic nerve compression.

HIGH-YIELD FACTS

Endocrine

Treatment

Administer **propranolol** for catecholamine symptoms followed by **radioablation.** Give **antithyroid drugs** (methimazole, carbimazole, propylthiouracil) for patients with mild thyrotoxicosis or goiter. **Thyroidectomy** is indicated for large goiters with postoperative levothyroxine to prevent hypothyroidism.

HYPOTHYROIDISM   UCV *IM1.23, 26*

A condition characterized by inadequate thyroid hormone in tissues. Hypothyroidism is most commonly caused by **Hashimoto's thyroiditis;** other causes include subacute or postpartum thyroiditis, drugs (e.g., iodide, amiodarone, sulfonamides, lithium), iatrogenic factors (radioablation or excision with inadequate supplementation), and pituitary dysfunction. Myxedema refers to severe hypothyroidism with deposition of mucopolysaccharides in the dermis. **Cretinism** refers to untreated congenital hypothyroidism leading to cognitive defects and physical abnormalities.

History

Patients present with weakness, fatigue, **cold intolerance, constipation,** weight gain, **depression,** menstrual irregularities, and **hoarseness.**

PE

Dry, cold, puffy skin, edema, thin eyebrows, **bradycardia,** and delayed relaxation of deep tendon reflexes.

Differential

Chronic fatigue, malnutrition, CHF, primary amyloidosis, depression.

Evaluation

Elevated TSH is the most sensitive measure. Also look for decreased serum T_4, decreased free T_4, and radioiodine uptake < 10% in 24 hours.

Antimicrosomal and anti-thyroglobulin antibodies are seen in patients with Hashimoto's thyroiditis.

Treatment

Administer **levothyroxine** for uncomplicated hypothyroidism. Levothyroxine plus hydrocortisone is indicated for myxedema coma.

Occurs in 0.1% of the population. Ninety percent of cases result from a single **adenoma;** 10% result from parathyroid hyperplasia. Parathyroid carcinoma accounts for < 1% of all cases.

History

Seventy percent of cases are **asymptomatic.**

PE

The following mnemonic describes common presenting symptoms and signs: **stones** (nephrolithiasis or nephrocalcinosis), **bones** (bone pain, muscle aches, arthralgias, fractures [osteitis fibrosa]), **groans** (PUD, pancreatitis), and **psychic overtones** (fatigue, depression, anxiety, irritability, sleep/concentration disturbances).

Differential

Same as for hypercalcemia (see "Hypercalcemia," p. 334 in Renal).

Evaluation

Hypercalcemia, hypophosphatemia, and hypercalciuria are the classic hallmarks. PTH will be elevated relative to ionized calcium.

Treatment

Treat with **parathyroidectomy** if symptomatic; administer bisphosphonates preoperatively. For acute hypercalcemia, give **IV fluids** and **loop diuretics** (once adequately hydrated).

A disorder caused by destruction of the adrenal cortices. **Autoimmune destruction** is the most common etiology and accounts for 80% of spontaneous cases. Addison's disease may be isolated or may occur as part of a polyglandular autoimmune syndrome (hypothyroidism, type I diabetes, vitiligo, premature ovarian failure, testicular failure, and pernicious anemia). Other causes include congenital enzyme deficiencies, hemorrhage (often bilateral), TB, and other infections.

> **AdD**ison's disease is due to **Ad**renocortical **D**eficiency.

History

Presenting symptoms include **weakness, weight loss, nausea,** and **vomiting.**

PE

Increased skin pigmentation, hypotension, and anorexia.

BRONZE

Differential

Anorexia nervosa, malabsorption states, occult malignancy, hypoparathyroidism, thyrotoxicosis, panhypopituitarism, hemochromatosis.

Evaluation

Findings include **elevated plasma ACTH** and low cortisol levels in response to ACTH challenge. Additional lab findings include **hyponatremia, hyperkalemia,** and **eosinophilia.**   (↓ MINERALOCORTICOIDS)

Treatment

Treat with replacement **glucocorticoids** and **mineralocorticoids.** Administer **stress-dose** steroids during periods of stress (e.g., major surgery, trauma, infection).

CUSHING'S SYNDROME   UCV IM1.19

A condition that refers to the manifestations of **hypercortisolism.** Cushing's syndrome is most commonly caused by **excessive** administration of corticosteroids. Non-iatrogenic causes include ACTH hypersecretion by the pituitary (70%) or by nonpituitary neoplasms (15%) such as small cell lung cancer, or cortisol secretion by an adrenal tumor or bilateral adrenal hyperplasia (15%).

History

Depression, oligomenorrhea, growth retardation, weakness, acne, and **excessive hair growth.** Symptoms of **diabetes** (e.g., polydipsia, polyuria, dysuria) may also be present secondary to decreased glucose tolerance.

PE

↑MINERALOCORTICOIDS

Hypertension, central obesity, muscle wasting, thin skin with easy **bruisability** and purple **striae,** psychological changes, **hirsutism, moon facies,** and "**buffalo hump.**"

Differential

Chronic alcoholism, depression, diabetes mellitus, exogenous steroid administration, adrenogenital syndrome.

Evaluation

- Screen for elevated **free urinary cortisol.**
- Administer **low-dose dexamethasone suppression test** (an abnormal result consists of persistently elevated cortisol levels after suppression the previous night).
- Localize the lesion; ACTH is high with an ectopic or pituitary source and is low or undetectable in the presence of an adrenal source. If high, a **high-dose dexamethasone suppression test** will suppress cortisol secretion in pituitary disease.
- CT (adrenal) or MRI (sphenoid) can further localize lesions.
- Other lab values suggestive of the diagnosis include **hyperglycemia,** glycosuria, and **hypokalemia.**

Treatment

Treat with **resection** of the hypersecretory source (pituitary, adrenal). Irradiation may be a consideration in pituitary disease. **Ketoconazole or metyrapone** may be used in adrenal carcinoma or small cell lung cancer (inhibits cortisol secretion).

Complications

Increased susceptibility to infection; vertebral compression fractures, avascular necrosis of the femoral head.

SAME SEQUELLAE AS EXOGENOUS CORTICOSTEROIDS

HEMOCHROMATOSIS **UCV** IM1.36

An **autosomal-recessive** disease that usually occurs in (males) and is rarely recognized before the (fifth) decade. Hemochromatosis is caused by hyperabsorption of iron with parenchymal hemosiderin accumulation in the liver, pancreas, heart, adrenals, testes, pituitary, and kidneys. Secondary hemochromatosis may occur with iron overload and is commonly seen in patients receiving **chronic transfusion therapy** and in **alcoholics** (alcohol increases GI absorption of iron). (β THALLAS)

MALE
FIFTY
↑Fe ABSORP
HEMOSIDERIN → PANC, HEART, ADRENAL, TESTES, PIT, K.D

PO TENT   PANC
PARENTS   PIT
ALWAYS   ADRENAL
LIKE   THE ART
ITALIE   LIVER
TEN   TESTES
KIDS   KIDNEYS

History

Patients may present with abdominal pain, **diabetic symptoms** (e.g., polydipsia, polyuria), and cirrhosis (e.g., **jaundice**). Patients may also have arthralgias and symptoms of endocrine dysfunction (e.g., **hypogonadism**).

2° LIVER FAILURE   2° PANC FAILURE

2° TESTICULAR Dz

PE

Bronze skin pigmentation, pancreatic dysfunction **(diabetes), cardiac dysfunction** (CHF). Hepatomegaly and testicular atrophy may also be present.

Differential

Other causes of cirrhosis, CHF, or hypopituitarism; diabetes mellitus.

Evaluation

↑Fe   ↑ TRANSFERRIN SAT   ↑Ferritin

Look for **elevated serum iron,** percentage saturation of iron, and ferritin. Serum transferrin levels are decreased. Other indicators include **glucose intolerance** as well as mildly elevated AST and alkaline phosphatase. Perform a **liver biopsy** (to determine hepatic iron index) or hepatic MRI.

Treatment   DONATE BLOOD

Weekly phlebotomy. Once serum iron levels decline, patients are placed on maintenance phlebotomy (every 2–4 months). Intramuscular deferoxamine (an iron chelator) may also be used for maintenance therapy.

Complications

Cirrhosis, hepatocellular carcinoma, cardiomegaly leading to CHF and/or conduction defects, diabetes, impotence, arthropathy, hypopituitarism.

WILSON'S DISEASE (HEPATOLENTICULAR DEGENERATION)   UCV Ped.9

COPPER → LIVER → ALFTS
          → BRAIN → Ψ

A rare **autosomal-recessive** disorder characterized by **excessive deposition of copper** in the liver and brain. Wilson's disease usually occurs in patients < 30 years old. The defect involves a copper-transporting protein and is linked to a defect on chromosome 13.

History

Patients present with **liver abnormalities** (e.g., jaundice secondary to hepatitis/cirrhosis) as well as neurologic and **psychiatric abnormalities.** Neurologic findings include loss of coordination, **tremor,** and dysphagia. Psychiatric abnormalities include psychosis, anxiety, mania, and depression.

PE

Kayser–Fleischer rings in the cornea (green-to-brown deposits of copper in Descemet's membrane; Figure 2.3–2), jaundice, hepatomegaly, parkinsonian tremor, and rigidity.

Differential

Other causes of hepatitis, cirrhosis, psychiatric and neurologic disturbances.

Wilson's disease—

ABCD
Asterixis (LIVER)
Basal ganglia (BRAIN) deterioration
Ceruloplasmin ↓, **C**irrhosis, **C**opper, **C**arcinoma (hepatocellular), (LIVER) **C**horeiform (BRAIN) movements
Dementia (BRAIN)

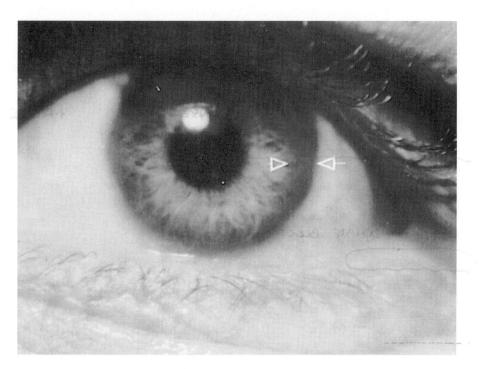

FIGURE 2.3–2. Kayser–Fleischer ring in Wilson's disease. The golden-brown corneal ring (arrows) is due to copper deposition in Descemet's membrane.

Evaluation

Decreased serum ceruloplasmin, elevated urinary copper excretion, and elevated hepatic copper.

↓CERULOPLASMIN

Treatment

Begin with **dietary copper restriction** (shellfish, liver, legumes). **Penicillamine** (a copper chelator that increases urinary copper excretion; administer with pyridoxine) and oral zinc (increases fecal excretion) can be used for maintenance therapy.

PENICILLAMINE
↓ COPPER
URINE

ZINC
↓ COPPER
FECES

PRIMARY HYPERALDOSTERONISM   **UCV** *Surg.7*

A condition that most commonly results from a unilateral adrenal tumor **(Conn's syndrome).** The remaining cases (30%) result from bilateral adrenocortical hyperplasia.

CONN TOP OF THE KIDNEY

History

↑Na RESORP   2° HTN

Patients present with **hypertension, headache, polyuria** (secondary to hypokalemic nephropathy), and **muscle weakness** (secondary to hypokalemia).

Hyper ALD
Hyper Tens
Head Ache
Hyper Urine
Hypo K

127

PE

Hypertension, tetany (secondary to hypokalemia), paresthesias, and, in severe cases, peripheral edema.

↘ Na RESORPTION

Differential

Essential hypertension, diuretic toxicity, nephrogenic diabetes insipidus, secondary hyperaldosteronism (renal artery stenosis, CHF, cirrhosis, renal failure associated with high plasma renin).

Evaluation

↓K   ↑ Na   ↑BICARB

Look for **hypokalemia, hypernatremia,** metabolic alkalosis, **low plasma renin,** and **elevated 24-hour urine aldosterone;** obtain CT or MRI to look for adrenal mass.

Treatment

Treat with laparoscopic or open **adrenalectomy** for Conn's syndrome and with **spironolactone** (an aldosterone receptor antagonist) for bilateral hyperplasia.

SPIRONOLACTONE = ANTI-ALDOSTERONE

Epidemiology

Length Bias

The tendency of a screening test to detect a disproportionate number of slowly progressive diseases and to miss rapidly progressive ones (which have a small window of detection, since afflicted individuals are present in the population only briefly). Length bias may lead to **overestimation of the effectiveness of screening.**

Lead-Time Bias

Lead-time bias occurs when screening advances the time of diagnosis, thereby prolonging the period of time between diagnosis and death without actually prolonging true survival. Since a disease is identified earlier but its natural course is not altered, survival will only **appear** to be greater.

Enrollment Bias

One example of an enrollment bias is the assignment of sicker patients to the intervention group than to the placebo group. This is an important reason for randomizing a study.

Self-Selection

Patients who choose to enroll in a study or respond to a survey may introduce **confounding variables** to that study; for example, some may enroll because their disease has been resistant to conventional therapy.

Observational Bias

Participants' responses to subjective questions may be affected by their awareness of the particular leg of the study in which they are enrolled. An observer's evaluation of a participant's clinical status may also be affected by such information. This is an important **reason for blinding a study.**

129

Recall Bias

Confounders may be introduced (e.g., in case-control studies) through **errors of memory** on the part of participants, since they may be asked to recall past events and exposures.

SENSITIVITY

PID = Positive In Disease (note that PID is a sensitive topic).

Sensitivity is the probability that a diseased patient will have a positive test result (number of true positives divided by the number of all people with the disease; Figure 2.4–1). False negative ratio is 1 − sensitivity. High sensitivity is desirable for a **screening test.**

SPECIFICITY

NIH = Negative In Health.

Specificity is the probability that a healthy patient will have a negative test result (number of true negatives divided by the number of all people without the disease; Figure 2.4–1). False positive ratio is 1 − specificity. High specificity is desirable for a **confirmatory test.**

POSITIVE PREDICTIVE VALUE (PPV)

Positive predictive value is the probability that a patient with a positive test result has the disease (true positives divided by the total number who tested positive). A test will have higher positive predictive value for diseases with a higher prevalence. **Both positive and negative predictive value are affected by the prevalence of the disease.**

NEGATIVE PREDICTIVE VALUE (NPV)

Negative predictive value is the probability that a patient with a negative test result is disease-free. A test will have a higher negative predictive value for diseases with a low prevalence.

	Patient Has Disease	*No Disease*	
Positive test	a	b	$PPV = a\,/\,(a+b)$
Negative test	c	d	$NPV = d\,/\,(c+d)$
	Sensitivity = a / (a + c)	Specificity = d / (b + d)	

FIGURE 2.4–1. Sensitivity, specificity, PPV, and NPV.

RELATIVE RISK (RR)

Used in **prospective studies,** relative risk compares the risk of disease in a group exposed to a particular factor with the risk in the unexposed group (Figure 2.4–2).

ODDS RATIO (OR)

The odds ratio is used in **retrospective studies** (e.g., case-control studies) and describes the odds of exposure in diseased individuals compared with those without the disease (Figure 2.4–2). For rare diseases, the odds ratio approximates the relative risk.

CASE CONTROL STUDY

An observational study, usually **retrospective,** in which cases (with disease) and controls (without disease) are identified. Information collected about past exposure to possible etiologic factors is used to calculate an OR.

- **Advantages:** Studies can use smaller study groups, are less costly, focus on **rare diseases,** and examine multiple potential etiologic factors.
- **Limitations:** Data may be inaccurate due to **recall bias** (exposures happened in the past) and **survivorship bias** (many of those with disease have already died) and cannot be used to calculate RR.

COHORT STUDY

An observational study that is usually **prospective.** A sample group (cohort) with matched controls (selected based on the presence or absence of exposure to a factor of interest) is **followed to see if disease develops.** A **relative risk** is calculated from these data.

- **Advantages:** Data are often more accurate, since they can be collected as the exposures occur (not based on recall of past events). Studies can examine the effects of **rare exposures** and multiple outcomes for the same exposure.

	Patient Developed Disease	No Disease	
Exposure	a	b	$RR = \dfrac{a/(a+b)}{c/(c+d)}$
No exposure	c	d	$OR = ad/bc$

FIGURE 2.4–2. Odds ratio and relative risk.

■ **Limitations:** Studies take a long time to complete and may be costlier. Confounders may be introduced (since exposure is not randomly distributed), rare diseases cannot be studied, and cases may be lost to follow-up.

CLINICAL TRIAL

An experimental, **prospective** study in which subjects are assigned to a treatment group or a control group. Studies are usually **randomized** to eliminate selection bias and to balance prognostic factors, as well as **double-blinded** to prevent observer bias on the part of those performing the study (since they often have a vested interest in the outcome). A new therapy should be compared to the established standard of care if this standard of care has been shown to be preferable to placebo.

■ **Advantages:** Highest-quality study; can control for many potential confounders with careful inclusion/exclusion criteria; can potentially prove causality.

■ **Limitations:** Very costly; can take a long time to complete.

CROSS–SECTIONAL SURVEYS

A survey of the population at a single point in time.

■ **Advantages:** Can be used to estimate disease prevalence and for hypothesis formation.

■ **Limitations:** Risk factors and presence of disease are collected simultaneously; thus, a cause-and-effect relationship cannot be established.

META-ANALYSIS

Pooling together data from several studies (often via literature search).

■ **Advantages:** Can achieve greater statistical power. Can be used to resolve controversial issues in the clinical literature (conflicting studies).

■ **Limitations:** Cannot overcome limitations of different studies. There are methodologic and statistical issues in combining means and variances in different studies.

CONFOUNDING VARIABLES

Confounding variables are variables in a study that are associated with both the exposure of interest and the disease and may thus disrupt the relationship between these two variables, leading to erroneous conclusions. Confounders such as socioeconomic status, gender, or age can be controlled for by design (matching for case control; stratification) or by analysis (multivariate analysis; adjustment).

132

Ethics

PATIENT RIGHTS UCV *Psych.22*

All competent patients have the right to refuse care. For example, **Jehovah's witnesses can refuse blood products.** However, a patient who has been deemed incompetent, such as an acutely intoxicated patient with altered mental status, cannot refuse treatment.

Incompetent patients cannot refuse treatment.

DISCLOSURE

Physicians must be honest and open with patients. Patients have a right to know about their medical status, their prognosis, and all potential treatment options **(full disclosure). Physicians are obligated to inform patients of mistakes made in their medical treatment.** A patient's family cannot make a physician withhold information from the patient. In the rare situation where disclosure would harm the patient or potentially undermine his or her decision-making capacity, it may be ethically acceptable to withhold information **(therapeutic privilege).**

INFORMED CONSENT

Before any procedure or medical therapy, a patient must be told the **indications** for that intervention, its **risks and benefits,** the potential **alternatives** (including the likely outcome of undergoing no treatment), and a **description** of the intervention. This information must be provided in a manner that the patient can understand. Patients cannot be coerced into giving **informed consent** and may change their minds at any time. Exceptions are as follows:

- In cases where treatment is needed emergently and the individual is unable to give consent, **consent to treatment is implied.** Likewise, it is not necessary to wait for parental consent (unless parents are present) before initiating emergent treatment on minors (implied consent).

- For patients lacking decision-making capacity, consent should be obtained from the **designated surrogate** decision maker or closest relative.
- Patients who have signed a waiver to the right of informed consent.

HIGH-YIELD FACTS

Ethics

CONFIDENTIALITY · UCV *Psych.23*

When in doubt, always maintain patient confidentiality.

Any information disclosed by a patient to his or her physician, as well as any information about a patient's medical condition, is considered to be **confidential** and should not be divulged without the expressed consent of the patient. When in doubt, always maintain patient confidentiality. However, it is ethically and legally **necessary to override confidentiality in order to prevent harm to a third party** (e.g., in cases involving child/elder/spousal abuse or threats against an individual that you feel the patient has the potential to carry out) as well as in specific legally defined situations (e.g., mandatory reporting of gunshot and knife wounds, intoxicated automobile drivers, and reportable diseases).

MINORS · UCV *Psych.20*

Parental consent is not necessary for pregnant minors or those requesting treatment for STDs or substance abuse.

Parental consent is not necessary in emergent life-threatening situations, since consent to treat is implied. For minors needing medical care **during pregnancy** or those requesting **treatment for STDs or substance abuse,** parental consent is not necessary, and confidentiality with the patient should be maintained. Confidentiality in such situations can be broken only with the patient's expressed permission, even if a parent requests information. Also remember that **confidentiality can be broken if a minor is a danger to himself or to others** (e.g., in instances where a minor expresses suicidal or homicidal intent).

DURABLE POWER OF ATTORNEY (DPOA) · UCV *Psych.19*

Durable power of attorney (DPOA) is a written advance directive that legally designates an individual as the surrogate health care decision maker if a patient loses decision-making capability. This is **more flexible** than a living will. The designated individual should make decisions consistent with the patient's stated wishes whenever possible.

LIVING WILL · UCV *Psych.19*

DNR/DNI orders do not imply "do not treat."

A living will is a written advance directive addressing the patient's wishes in limited, specific medical situations. Examples include **DNR** ("do not resuscitate") and **DNI** ("do not intubate") directives. Note: DNR/DNI orders do not imply "do not treat"; patients with such orders should still receive the maximal medical intervention available short of resuscitation and/or intubation.

SURROGATE

When patients are unable to make decisions regarding their health care and no living will or DPOA exists, decisions should be made by **close family members, friends,** or **personal physicians,** in that order. In such situations, the individuals in question will make decisions consistent with what they believe to be the patient's wishes.

END-OF-LIFE ISSUES   UCV *Psych.25*

Patients and their decision makers have the right to forgo life-sustaining treatments even when this requires the withdrawal of care. This includes mechanical ventilation, IV hydration, parenteral/enteral nutrition, and the administration of medications, including antibiotics. It is important to know that from an ethical perspective, **there is no distinction between the withholding and the withdrawal of life-sustaining interventions.** It is also ethical to provide palliative treatment to relieve pain and suffering even though it may hasten a patient's death.

It is ethical to provide palliative treatment even though it may hasten the patient's death.

FUTILITY

Physicians are not ethically obligated to provide treatment when:

- There is no pathophysiologic rationale for treatment.
- Maximal intervention is currently failing.
- A given intervention has already failed.
- Treatment will not achieve the goals of care.

In such circumstances, physicians are permitted to **refuse** a family's request for further intervention.

EUTHANASIA

Euthanasia is the administration of a **lethal agent** with the intent of **relieving suffering.** This is a highly controversial issue that is currently the subject of intense debate both in court and in the media. The AMA Code of Medical Ethics currently **opposes** such practices. **Inadequate pain control** or comorbid depression are common causes for requests for euthanasia.

HIGH-YIELD FACTS

Ethics

HIGH-YIELD FACTS

Ethics

Gastrointestinal

GASTROESOPHAGEAL REFLUX (GERD) $\boxed{\text{UCV}}$ *IM1.35*

Symptomatic reflux of gastric contents into the esophagus. **Transient lower esophageal sphincter (LES) relaxation** is the most common etiology of GERD. GERD can be due in part to an incompetent LES, abnormally acidic gastric contents, and hiatal hernia. Risk factors include obesity, pregnancy, and scleroderma/Raynaud's disease. Alcohol, caffeine, nicotine, chocolate, and fatty foods can reduce LES tone.

Risk factors for GERD include hiatal hernia, obesity, and pregnancy.

↑ ACID IN ESOPHAGUS

History

Patients present with **"heartburn"** (substernal burning) that commonly occurs 30–90 minutes **after a meal,** frequently **worsens with reclining,** and often improves with antacids, standing, or sitting. Other symptoms include sour taste ("water brash"), regurgitation, dysphagia, and cough/wheezing/dyspnea (symptoms may mimic or exacerbate asthma).

GERD may mimic asthma.

PE

Usually **normal** unless there is evidence of associated systemic disease (e.g., Raynaud's disease/scleroderma).

Differential

PUD, CAD, infectious (CMV, candidal) or chemical esophagitis, gallbladder disease, achalasia, esophageal spasm, pericarditis.

PEPTIC ULCER
CORONARY ARTERY DISEASE
ESOPHAGITIS
G BLADDER Dz
ACHALASIA

Evaluation

Diagnosis is based primarily on history. Upper endoscopy should be performed if the patient has long-standing symptoms (to look for Barrett's esophagus and adenocarcinoma). Evaluation may include abdominal x-ray (AXR), chest x-ray (CXR), barium swallow (of limited usefulness, but can diagnose associated hiatal hernia), and esophageal manometry/pH monitoring.

Treatment

- **Lifestyle:** Lifestyle modifications include weight loss, elevation of the head of the bed, and avoidance of nocturnal meals and substances reducing LES tone.
- **Pharmacologic:** Start with **antacids** in patients with mild to moderate disease; use **H₂ receptor antagonists** (cimetidine, ranitidine) or **proton pump inhibitors** (omeprazole, lansoprazole) in patients with severe or refractory disease. For patients who have problems with LES function, a **pro-motility agent** (cisapride) may be beneficial.
- **Surgical:** For refractory or severe disease, **Nissen fundoplication** or hiatal hernia repair may offer significant relief.
- **Health maintenance:** Monitor for Barrett's esophagus and esophageal adenocarcinoma with **serial endoscopy/biopsy.**

Complications

Esophageal ulceration, esophageal stricture, aspiration of gastric contents, upper GI bleeding, and **Barrett's esophagus** (columnar metaplasia) of the distal esophagus secondary to chronic acid irritation; associated with an increased risk of esophageal **adenocarcinoma**).

PEPTIC ULCER DISEASE (PUD)

UCV *IM1.40, Surg.30*

Damage to the gastric or duodenal mucosa caused by a combination of impaired mucosal defense and acidic gastric contents. **H. pylori** plays a causative role in > 90% of duodenal ulcers as well as in many gastric ulcers. Patients on chronic NSAID therapy are at particular risk for gastric ulcers. Ulcers are more common in the **duodenum** than in the stomach. Other risk factors include **corticosteroid and tobacco** use. Males are affected more often than females.

History

Patients present with chronic/periodic, **dull/burning/aching epigastric pain** (dyspepsia) that **improves with meals** (especially duodenal ulcers), worsens 2–3 hours after eating, and can radiate to the back. Patients may also complain of nausea, hematemesis ("coffee-ground" emesis), and blood in the stool (melena or hematochezia).

PE

Varying degrees of **epigastric tenderness** and **positive stool guaiac** if there is active bleeding. An acute perforation will commonly present with a rigid abdomen, rebound tenderness, guarding, or other signs of peritoneal irritation.

Differential

GERD, CAD, gastritis, pancreatitis (acute or chronic), cholecystitis, Zollinger–Ellison syndrome, aortic aneurysm, and other causes of acute abdomen, depending on the severity of the pain and on physical findings (severe pain suggests perforation).

Evaluation

AXR to **rule out perforation** (free air under the diaphragm) and CBC to assess for GI bleeding (low or falling hematocrit). **Upper endoscopy** to confirm the diagnosis and to rule out active bleeding. PUD can also be diagnosed with a barium **upper GI study. Biopsy** of the ulcer with histologic evaluation/rapid urease testing can be used to rule out gastric adenocarcinoma and to detect *H. pylori* infection. **ELISA** (to detect IgG antibodies against *H. pylori*) offers a noninvasive test for *H. pylori* exposure. Elevated amylase suggests pancreatic involvement. In recurrent or refractory cases, serum gastrin should be measured to screen for Zollinger–Ellison syndrome.

GASTRINOMA ↑GASTRIN

Rule out Zollinger–Ellison syndrome with serum gastrin levels in cases of GERD and PUD that are refractory to medical management.

Treatment

- **Acute:** Rule out active bleeding with nasogastric lavage, stool guaiac, and serial hematocrits. If perforation is likely (based on exam and AXR), **surgery** is usually indicated. For GI bleeding, carefully monitor the patient's hematocrit and BP and initiate IV hydration, transfusion, endoscopy, and surgery as needed.

  NG LAVAGE HOME OCCULT SERIAL CBC

- **Pharmacologic:** Patients with confirmed *H. pylori* infection should receive a course of **antibiotic treatment** (e.g., metronidazole + clarithromycin or bismuth salicylate/amoxicillin) plus treatment with a proton pump inhibitor (e.g., omeprazole) for at least 1–3 weeks, followed by proton pump inhibitor or H_2 receptor antagonist therapy for 1–2 months. If *Helicobacter* infection is not likely or proves difficult to eradicate, symptomatic treatment with a **proton pump inhibitor** or an H_2 **receptor antagonist** (e.g., ranitidine, cimetidine) may suffice. The addition of sucralfate for mucosal defense may be helpful. For NSAID-induced ulcers, **discontinue NSAID use.** Misoprostol (a prostaglandin analog) can be used in patients with a history of PUD who require NSAID therapy. Patients with recurrent or severe disease may require chronic symptomatic therapy; mild disease can be treated with antacids.

  FLAGYL or BISMUTH CLARRITHRO AMOX + PROT PUMP INHIB

  Misoprostol can help patients with PUD who require NSAID therapy (e.g., patients with arthritis).

- **Surgery/endoscopy:** All patients with gastric (but not duodenal) ulcers for **> 2 months** must undergo biopsy to rule out malignancy. Truly refractory cases may require a surgical procedure such as **parietal cell vagotomy** (most selective; preferred) or antrectomy/vagotomy.

GASTRIC → R/O MALIGNANCY

Complications

Hemorrhage (especially with posterior ulcers that erode into the gastroduodenal artery), gastric outlet obstruction, perforation (usually anterior ulcers; look for a perforated viscus on x-rays), and intractable disease. Long-standing gastric ulcers that are unresponsive to medical therapy require serial endoscopy with biopsy to monitor for gastric adenocarcinoma.

DIVERTICULAR DISEASE UCV *IM1.34, Surg.33*

Outpouchings of mucosa/submucosa (false diverticula) that herniate through the colonic muscle layers. Diverticular disease is asymptomatic unless complicated by diverticulitis or hemorrhage. **Diverticulitis** is the microscopic or macroscopic perforation of a diverticulum secondary to obstruction, infection, inflammation, or increased luminal pressure. Diverticular bleeding is due to the erosion of a diverticulum into a colonic blood vessel. Intestinal diverticula most commonly occur in the **sigmoid colon** because of increased intraluminal pressure; risk factors include a **low-fiber and high-fat diet,** Western ancestry (probably due to diet), old age (65% occur in those > 80 years old), Ehlers–Danlos syndrome, and Marfan's syndrome. Diverticular disease is the most common cause of acute lower GI bleeding in patients > 40 years of age.

Diverticular disease is the most common cause of acute lower GI bleeding in patients > 40 years old.

History

Diverticular disease is often **asymptomatic** but can manifest as constipation, **lower abdominal pain,** and **abnormal bowel habits.** Diverticulitis presents as acute, mild to severe, steady or cramping lower abdominal pain that is commonly localized to the **LLQ** (but can be suprapubic or in the RLQ) accompanied by fever and nausea/emesis. Diverticular bleeding presents as melena/hematochezia and symptoms of anemia (fatigue, light-headedness, dyspnea on exertion).

PE

Diverticular disease without complications usually does not have any physical findings. Findings consistent with diverticulitis include low-grade **fever,** a palpable lower abdominal **mass,** a positive stool guaiac test, and generalized abdominal tenderness with peritoneal signs in the presence of free perforation. Diverticular bleeding presents as a **lower GI bleed.**

Differential

Diverticular disease should be distinguished from colon cancer.

Diverticulitis should be distinguished from **colorectal cancer** with perforation, Crohn's disease, mesenteric ischemia, appendicitis, and gynecologic disease (e.g., ovarian cyst). Diverticular bleeding must be distinguished from **AVMs** and colorectal cancer.

Evaluation

[handwritten: → DIVERTICULITIS]

CBC (look for **leukocytosis**) and AXR. Diagnosis is based on AXR, colonoscopy, or barium enema. In patients with severe disease or those who show lack of improvement, CT scans may reveal abscess or free air.

Treatment

- **Diverticular disease without complications:** Patients can be followed and placed on a high-fiber diet or fiber supplements.
- **Diverticulitis:** Treat with **bowel rest** (no enteric feeds), NG tube, and **broad-spectrum antibiotics** (metronidazole and second- or third-generation cephalosporin) if the patient is stable. In the presence of free perforation, perform immediate surgical resection of diseased bowel along with anastomosis or temporary colostomy and a Hartmann's pouch/mucous fistula.
- **Diverticular bleeding:** Bleeding usually stops spontaneously; transfuse/hydrate as needed. If bleeding does not stop, angiography with embolization or **surgery** is indicated.

Complications

Diverticular bleeding and diverticulitis. Diverticulitis may also lead to abscess formation, intestinal perforation, **fistula formation** (into the bladder, skin, or vagina), hepatic abscess, retroperitoneal fibrosis, and sepsis.

APPENDICITIS

Inflammation of the appendix that leads to infection (abscess) and/or perforation if not recognized and treated appropriately. Appendicitis occurs most frequently in people aged 10–30 years and is more common in the U.S. than in parts of Africa and Asia (due to the low-fiber diet in the U.S.). It is the most common abdominal emergency among those < 35 years of age. The most common etiologies of appendicitis in the U.S. are **lymphoid hyperplasia** (60%) and **fecalith obstruction** (35%).

[handwritten: PU → RLQ]

History

Commonly begins as **dull periumbilical pain** that waxes and wanes followed by **nausea,** emesis, and **anorexia.** Classically, **pain then shifts to the RLQ** (secondary to peritoneal irritation) and becomes sharp, continuous, localized, and increasingly severe. With perforation, abdominal pain may worsen and distention may develop (acute abdomen).

[margin right, top] Avoid flexible sigmoidoscopy and barium enemas in the initial stages of diverticulitis because there is a risk of perforation.

[margin right, vertical black tab] **HIGH-YIELD FACTS**

[margin right, vertical black tab] **Gastrointestinal**

[margin right, bottom] If a patient has pain that moves from the periumbilical area to the RLQ, think appendicitis.

PE

Localized tenderness at McBurney's point, mild to moderate rebound tenderness, pain with cough, **psoas/obturator signs, Rovsing's sign** (RLQ pain on palpation of the LLQ), and low-grade fever. Patients often present before the pain has localized to the RLQ. Perform a **rectal exam** (tenderness suggests an inflamed posterior appendix).

Differential

PID, ovarian torsion, other gynecologic disorders **(always do a gynecologic exam),** volvulus, gastroenteritis, ruptured ectopic pregnancy, pyelonephritis, diverticulitis, colon cancer with perforation, Crohn's disease, perforated peptic ulcer, cholecystitis, mesenteric ischemia, pneumonia, Meckel's diverticulum.

Evaluation

Always perform a pregnancy test in women of childbearing age with abdominal pain.

The diagnosis is **clinical** and based on careful observation and serial abdominal examinations. Look for leukocytosis with a left shift on CBC; also obtain an AXR. **Appendiceal fecalith** on AXR is suggestive of the diagnosis but not pathognomonic. Look for **free air,** which would suggest perforation. CXR may rule out right middle/lower lobe **pneumonia. Ultrasound/CT** is used in unusual or difficult cases. A β-HCG test to rule out ectopic/uterine pregnancy is essential in women of childbearing age.

Treatment

Appendectomy. With free perforation, emergency surgery is necessary. If the patient has an abscess but is clinically stable, **CT-guided drainage** followed by nonurgent appendectomy may be preferable. A 20% negative appendectomy rate (i.e., removal of a normal appendix) is acceptable to minimize the number of missed cases.

Complications

Abdominal abscess, appendiceal perforation, wound infection, hepatic abscess, and septic pylephlebitis.

INFLAMMATORY BOWEL DISEASE (IBD) UCV *IMI.33, 42*

IBD consists primarily of **Crohn's disease** and **ulcerative colitis** (Figure 2.6–1 A and B). Rarer forms of IBD include mixed forms and microscopic IBD. These diseases are characterized by inflammation of the GI tract with subsequent tissue damage. Patients in families with a history of one type of IBD are at risk for both. It is most common in whites and **Ashkenazi Jews** and often presents in patients in their teens or early 20s. Table 2.6–1 presents features of ulcerative colitis and Crohn's disease.

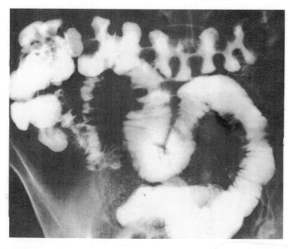
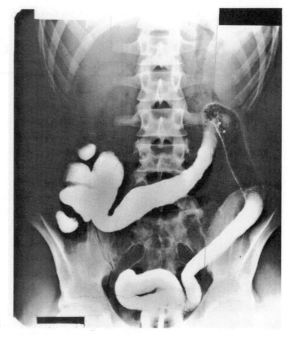

FIGURE 2.6–1. Inflammatory bowel disease. (A) Crohn's disease. Barium enema x-ray reveals deep transverse fissures, ulcers, and edema of the bowel. (B) Ulcerative colitis. Barium enema x-ray demonstrates shortening of the colon, loss of haustra ("lead pipe" appearance), and fine serrations at the bowel edges from small ulcers.

IRRITABLE BOWEL SYNDROME

— SLEEP WELL

UCV *IM1.39*

An idiopathic functional disorder characterized by abdominal pain and irregular bowel habits. Patients most commonly present in their teens and 20s, but since this syndrome is chronic, patients can present at any age. Half of all patients with this disorder who seek medical care have **comorbid psychiatric disorders** (e.g., depression, anxiety).

Half of all patients with irritable bowel syndrome have psychiatric disorders.

History

Patients present with **abdominal pain,** irregular bowel habits (including **alternating diarrhea and constipation**), and abdominal distention. Irritable bowel syndrome rarely awakens patients from sleep.

PE

Usually **unremarkable** except for mild abdominal tenderness.

Differential

Crohn's : SIMILAR AGE, Sx, SITES

Crohn's disease/ulcerative colitis, mesenteric ischemia, diverticulitis, gastric/duodenal ulcer, colonic neoplasia, infectious/pseudomembranous colitis, gynecologic disorders.

TABLE 2.6–1. Ulcerative Colitis vs. Crohn's Disease.

	Ulcerative Colitis	Crohn's Disease
Site of involvement	The rectum is always involved. May extend proximally in a **continuous fashion** to involve some or all of the colon. Inflammation and ulceration are limited to the mucosa and submucosa.	May involve **any portion** of the GI tract, particularly the ileocecal region, in a **discontinuous pattern.** The rectum is often spared. Inflammation is transmural.
Symptoms and signs	Bloody diarrhea, lower abdominal cramps, and urgency. Exam may reveal orthostatic hypotension, tachycardia, abdominal tenderness, frank blood on rectal exam, and extraintestinal manifestations (see below).	Abdominal pain, abdominal mass, low-grade fever, weight loss, watery diarrhea. Exam may reveal fever, abdominal tenderness or mass, **perianal fissures, fistulas,** and extraintestinal manifestations (see below).
Extraintestinal manifestations	Aphthous stomatitis, episcleritis/uveitis, arthritis, sclerosing cholangitis, erythema nodosum, and pyoderma gangrenosum.	In addition, nephrolithiasis and fistulas to the skin, biliary tract, urinary tract, or between bowel loops.
Differential	Crohn's disease, infectious colitis (e.g., bacterial, amebic, C. difficile), ischemic colitis, proctitis secondary to radiation therapy or STDs.	Ulcerative colitis, ischemic colitis, irritable bowel syndrome, appendicitis, intestinal lymphoma, diverticulitis.
Workup	CBC, AXR, stool cultures, ova and parasites, stool assay for C. difficile, and barium enema/colonoscopy. Colonoscopy shows diffuse and continuous rectal involvement, friability, edema, and pseudopolyps. Definitive diagnosis can be made by biopsy.	Crohn's has the same laboratory workup as colitis. Colonoscopy may show aphthoid, linear, or stellate ulcers, strictures, "cobblestoning," and "skip lesions."
Treatment	**Sulfasalazine** or **5-aminosalicylate** (mesalamine). Corticosteroids and immunosuppressants are reserved for refractory disease. **Total colectomy is curative** (done for long-standing or fulminant colitis or toxic megacolon).	**Sulfasalazine,** corticosteroids and immunosuppression are indicated if disease does not improve. If perforation is likely, surgical resection may be necessary, although **Crohn's disease may recur** elsewhere in the GI tract.
Incidence of cancer	Markedly increased risk of **colon cancer** in long-standing cases (monitor with fecal occult blood screening, colonoscopy).	Incidence of secondary malignancy much lower than in ulcerative colitis.

Evaluation

Irritable bowel syndrome is a diagnosis of exclusion.

A **diagnosis of exclusion** based on clinical history and evaluation, so rule out other causes of GI disease. Tests can include CBC and electrolytes, stool cultures, abdominal films, and barium contrast studies. Some physicians use manometry to assess sphincter function.

Treatment

- **Psychological:** Patients need **assurance** from their physicians. Do not tell patients that their symptoms are "all in their head."
- **Dietary:** A high-fiber diet or **fiber supplements** may help.
- **Pharmacologic:** Treat with **antidiarrheal** (loperamide), **antispasmodic** (dicyclomine, anticholinergics), and **psychiatric** medications as indicated.

[handwritten margin notes: ANTI DIARRHEAL / LOPERAMIDE / ANTISPASMODIC / ANTICHOLINERGICS / PSYCHIATRIC]

Table 2.6–2 lists the important features of acute and chronic pancreatitis.

TABLE 2.6–2. Acute and Chronic Pancreatitis.

	Acute Pancreatitis	Chronic Pancreatitis
Pathophysiology	Leakage of pancreatic enzymes from the biliary system to pancreatic and peripancreatic tissue, often secondary to gallstone disease or alcoholism.	Obstruction and/or dysfunction of the pancreatic system.
Time course	Abrupt onset, severe.	Persistent, recurrent.
Risk factors	**Gallstones, alcoholism,** hypercalcemia, hypertriglyceridemia, trauma, drug side effects (including diuretics), viral infections, and post-ERCP.	**Alcoholism,** pancreatolithiasis, hyperparathyroidism, congenital malformation (pancreas divisum). May also be idiopathic.
Symptoms	Severe **epigastric pain** (radiating to the back), nausea, vomiting, weakness, fever, shock.	Persistent **epigastric pain,** anorexia, nausea, constipation, flatulence, steatorrhea.
Workup	↑ amylase, ↑ lipase, ↓ Ca⁺⁺ if severe; "sentinel loop" or "colon cutoff" sign on x-ray. Peripancreatic fluid, pseudocyst, and phlegmon on CT (see Figure 2.6–2).	↑ amylase, ↑ lipase, glycosuria, calcifications and mild ileus on x-ray and CT.
Management	Bowel rest, NG suction, surgical debridement, antibiotics, volume support, nutritional support, possible respiratory support, analgesia, removal of offending agent if possible (stone, drugs, etc.).	No alcohol, low-fat diet, pancrease, analgesia, surgery for structural causes.
Prognosis	Poor (patients may require ICU treatment and may die).	Fair (patients may have chronic pain and pancreatic exocrine/endocrine dysfunction).
Complications	Death, pancreatic **pseudocyst,** relapse, fistula formation, chronic pancreatitis, sepsis.	Pancreatic insufficiency (exocrine/endocrine), **chronic pain,** malnutrition, PUD.

[handwritten margin notes: ↑Ca / ↑TG beside Risk factors; ↑ PTH (TG) beside chronic column]

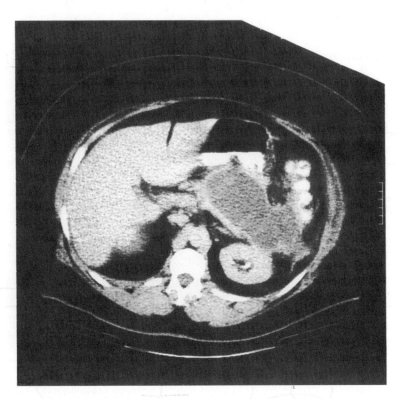

FIGURE 2.6–2. Pancreatic pseudocyst. The large pseudocyst impinges on the posterior wall of the stomach (filled with contrast) on CT scan.

CHOLELITHIASIS AND BILIARY COLIC

Symptoms of gallstones are due to transient cystic duct blockage from impacted stones. Risk factors include the **"5 F's"**: female, fat, fertile, forty, and flatulent—although the disorder is common and can occur in any patient. Other risk factors include oral contraceptive use, rapid weight loss, chronic hemolysis (pigment stones), small bowel resection, and total parenteral nutrition.

History

Patients present with postprandial abdominal pain (usually in the RUQ) radiating to the right subscapular area or epigastrium. Pain is of abrupt onset followed by gradual relief and is often associated with **nausea and vomiting**. Presenting symptoms may also include fatty food intolerance, dyspepsia, and flatulence. Gallstones may be asymptomatic in up to 80% of patients.

PE

RUQ tenderness and palpable gallbladder.

Patients with gallstones—

The 5 F's
Female
Fat
Fertile
Forty
Flatulent

Differential

Acute cholecystitis, PUD, MI, acute pancreatitis, GERD, hepatitis, appendicitis.

Evaluation

RUQ ultrasound may show gallstones (95% sensitive). Consider upper GI series to rule out hiatal hernia or ulcer.

Treatment

Cholecystectomy is both definitive and curative and can be performed on an elective basis. For patients who are not surgical candidates, treat with **dietary modification** (avoid triggering substances like fatty foods) and **pharmacologic dissolution** (with bile salts) with or without **lithotripsy** (associated with a high recurrence rate).

Complications

Recurrent biliary colic, acute cholecystitis, choledocholithiasis, gallstone ileus, and gallstone pancreatitis.

ACUTE CHOLECYSTITIS
UCV *Surg.11*

Prolonged blockage of the cystic duct by an impacted stone, resulting in post-obstructive distention, inflammation, superinfection, and, in extreme cases, gangrene of the gallbladder. In chronically debilitated patients, those on TPN, and trauma or burn victims, acute cholecystitis may occur in the absence of cholelithiasis **(acalculous cholecystitis).**

TPN → GB PROBS ∅STONES

History

Patients present with RUQ pain, nausea, and vomiting similar to that seen in biliary colic, but typically more severe and of longer duration.

PE

RUQ tenderness, inspiratory arrest during deep palpation of the RUQ **(Murphy's sign),** low-grade fever, mild icterus, and possibly guarding or rebound tenderness.

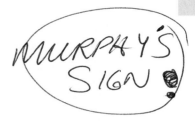

MURPHY'S SIGN

Differential

Biliary colic, cholangitis, GERD, hepatitis, acute pancreatitis, MI, acute appendicitis, renal colic, Fitz–Hugh–Curtis syndrome (acute gonococcal perihepatitis), PUD, pneumonia.

c̄ PID

Evaluation

CBC (leukocytosis), amylase, and LFTs (normal or elevated). Ultrasound may demonstrate stones, bile sludge, pericholecystic fluid, a thickened gallbladder wall, and gas in the gallbladder (Figure 2.6–3). Obtain a **HIDA scan** when ultrasound is equivocal (Figure 2.6–4); absence of the gallbladder on HIDA scan suggests acute cholecystitis. Diagnosis is made on the basis of clinical suspicion and imaging modalities.

HIDA IS SORTA LIKE IVP OF BIL TRACT

Treatment

In patients with significant medical problems (including diabetes), delay cholecystectomy until acute inflammation resolves.

Hospitalize patients, administer **IV antibiotics** and **IV fluids,** and replete electrolytes. Perform **early cholecystectomy** (within 72 hours of onset of symptoms) in patients without significant operative risk factors along with an **intraoperative cholangiogram** to rule out common bile duct stones. An expectant approach should be taken toward patients with significant medical problems (especially diabetes). Since 50% of cases resolve spontaneously, such patients can be treated medically as long as there is no deterioration in their condition, with a four- to six-week delay in surgical treatment.

Complications

Gangrene, empyema, perforation, fistulization, sepsis, or abscess formation.

CHOLANGITIS
UCV EM.12, Surg.16

An infection/inflammation of the biliary tree that commonly occurs secondary to obstruction, usually from **gallstones or malignancy.** Sclerosing cholangitis is due to progressive inflammation of the biliary tree and occurs most commonly in patients with choledocholithiasis or IBD. Other risk fac-

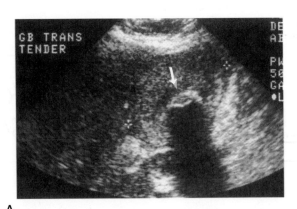
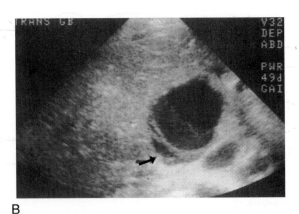

A   B

FIGURE 2.6–3. Acute cholecystitis, ultrasound. (A) Note the sludge-filled, thick-walled gallbladder with a hyperechoic stone and acoustic shadow (arrow). (B) This patient exhibits sludge and pericholecystic fluid (arrow) but no gallstones.

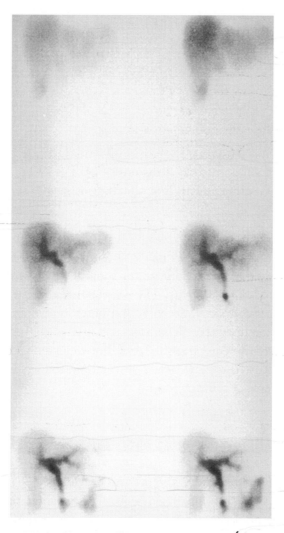

FIGURE 2.6–4. Acute cholecystitis, HIDA scan. Intravenous dye is taken up by hepatocytes, conjugated, and excreted into the common bile duct. The gallbladder is not visualized, although activity is present in the liver, common duct, and small bowel, suggesting cystic duct obstruction due to acute cholecystitis.

tors include bile duct stricture, ampullary carcinoma, and pancreatic pseudocyst. The organisms most commonly associated with cholangitis are gram-negative enterics (e.g., *E. coli, Enterobacter, Pseudomonas*).

History

Patients present with Charcot's triad: **RUQ pain, jaundice,** and **fever/chills.**
Reynold's pentad (Charcot's triad plus **shock** and **altered mental status**) may
be present in acute suppurative cholangitis.

PE

RUQ tenderness, jaundice, and **fever/chills.**   *Charcot's*

Differential

Pancreatic cancer, cholangiocarcinoma, carcinoma of the bile ducts, metastatic carcinoma, hepatitis, primary biliary cirrhosis *(IM1.41)*, cholecystitis, pancreatitis, sepsis, liver abscess.

Workup

Look for leukocytosis, increased bilirubin, and increased alkaline phosphatase. Obtain blood cultures. **Ultrasound** or CT may be a useful adjunct, but diagnosis is often clinical. **ERCP** is the diagnostic gold standard.

Treatment

This is a serious, life-threatening disease. Patients often require **ICU admission** for monitoring and hydration/pressor support along with aggressive **IV antibiotic treatment.** Patients with acute toxic cholangitis require **emergent bile duct decompression** via endoscopic sphincterotomy, percutaneous transhepatic drainage, or operative decompression. After the acute episode has been managed, percutaneous transhepatic cholangiography or ERCP should be performed to locate the cause of the obstruction, followed by stone extraction, stent placement, or sphincterotomy.

PORTAL HYPERTENSION

UCV *IM1.37, Surg.32*

Portal pressure > 5 mmHg above the pressure in the IVC. Causes are divided into presinusoidal (splenic vein thrombosis, schistosomiasis), sinusoidal (cirrhosis), and postsinusoidal (right heart failure, constrictive pericarditis, hepatic vein thrombosis).

History

Patients can present with ascites, bacterial peritonitis (fever, abdominal pain), **hepatic encephalopathy** (asterixis, delirium), **esophageal varices** (hematemesis, GI bleed), and renal dysfunction.

PE

Abdominal fluid wave, shifting dullness, and splenomegaly. Patients with cirrhosis may have easy bruising, spider angiomata, dilated abdominal veins (**caput medusae**), gynecomastia, and testicular atrophy.

Evaluation

Evaluation should include LFTs, alkaline phosphatase, bilirubin, albumin, and PT/PTT to assess hepatic function, and other tests to determine the cause of liver disease (serum ferritin for hemochromatosis, CT scan for Budd–Chiari syndrome). Diagnosis can be made on the basis of clinical findings plus laboratory tests that show evidence of hepatic or other dysfunction. Indirect hepatic vein wedge pressure (a measure of portal pressure) is increased.

Gastrointestinal

Treatment

Treatment is aimed at ameliorating the complications of portal hypertension.

- **Ascites: Sodium restriction and diuretics** (furosemide and spironolactone); rule out infectious/neoplastic causes (perform paracentesis to obtain serum ascites albumin gradient [SAAG], WBC, cultures); treat underlying liver disease if possible.
- **Spontaneous bacterial peritonitis:** Check peritoneal fluid if there is a question of infection (PMNs > 250 with clinical signs and PMNs > 500 in an asymptomatic patient). Treat with **IV antibiotics** to cover both gram-positive and gram-negative organisms until a causative organism is identified.
- **Hepatorenal syndrome:** This is difficult to treat, often requires dialysis, and may be fatal.
- **Hepatic encephalopathy:** Decrease protein consumption; treat with **lactulose** and/or **neomycin.**
- **Esophageal varices:** Monitor for GI bleeding; treat endoscopically or surgically if necessary.
- In some cases a hepatic shunt can be performed surgically or by transjugular intrahepatic portacaval shunt (TIPS), but this is normally a short-term bridge to transplant and may worsen hepatic encephalopathy.

SERUM ASCITES ALB GRADIENT

Spontaneous bacterial peritonitis is diagnosed by > 500 PMNs/μL in the ascitic fluid.

DYSPHAGIA

Difficulty swallowing due to difficulty getting food into the esophagus **(oropharyngeal dysphagia)**, difficulty getting it through the esophagus **(esophageal dysphagia)**, or pain with swallowing **(odynophagia).**

History

Oropharyngeal dysphagia usually involves liquids more than solids and may be accompanied by dysarthria or dysphonia. Esophageal dysphagia usually involves both liquids and solids and is generally progressive.

PE

Examine for masses (goiter, tumor) and anatomic defects.

Differential

- **Oropharyngeal dysphagia:** Neurologic disorders (e.g., cranial nerve disease or bulbar injury), muscular disease, thyroid disease, sphincter dysfunction, Zenker's diverticulum, neoplasm, post-surgery/radiation.
- **Esophageal dysphagia:** Schatzki's ring, neoplasm *(Surg.15)*, achalasia *(Surg.9)*, spasm, peptic stricture, scleroderma (Table 2.6–3).
- **Odynophagia:** Infectious agents (in HIV+ patients, consider *Candida*, CMV, and herpesvirus), chemical agents (lye ingestion or pill-induced).

Diagnostic hints:
Patient who smokes and drinks: esophageal cancer.
Patient with iron deficiency anemia: esophageal webs.
Patient with AIDS: Candida esophagitis.

Evaluation

- **Oropharyngeal dysphagia:** Videoesophagography.
- **Esophageal dysphagia:** Barium swallow followed by endoscopy, manometry, or pH monitoring. If an obstructive lesion is suspected, proceed straight to endoscopy.
- **Odynophagia:** Barium study or endoscopy.

Treatment

Treat the underlying disease. Viscous lidocaine may relieve odynophagia.

ILEUS

Anticholinergics and opioids slow GI motility.

Loss of peristalsis **without structural obstruction.** Risk factors include recent surgery/GI procedures, severe medical illness, hypothyroidism, diabetes, or medications that slow GI motility (e.g., anticholinergics, opioids). The condition is commonly seen in elderly patients on opioids.

History

Presenting symptoms include diffuse, constant, moderate abdominal discomfort; **nausea/emesis,** especially with feeding; **abdominal distention;** and an absence of **flatulence or bowel movements.**

PE

Mild, diffuse tenderness and **abdominal distention** with **no peritoneal signs** (no guarding or rebound) along with **reduced or absent bowel sounds.**

TABLE 2.6–3. Causes of Esophageal Dysphagia.

Cause	Clues
Mechanical obstruction	Solid foods worse than liquids
Schatzki's ring	Intermittent dysphagia; not progressive
Peptic stricture	Chronic heartburn; progressive dysphagia
Esophageal cancer	Progressive dysphagia; age > 50
Motility disorder	Solid and liquid foods
Achalasia	Progressive dysphagia
Diffuse esophageal spasm	Intermittent; not progressive; may have chest pain
Scleroderma	Chronic heartburn; Raynaud's phenomenon

Differential

Partial obstruction of the small intestine or colon, appendicitis, gastroenteritis, pancreatitis, neoplasm.

Evaluation

Obtain supine and upright plain films of the abdomen to **rule out perforation or obstruction,** as well as CBC/electrolytes. Diagnosis is based on **distended small and large bowel** on AXR and **air-fluid levels;** barium study may be performed to rule out partial obstruction. Obtain CT to rule out obstructing masses. Rule out thyroid disease with TSH.

Look for air throughout the small and large bowel on AXR.

Treatment

- Decrease use of narcotics and any other drugs that **inhibit bowel motility.**
- Reduce or discontinue oral feeds.
- Initiate **NG suction/parenteral feeds** as necessary.
- Replete electrolytes as needed.

GASTROINTESTINAL BLEEDING

UC**V** *Surg.21, 22*

Bleeding from the GI tract that presents as hematemesis, blood in the stool (hematochezia, melena), or both (see Table 2.6–4).

High-Yield Facts

Gastrointestinal

TABLE 2.6–4. GI Bleeding.

	Upper GI Bleeding	Lower GI Bleeding
History/PE	Hematemesis or coffee-ground emesis, melena > hematochezia, depleted volume status (e.g., lightheadedness, hypotension).	Hematochezia > melena, but can be either (upper or lower GI bleed can cause either symptom).
Evaluation	NG tube/lavage, endoscopy if stable.	Colonoscopy if stable. Rule out upper GI bleed with NG tube/lavage.
Common causes	PUD, Mallory–Weiss tear, esophageal varices, vascular abnormalities, neoplasm, esophagitis, gastritis.	Diverticulosis, AVMs, neoplasm, IBD, anorectal disease, mesenteric ischemia..
Initial management	Ensure that the airway is protected. Two **large-bore IV lines ASAP.** Stabilize patient with fluids, blood (hematocrit is not an accurate measure of acute blood loss).	Similar to upper GI bleed.
Management	Endoscopy followed by therapy directed at underlying cause (e.g., H₂ blockers or omeprazole if PUD; sclerotherapy for varices).	Rule out upper GI bleed; then anoscopy or sigmoidoscopy; then colonoscopy; then management of cause of bleeding (resect tumor or diverticula, medical therapy for IBD, etc.).

153

Acute or chronic **liver inflammation** due to a variety of agents, most notably viral infection by one of the **hepatitis viruses** or **alcohol** use. Risk factors include IV drug use (hepatitis B/C), alcohol use (alcoholic hepatitis), and travel to developing countries (hepatitis A and E).

- **Hepatitis A virus:** HAV, an RNA picornavirus, can cause **acute hepatitis.** HAV is spread by fecal-oral transmission (e.g., contaminated food, water, and **shellfish**) and can lead to epidemics. Acute HAV infection is diagnosed by IgM antibody serology; the presence of IgG antibodies indicates exposure. It does not cause chronic hepatitis.
- **Hepatitis B virus:** HBV can cause **acute hepatitis** (1% of patients suffer fulminant or even fatal acute hepatitis) or **chronic hepatitis** (frequently with neonatal infection) and is a major cause of **hepatocellular carcinoma** worldwide. HBV is spread by **blood-borne transmission.** HBsAg is present before and during clinical disease, whereas anti-HBs antibodies indicate disease resolution or vaccination. **Anti-HBc antibodies are never seen after vaccination** (Table 2.6–5).
- **Hepatitis C virus:** HCV causes **acute** and/or **chronic** hepatitis. It is a major cause of cirrhosis and a major cause of **post-transfusion hepatitis.** It is often associated with IV drug abuse and is spread by **blood-borne** transmission.
- **Hepatitis D virus:** HDV causes disease only in association with HBV (coinfection or superinfection). HDV can cause **acute** or **chronic** (often severe) hepatitis and is spread by **blood-borne** transmission.
- **Hepatitis E virus:** HEV normally causes self-limited disease but can be severe (fatal) in **pregnant** women. Commonly seen in Asia and third-world countries; spread by fecal-oral transmission.
- **Alcoholic hepatitis:** Acute or chronic disease secondary to years of alcohol use; varies in severity.

TABLE 2.6–5. Common Serologic Patterns in Hepatitis B Virus Infection.

HBsAg	Anti-HBs	Anti-HBc	HBeAg	Anti-HBe	Interpretation
+	−	IgM	+	−	Acute hepatitis B
+	−	IgG	+	−	Chronic hepatitis B with active viral replication
+	−	IgG	−	+	Chronic hepatitis B with low viral replication
+	+	IgG	+/−	+/−	Chronic hepatitis B with heterotypic anti-HBs (10% of cases)
−	−	IgM	+/−	−	Acute hepatitis B
−	+	IgG	−	+/−	Recovery from hepatitis B (immunity)
−	+	−	−	−	Vaccination (immunity)

- **Autoimmune hepatitis:** Usually causes chronic hepatitis in young women and can lead to cirrhosis requiring transplantation. Treat with ~~prednisone +/– azathioprine.~~
  IMURAN

ACUTE HEPATITIS

History

Acute hepatitis often starts with a viral prodrome of (nonspecific) symptoms (**malaise,** joint pain, fatigue, URI symptoms, **nausea, vomiting,** changes in bowel habits) followed by **jaundice,** fatigue, and other symptoms. There is then a convalescent period followed by recovery.

PE

Jaundice, scleral icterus, **tender hepatomegaly,** possible splenomegaly, and lymphadenopathy.

Differential

Mononucleosis and other systemic viral illnesses (CMV), toxoplasmosis, rickettsial diseases (Q fever, Rocky Mountain spotted fever), drug-induced hepatitis, autoimmune hepatitis, "shock liver" secondary to hypoperfusion (e.g., MI or trauma), neoplasm, alcohol use.

An AST:ALT > 2 suggests alcoholic hepatitis.

Evaluation

Elevated WBC, dramatically **elevated ALT/AST,** and elevated bilirubin/alkaline phosphatase. Diagnosis is made on the basis of **hepatitis serology.** Liver biopsy may be performed in severe cases.

Treatment

- Rest and wait for resolution of symptoms.
- **Look for sick contacts.**
- Administer **alpha-interferon for HBV and HCV** to decrease the likelihood of chronic hepatitis.
- **Steroids** for severe alcoholic hepatitis.

α INTERFERON

CHRONIC HEPATITIS

History/PE

Chronic hepatitis usually gives rise to symptoms indicative of chronic liver disease (jaundice, cirrhosis). At least 70% of those infected with HCV and 10% of those with HBV will develop chronic hepatitis.

Seventy percent of patients infected with HCV will develop chronic hepatitis.

155

Differential

HBV, HCV, HDV, autoimmune hepatitis, alcoholic hepatitis (IM1.38), drug-induced disease ((INH) or methyldopa), Wilson's disease, hemochromatosis, alpha-1-antitrypsin deficiency, neoplasms.

Evaluation

Findings include an **elevated ALT/AST** and a rise in bilirubin/alkaline phosphatase. In severe cases, PT will be prolonged (most clotting factors are produced by the liver). Diagnosis is made on the basis of **hepatitis serologies** and **liver biopsy,** which may show inflammation, fibrosis, and necrosis involving hepatocytes. Additional evaluation may include ANA (autoimmune hepatitis) and antimitochondrial antibody.

Treatment

- For autoimmune hepatitis, **immunosuppression** with steroids and other agents (azathioprine) is standard of care. **Alpha-interferon** and lamivudine (3TC) have proven efficacy in chronic HBV infection. Treat HCV infection with **alpha-interferon** and ribavirin.
- **Liver transplantation** (if available) is the treatment of choice for patients with end-stage liver failure.

Complications

Chronic HBV infection carries a risk of **cirrhosis,** liver failure, and **hepatocellular carcinoma,** and about half of patients die within five years of onset of symptoms. Chronic HCV infection is more indolent and subclinical but can also lead to eventual liver failure or **hepatocellular carcinoma.**

Sequelae of chronic hepatitis include cirrhosis, liver failure, and hepatocellular carcinoma.

DIARRHEA

Increased **frequency of bowel movements** or **increased stool liquidity.** Risk factors include viral infection, systemic infection, sick contacts, and recent travel.

History/PE

Acute diarrhea is usually infectious.

- **Acute diarrhea:** Acute diarrhea is characterized by acute onset with < 3 weeks of symptoms and is usually **infectious.** Causes include E. coli, Salmonella, Shigella, post-antibiotic pseudomembranous colitis (C. difficile), HIV-related diseases (cryptosporidium, Isospora), bacterial toxins (S. aureus), and food poisoning (Salmonella, Campylobacter, cholera, giardiasis, amebiasis).
- **Chronic diarrhea:** Chronic diarrhea is characterized by more long-standing symptoms and is due to such factors as **lactose intolerance,**

malabsorption (mucosal disease, Whipple's disease, neoplasm, malnutrition), IBD, and **motility disorders.**

- **Pediatric diarrhea:** Pediatric diarrhea is most commonly due to **rotavirus infection,** bacterial infection (*E. coli, Shigella, Salmonella, Campylobacter*), post-antibiotic disease (*C. difficile*), or immunosuppression.

Evaluation

Acute diarrhea usually does not require laboratory investigation unless the patient has a high fever, bloody diarrhea, or diarrhea > 4–5 days. In this case, send stool for fecal leukocytes, bacterial culture, *C. difficile* toxin, and ova and parasites. Consider sigmoidoscopy in patients with severe proctitis, bloody diarrhea, or possible *C. difficile* colitis. See Figure 2.6–5 for the evaluation of chronic diarrhea.

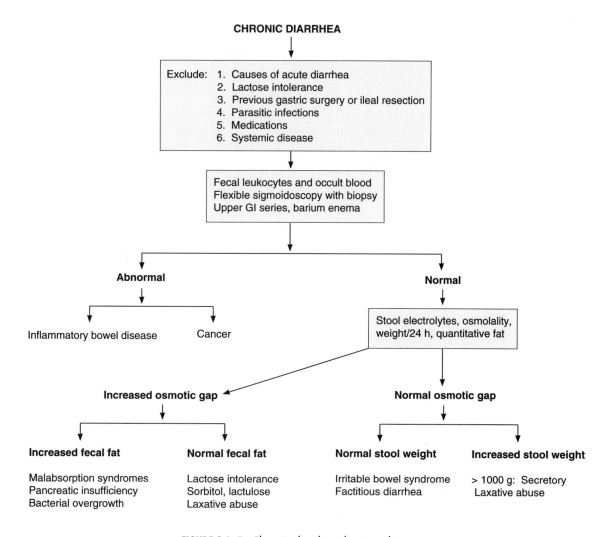

FIGURE 2.6–5. Chronic diarrhea decision diagram.

Treatment

Avoid antimotility agents in patients with bloody diarrhea, high fever, or systemic toxicity.

- **Acute diarrhea:** Treat with oral or IV **fluids** and electrolyte replacement. **Antidiarrheal agents** such as loperamide or bismuth salicylate may improve symptoms. If the patient has evidence of systemic infection (fever, bloody stool, chills, malaise), antibiotics may be started.
- **Chronic diarrhea:** Treatment should be aimed at the underlying cause and can also include loperamide, opioids, clonidine, octreotide, and cholestyramine.
- **Pediatric diarrhea:** For a child who cannot take medication and PO fluids, hospitalize, give IV fluids, and treat the underlying cause.

ACUTE ABDOMEN

Acute-onset abdominal pain that may require immediate surgical intervention. The approach to the patient with an acute abdomen is as follows:

History

PID is a common cause of acute abdominal pain in women.

- Character of pain: sharp pain implies parietal (peritoneal) pain; dull, diffuse pain is commonly visceral (organ) pain. Note location (and whether it shifts or radiates), onset (sudden vs. gradual), severity, the exacerbating and ameliorating factors, and temporal nature (constant vs. colicky).
- GI and systemic symptoms (e.g., anorexia, nausea/emesis); ask about constipation, bloody diarrhea, or hematochezia.
- Hematuria (GU disorders), STD risk factors (PID is a common cause of acute abdominal pain in women), and fever/chills.
- Note the patient's menstrual history, family history (acute intermittent porphyria, familial Mediterranean fever), and past medical and surgical history (vasculitis, SLE, sickle cell disease).

PE

All abdominal pain is not GI pain (PID, pyelonephritis).

- Low BP and high HR are signs of shock or impending shock. High fever in the presence of abdominal pain is a concern.
- **Abdominal distention** suggests a surgical abdomen.
- Manipulate the lower extremity to elicit abdominal pain (suggestive of appendicitis), and check for **CVA tenderness** (pyelonephritis).

Differential

Figure 2.6–6 differentiates the causes of acute abdominal pain by quadrant.

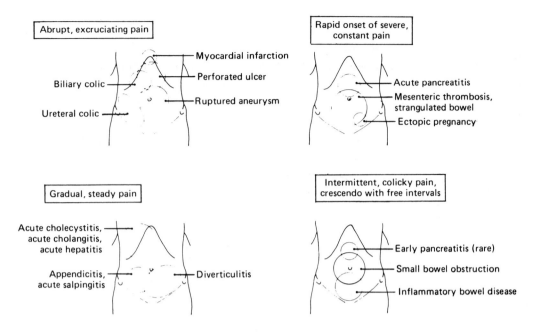

FIGURE 2.6–6. Acute abdomen. The location and character of pain are helpful in the differential diagnosis of the acute abdomen.

Evaluation

Evaluation should include CBC/electrolytes, amylase, ABG if the patient is hypoxic or unstable, lactate, LFTs, PT/PTT, UA/culture, and stool guaiac. **All women of childbearing age should have a β-HCG test to rule out ectopic/uterine pregnancy.** Obtain abdominal plain x-rays followed by appropriate studies based on clinical suspicion. Contrast studies are often performed, but do not use barium if an LBO is suspected, as it may worsen the patient's condition. If RUQ pain is present, perform an ultrasound/HIDA scan to detect cholecystitis. Paracentesis may be diagnostic if there is ascites.

In patients with acute abdomen, always assess for surgical emergencies.

Treatment

Determine whether emergent surgical intervention is necessary (Table 2.6–6). Discontinue oral feeds; insert NG tube if obstruction is suspected or in cases of impending surgery; provide analgesia and supportive care (IV fluids). Type and cross all patients.

TABLE 2.6–6. Indications for Urgent Operation in Patients With Acute Abdomen.

Physical findings

Involuntary guarding or rigidity, especially if spreading

Increasing or severe localized tenderness

Tense or progressive distention

Tender abdominal or rectal mass with high fever or hypotension

Rectal bleeding with shock or acidosis

Equivocal abdominal findings along with—

Septicemia (high fever, marked or rising leukocytosis, mental changes, or increasing glucose intolerance in a diabetic patient)

Bleeding (unexplained shock or acidosis, falling hematocrit)

Suspected ischemia (acidosis, fever, tachycardia)

Deterioration on conservative treatment

Radiologic findings

Pneumoperitoneum

Gross or progressive bowel distention

Free extravasation of contrast material

Space-occupying lesion on scan with fever

Mesenteric occlusion on angiography

Endoscopic findings

Perforated or uncontrollably bleeding lesion

Paracentesis findings

Blood, bile, pus, bowel contents, or urine

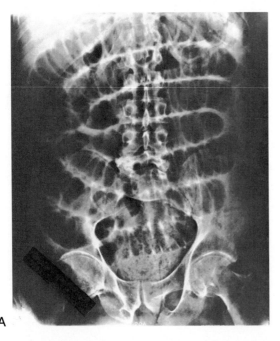

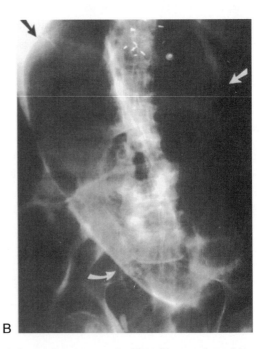

A

B

FIGURE 2.6–7. Bowel obstruction. (A) Small bowel obstruction. Supine abdominal x-ray reveals dilated loops of small bowel in a ladder-like pattern. Air-fluid levels may be apparent on an upright x-ray. (B) Sigmoid volvulus. Abdominal x-ray reveals the distinctive U-shaped appearance of the air-filled dilated sigmoid colon (arrows). Sigmoid volvulus is a common cause of large bowel obstruction.

Table 2.6–7 describes features that distinguish small and large bowel obstruction.

TABLE 2.6–7. Small and Large Bowel Obstruction.		
Variable	**Small Bowel Obstruction (SBO)**	**Large Bowel Obstruction (LBO)**
History	Moderate to severe abdominal pain; **copious emesis.** Cramping pain with distal SBO. Fever and signs of dehydration/low BP may be seen.	Constipation/obstipation, deep and cramping abdominal pain, abdominal distention, nausea and emesis (less than SBO but more commonly **feculent**).
PE	**Abdominal distention** (distal SBO), abdominal tenderness, visible peristaltic waves, fever, hypovolemia; look for **surgical scars and hernias** and perform rectal exam. **High-pitched "tinkly" bowel sounds,** peristaltic rushes, or absence of bowel sounds.	**Abdominal distention,** tympany, tenderness; look for peritoneal irritation; feel for palpable mass; signs of shock or fever indicate possible perforation/peritonitis vs. ischemia/ strangulation. **High-pitched "tinkly" bowel sounds,** peristaltic rushes, or absence of bowel sounds.
Causes	**Adhesions** (postsurgery), hernias, neoplasm, intussusception, volvulus, gallstone ileus, foreign body, Crohn's disease, CF, stricture, hematoma.	**Colon cancer,** diverticulitis, volvulus (Figure 2.6–7), fecal impaction, benign tumors. **Assume colon cancer until proven otherwise.**
Differential	LBO, paralytic ileus, gastroenteritis, pseudo-obstruction.	SBO (more acute onset, less cramping pain, more emesis, less distention), ileus, pseudo-obstruction (Ogilvie's syndrome), appendicitis, IBD.
Evaluation	Obtain CBC, lactic acid, electrolytes, **abdominal plain films** (Figure 2.6–7); perform contrast studies (determine if it is partial or complete), CT scan.	Obtain CBC, electrolytes, lactic acid, **abdominal films** (unlike the small bowel, the haustra of the colon do not cross the entire lumen; see Figure 2.6–7), CT scan; obtain barium or water contrast enema (if perforation is suspected); perform sigmoidoscopy/colonoscopy if stable.
Treatment	Hospitalize. Partial SBO can be treated conservatively with **nasogastric decompression,** but complete SBO should be managed aggressively. Make patient NPO, insert NG tube, give IV fluids to rehydrate, and **operate.**	Hospitalize. In some cases, obstruction can be opened colonoscopically or with a **rectal tube,** but **surgery** is usually required. Gangrenous colon requires partial colectomy with a diverting colostomy unless all bowel is well perfused at surgery. Treat underlying cause (e.g., neoplasm).

HIGH-YIELD FACTS

Gastrointestinal

Hematology

Low hematocrit and/or hemoglobin relative to the sex and age of the patient (check normal values). Risk factors include neoplasia, family history, drug exposure, GI bleeding, vegan diet, alcoholism, black race (sickle cell disease), and Mediterranean descent (thalassemia).

Normal hematocrit depends on age and sex.

History

Patients often present with **weakness** or fatigue, headache, and **dyspnea on exertion.** Severe anemia can cause **angina** or syncope. Patients with iron deficiency anemia may also have **pica** (strange cravings for clay, ice chips, etc.).

Anemia may cause angina.

PE

Pallor (skin and conjunctiva), **tachycardia,** tachypnea, increased pulse pressure, **systolic flow murmur,** jaundice (hemolytic anemia), and positive stool guaiac (GI bleed).

Fe T A L S
↓ SIDERO
↓ LEAD POIS
AN OF CHRONIC Dz
→ THALLASS
→ IRON DEF

Differential

The differential diagnosis is broad and may be organized by MCV:

- **Microcytic (MCV < 80):**
  - Iron deficiency anemia (low ferritin, low serum iron, high TIBC; Figure 2.7–1)
  - Anemia of chronic disease (normal/high ferritin, low serum iron, normal/low TIBC) *Ferritin present, not utilized*
  - Sideroblastic anemia (high ferritin, high serum iron, low TIBC) *IRON OVERLOAD*
  - Other: lead poisoning, thalassemia
- **Macrocytic (MCV > 100):**
  - B_{12}/folate deficiency (Figure 2.7–2) *(IM1.56)*
  - Hemolytic anemia (increased reticulocyte count, mechanical [e.g., heart valve; Figure 2.7–3] vs. immunologic [positive Coombs' test])

Causes of micro-cytic anemia—

TICS
Thalassemia
Iron deficiency
Chronic disease
Sideroblastic anemia

EtOH OR LEAD
Can cause sideroblastic

163

- Drug exposure (MTX, phenytoin, phenobarbital, etc.)
- Other: alcohol use, liver disease, hypothyroidism
■ **Normocytic (MCV 80–100):**
  - Hemorrhage
  - Intravascular hemolysis (G6PD, microangiopathic hemolysis)
  - Extravascular hemolysis (hereditary spherocytosis [Figure 2.7–4] *(IM1.48)*, cold agglutinins, hypersplenism)
  - Infection (osteomyelitis, HIV, *Mycoplasma*, EBV)
  - Bone marrow disease (leukemia, lymphoma, metastatic cancer, myelodysplasia)
  - Renal failure
  - Any cause of microcytic/macrocytic anemia

Evaluation

Decreased serum haptoglobin indicates intravascular hemolysis.

Assess hematocrit, **MCV** (to distinguish microcytic from normocytic/macrocytic), and **reticulocyte count;** obtain **peripheral blood smear.** Then evaluate as follows:

- **Microcytic (low MCV):** Ferritin, iron, TIBC.
- **Macrocytic (high MCV):** RBC folate, serum B$_{12}$, HAPTOGLOBIN, COOMBS
- **Normocytic (normal MCV):** Coombs' test, iron studies, bilirubin.

Obtain serum bilirubin, LDH, and haptoglobin levels if hemolysis is suspected. If diagnosis is not certain or mixed anemia is suspected, perform all these tests (a classically microcytic anemia can present as macrocytosis). Consider bone marrow biopsy and immunologic tests; **screen for malignancy.**

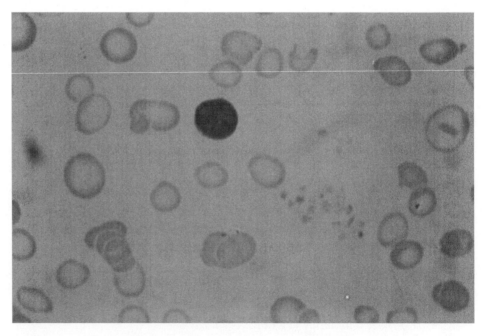

FIGURE 2.7–1. Iron deficiency anemia. Note the microcytic, hypochromic red blood cells ("doughnut cells") with enlarged areas of central pallor.

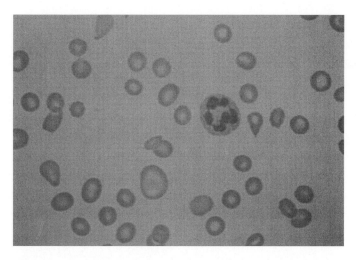

FIGURE 2.7–2. Hypersegmentation. The nucleus of this hypersegmented neutrophil has six lobes (six or more nuclear lobes are required). This is a characteristic finding of megaloblastic anemia.

Right-sided colon cancer can present as a hypochromic, microcytic anemia in an otherwise asymptomatic elderly patient, so perform a hemoccult test to rule out occult GI blood loss.

Treatment

- Treat the underlying disease.
- If iron-deficiency anemia, **search for the source** of bleeding (e.g., GI cancer, menstruation, trauma) or cause of iron malabsorption (e.g., diet, malabsorption).
- Treat iron-deficiency anemia with oral **ferrous sulfate** or gluconate.

Iron-deficiency anemia in an elderly patient is colon cancer until proven otherwise.

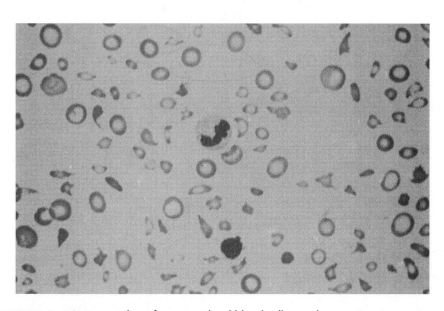

FIGURE 2.7–3. Schistocytes. These fragmented red blood cells may be seen in microangiopathic hemolytic anemia and mechanical hemolysis.

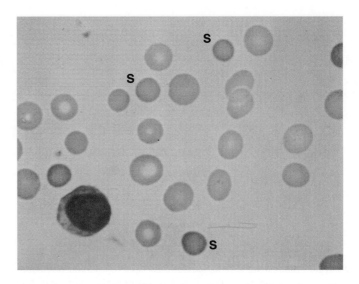

FIGURE 2.7–4. Spherocytes. These RBCs (S) lack areas of central pallor. Spherocytes are seen in autoimmune hemolysis and hereditary spherocytosis.

Administer monthly B_{12} injections for B_{12} deficiency due to pernicious anemia. Transfuse in the presence of severe symptoms or worsening status. Be aggressive in patients with CAD, as anemia can provoke or worsen myocardial ischemia.
- Anemic patients with renal failure should receive exogenous erythropoietin.

THALASSEMIA UCV *IM1.54*

A group of disorders resulting from reduced synthesis of alpha- or beta-globin protein subunits.

Alpha-globin disorders most frequently affect Asians and blacks and can be classified into the following categories:

- **Hydrops fetalis:** No alpha-globin genes; results in stillborn fetus.
- **Hemoglobin H disease:** One alpha-globin gene; associated with **chronic hemolytic anemia, pallor,** and **splenomegaly;** may require occasional transfusion (e.g., during infection).
- **Thalassemia minor:** Two alpha-globin genes; associated with **mild microcytic anemia** and normal life expectancy.
- **Carrier:** Three alpha-globin genes; children of carriers are at risk for thalassemia if the other parent is affected or is a carrier.

Beta-globin disorders most frequently affect people of Mediterranean origin, Asians, and blacks and are classified as follows:

- **Thalassemia major:** No beta-globin production (homozygous); presents in the first year of life as HbF expression declines. Characterized by growth retardation, bony deformity/pathologic fracture, hepatospleno-

Handwritten notes in left margin:
$\phi \alpha$ = DEATH IN UTERO (BART'S)
1α = Hb H
2α = α Thal minor
3α = α Thal carrier

$\phi \beta$ = β Thal major
1β = β Thal minor

Handwritten note at bottom: high levels of HbF

megaly, and jaundice. Symptoms may improve with transfusion therapy, but patients usually die from sequelae of **iron overload** (heart, liver failure) from multiple transfusions. Treat with **transfusions, splenectomy, folic acid,** and **bone marrow transplant** if possible and appropriate (this offers a chance of cure but has a high treatment-associated mortality).

- **Thalassemia minor:** Heterozygote, mild hypochromic/microcytic anemia. Presents similarly to iron deficiency anemia and alpha-thalassemia minor. Treat with folate, **no iron therapy,** and transfusions during severe anemia/pregnancy/stress.

2° HEMOCHROMATOSIS

Patients with thalassemia major usually die from the sequelae of iron overload.

G6PD DEFICIENCY

An **X-linked recessive** deficiency of the G6PD enzyme that causes episodic hemolytic anemia. Black males are most often affected. Mediterranean variants can cause severe hemolytic crises.

History

Usually asymptomatic but may present as acute, self-limited hemolytic anemia (fatigue, **jaundice, dark urine**) with RBC oxidative stress (e.g., from exposure to **fava beans** or to drugs such as dapsone, sulfonamides, quinine/quinidine, and primaquine).

Exposure to sulfonamides or antimalarial drugs may precipitate a hemolytic crisis in patients with G6PD deficiency.

PE

SNS ONLY DURING EPISODE

Usually **normal.** Jaundice and signs of anemia (pallor, tachycardia) are found during hemolytic episodes.

DARK URINE DUE TO HEMOGLOBIN URIA

Differential

Other causes of hemolytic anemia (e.g., hereditary spherocytosis), drug side effects, sickle cell disease, thalassemia.

Evaluation

During hemolytic episodes, look for a low hematocrit, high reticulocyte count, high indirect bilirubin, low serum haptoglobin, and **Heinz bodies** and "bite" cells on blood smear. A **quantitative G6PD enzyme test** is diagnostic.

Treatment

- Usually **self-limited;** avoid exposure to drugs that can cause hemolytic episodes.
- Transfuse if severe.

↑ RBC
wl or ↑ or ↓ WBC
wl or ↑ or ↓ PLT

A **myeloproliferative disease** marked by increased production of RBCs ± platelets and WBCs. Individuals > 60 years of age are at highest risk; males are affected more frequently than females. The most common cause of erythrocytosis is **chronic hypoxia** secondary to lung disease, not polycythemia vera.

History

Patients can present with malaise, fatigue, **pruritus** (typically after warm bath), tinnitus, blurred vision, headache, and **epistaxis.**

PE

Plethora, large retinal veins on fundoscopy, and **splenomegaly.**

Differential

Distinguish polycythemia vera from secondary causes with normal oxygen saturation, low EPO level, and elevated RBC mass.

Secondary polycythemia due to hypoxia (high altitudes, lung disease), smoking (carboxyhemoglobin), erythropoietin (EPO)-producing renal cyst or mass (e.g., renal cell carcinoma), CML, other myelodysplasias, spurious finding (dehydration).

Evaluation

Assessment should include **RBC mass (↑), hematocrit (> 50%), EPO level (↓),** WBCs/platelets (normal or ↑), peripheral blood smear (normal RBCs; basophilic WBCs), and bone marrow biopsy (hypercellular).

Treatment

Hru for PV

- **Serial phlebotomy.**
- Myelosuppressive agents (e.g., **hydroxyurea**) may be used if necessary.
- Daily **aspirin** to prevent thrombotic complications.

Complications

There is a **risk of conversion** to CML, myelofibrosis, or AML.

Viruses transmitted through blood transfusions: HBV, HCV, HIV, CMV, HTLV-I and II.

Immunologic reactions to transfused blood, causing hemolysis and systemic symptoms. Occurs as a result of clerical errors, mislabeled specimens, or reactions to antigens not commonly tested. **Viral infections** can also be transmitted through blood transfusions, including hepatitis B and C, HIV, HTLV-I and II, and CMV.

HIGH-YIELD FACTS

Hematology

History

Severe chills and **high-grade fever** (chills and low-grade fever are common during transfusions); back, chest, or abdominal pain and **dark urine** (hemoglobinuria). Reactions can progress to vascular collapse with shortness of breath and hypotension.

PE

Fever, chills, and back and abdominal tenderness. Severe cases may present with respiratory distress and shock.

Differential

Leukoagglutination reaction, anaphylaxis, gram-negative bacterial contamination, MI, **IgA deficiency,** sepsis, abdominal emergency.

Evaluation

Stop the transfusion and **then** investigate; **retype** the patient's blood against that of the donor; follow hematocrit; **assess creatinine** (renal failure); obtain D-dimer/coagulation studies (DIC). Culture the blood to rule out bacterial contamination.

Hemoglobinuria may lead to acute tubular necrosis and subsequent renal failure.

Treatment

- **Stop the transfusion** immediately.
- Check for hemoglobinemia (in plasma).
- **IV hydration and mannitol** for renal protection.

THROMBOTIC THROMBOCYTOPENIC PURPURA (TTP) UCV IM1.55

younger peeps

Microangiopathic hemolytic anemia, thrombocytopenia, neurologic abnormalities, fever, and **renal dysfunction.** Risk factors include pregnancy, OCP use, and HIV infection; individuals < 50 years of age are at greatest risk.

Features of TTP—

FAT RN
Fever
Anemia
Thrombocytopenia

Renal dysfunction
Neurologic abnormality

History

Patients can present with **fever,** symptoms of anemia, bleeding, **changes in mental status,** headache, aphasia, seizures, and hemiparesis. RENAL NEURO

PE

Fever, bleeding, pallor, **purpura/petechiae** (Figure 2.7–5), altered mental status, and splenomegaly.

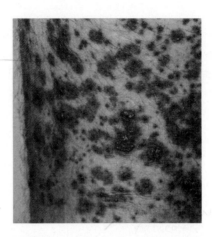

FIGURE 2.7–5. Palpable purpura. Note the round or oval pink to red macules or patches with overlying purple to red papules. Palpable purpura is associated with necrotizing vasculitides, including Henoch–Schönlein purpura, serum sickness, and essential mixed cryoglobulinemia.

Hemolytic-uremic syndrome is TTP without the fever and neurologic abnormalities.

HUS IS RAT
TTP IS FAT RN

Differential

DIC, hemolytic-uremic syndrome (HUS), ITP, mechanical hemolysis (e.g., "Waring blender" valve), Evans's syndrome, endocarditis, neoplasm (Table 2.7–1).

Evaluation

CBC (anemia, thrombocytopenia), peripheral blood smear (**schistocytes;** see Figure 2.7–6), **bilirubin (elevated indirect fraction), LDH (elevated),** Coombs' test (negative), creatinine (may be elevated), and coagulation studies (normal).

Treatment

- Immediate large-volume **plasmapheresis.**
- **Corticosteroids,** anti-platelet agents (aspirin, others), and dextran.
- **Splenectomy** if recurrent or refractory to plasmapheresis and corticosteroids.

TABLE 2.7–1. Causes of Microangiopathic Hemolytic Anemia.

Thrombotic thrombocytopenic purpura
Hemolytic-uremic syndrome
DIC
Prosthetic valve hemolysis
Metastatic adenocarcinoma
Malignant hypertension
Vasculitis

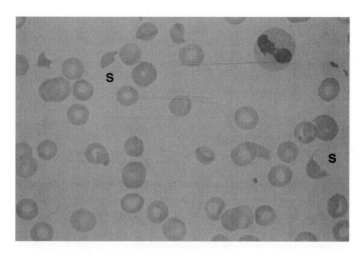

FIGURE 2.7–6. Thrombotic thrombocytopenic purpura (TTP). Note the schistocytes (S) and paucity of platelets.

IDIOPATHIC THROMBOCYTOPENIC PURPURA (ITP)   UCV *Ped.18*

An **autoimmune** platelet disorder. ITP includes pediatric (postviral, self-limited) and adult (chronic) forms. Females are affected twice as often as males, and individuals < 50 years old are at greatest risk. **Evans's syndrome** is ITP plus autoimmune hemolytic anemia. Diseases that are associated with ITP include Hodgkin's and non-Hodgkin's lymphoma, CLL, HIV, SLE, and RA.

IgG ANTI-PLT AUTOIMMUNE

EVAN'S = ITP + COOMB'S ANEMIA

History

Patients are afebrile (unlike TTP) and present with **mucosal bleeding** (epistaxis, oral bleeding, menorrhagia), **petechiae/purpura,** and easy bruising.

↓ Thrombocytes (PLT) ⇒ mucosal bleed

PE

Petechiae, purpura, ecchymoses, and oral hemorrhagic bullae, but **no splenomegaly** (unlike TTP).

∅ SPLENOMEGALY

Differential

ALL/CLL, myelodysplastic syndrome, SLE, drug side effects (e.g., ranitidine), DIC, alcoholism, HIV infection, aplastic anemia, TTP.

↓ PRODUCTION BONE MARROW

Evaluation

CBC (very low platelets, mild or no anemia), coagulation studies, bleeding time, peripheral blood smear (megathrombocytes, **no schistocytes**), DIC panel, bone marrow aspiration (relatively normal; possibly elevated megakaryocytes), and **platelet-associated IgG test.**

↓ PLT w/ nl H & H

Treatment

- In most pediatric patients the condition will resolve **spontaneously,** but the majority of adults require treatment.
- Initial treatment consists of **corticosteroids.**
- **IVIG** (for acute treatment) or **splenectomy** (curative) if refractory to steroids.
- Administer danazol, vincristine/vinblastine, cyclophosphamide, or azathioprine if still refractory.   CHEMO TX
- Give platelets for severe, uncontrollable bleeding.

ACQUIRED

DISSEMINATED INTRAVASCULAR COAGULATION (DIC)   UCV *IM1.47*

A systemic coagulation disorder with pathologic coagulation and a lack of physiologic coagulation. May occur secondary to sepsis, transfusion reaction, neoplasia, trauma (burns and head trauma), and obstetric complications (amniotic embolus, septic abortion, retained dead fetus).

History

Patients often present with **bleeding from venipuncture sites or incisional wounds,** epistaxis, hematemesis, and digital gangrene. DIC leads to systemic collapse and death without early identification and institution of supportive measures.

PE

Evidence of diffuse bleeding, digital cyanosis/gangrene, and vascular collapse with hypotension, tachycardia, tachypnea, and respiratory failure.

Differential

Severe liver disease, sepsis without DIC, vitamin K deficiency (normal fibrinogen), TTP.

Evaluation

Evaluation should include **fibrin split products (high),** D-dimer (high), **fibrinogen (low), PT/PTT (may be elevated),** platelets (very low), and hemocrit (low).

Treatment

- **Treat underlying disorder** (e.g., infection).
- Give **platelets** if < 30,000–50,000; give **cryoprecipitate** to replenish fibrinogen.
- Consider **heparin** (give FFP first to raise AT III) to treat thrombotic complications.

- If refractory, try aminocaproic acid (must be used with heparin) or tranexamic acid.

HEMOPHILIA UCV *Ped.15*

HEMOPHILIA A TE
(FACTOR 8)

An **X-linked recessive** (males affected) coagulopathy due to decreased factor VIII (hemophilia A) or factor IX (hemophilia B) activity.

History/PE

Patients may present with **hemarthroses,** intramuscular bleeding, GI bleeding, and excessive **bleeding in response to mild trauma/surgical/dental procedures.**

Hemophilia A and hemophilia B are clinically indistinguishable.

Differential

DIC, von Willebrand's disease, other coagulopathies.

Evaluation

↑PTT (FACT 8

Findings include **prolonged PTT but normal PT,** reduced factor VIII:C with normal vWF, or reduced factor IX levels. **Bleeding time is normal.**

Bleeding time and PT are normal in hemophilia, whereas PTT is elevated.

Treatment

- **Factor VIII** (hemophilia A) or **factor IX** concentrate (hemophilia B) as needed during bleeding episodes.
- Presupplement with factor VIII or factor IX before surgical and dental procedures.
- Supplement aggressively in cases of head trauma.
- In mild hemophilia A, **desmopressin** may be administered before minor surgical procedures to increase endogenous factor VIII production (bleeding after desmopressin treatment should be treated with aminocaproic acid).
- Think about **HIV** in older hemophiliacs who received replacement factors in the late 1970s to early 1980s.

A
RESPONDS
TO
DDAVP, CR40

B
K DEPENDANT
PROTEIN

VON WILLEBRAND'S DISEASE UCV *Ped.20*

AUTO DOM

An **autosomal-dominant** condition resulting in deficient or defective von Willebrand's factor (vWF). vWF, which is produced by megakaryocytes and endothelial cells, is the only clotting factor not synthesized by the liver.

History

Patients often present with **easy bruising** and **mucosal bleeding** (epistaxis, oral bleeding, menorrhagia), GI bleeding, and postincisional bleeding. Symptoms worsen with aspirin use.

PE

Mucosal/GI bleeding and bruises.

Differential

PLT DYSFXN
βRESPONSE TO ADP,

Hemophilia, drug side effects, Glanzmann's thrombasthenia.

Evaluation

Bleeding time is increased in von Willebrand's disease.

Assess bleeding time (↑), platelet count (normal), PT (normal), PTT (normal or elevated), **factor VIII antigen levels (↓),** ristocetin platelet study (abnormal), direct measurement of vWF (low).

Treatment

- Treat bleeding in mild disease with **desmopressin** (once per 24 hours) in all but type IIa.
- **Factor VIII concentrate** or **cryoprecipitate** (if concentrate is not available) should be given before surgery/dentistry.
- Tranexamic acid can be used as an adjunct to desmopressin.
- Avoid aspirin or aspirin-containing products.

SICKLE CELL DISEASE
UCV *EM.25, Ped.19*

An **autosomal-recessive** disorder due to abnormal hemoglobin. Homozygotes suffer from hematologic/systemic disease, whereas heterozygotes (sickle cell trait) are usually asymptomatic and are less susceptible to malarial infection (balanced polymorphism). Blacks are most commonly affected.

History

Sickle cell crises are precipitated by infection, dehydration, and hypoxia.

Acute episodes of bone/chest pain with fever (vaso-occlusive events) may be precipitated by infection, dehydration, or hypoxia. Patients may present with **strokes** or **priapism.** Up to 50% of affected children < 3 years old will develop **dactylitis** (painful swelling of the hands and feet).

PE

Splenomegaly (young children only), **jaundice,** pallor, fever, and **bone/joint tenderness;** dyspnea/tachypnea with chest pain ("chest syndrome") may be observed.

Differential

Thalassemia and other hemoglobinopathies, osteomyelitis, pneumonia, rheumatic fever, acute abdomen.

Evaluation

Diagnose by hemoglobin electrophoresis. Obtain CBC (normocytic anemia), reticulocyte count (high), **peripheral blood smear** (sickling; Figure 2.7–7), and CXR (for chest syndrome). **"Fish-mouth vertebrae"** may be seen on radiographs of the lumbar spine.

Treatment

- **Hydration, oxygen,** and **analgesia** during an acute vaso-occlusive attack; **exchange transfusion** or simple transfusion may be necessary for severe attacks or for chest syndrome with respiratory distress.
- Chronic hydroxyurea therapy may decrease the frequency of crises.
- **Pneumococcal vaccine** to prevent pneumococcal sepsis; be alert for infection by encapsulated organisms.

Complications

Salmonella osteomyelitis, MI, liver disease, gallbladder disease, infection with encapsulated organisms (secondary to functional asplenia), aplastic crisis (with parvovirus B19 infection), retinopathy, renal disease, strokes, priapism, avascular necrosis of the femoral head.

Sickle cell patients are at increased risk of infection by encapsulated organisms due to functional asplenia.

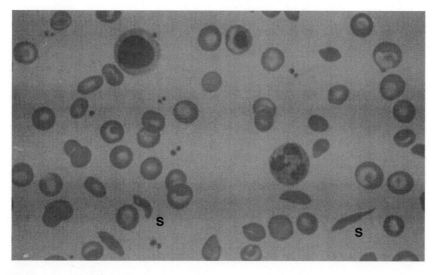

FIGURE 2.7–7. Sickle cells. Sickle-shaped RBCs (S) may appear during infection, dehydration, or hypoxia. Anisocytosis, poikilocytosis, target cells, and nucleated RBCs are also seen in sickle cell disease.

Oncology

UCV OB.3

Risk factors include breast cancer in first-degree relatives, personal history of breast cancer, history of benign breast disease with atypia, nulliparity, early menarche, and late menopause; women who have their first child at age 35 or older are at greater risk. Risk is decreased by late menarche. Breast cancer is rarely seen in males. BRCA1 and BRCA2 mutations are associated with multiple/early-onset breast and ovarian cancer.

Increased exposure to estrogen (early menarche, late menopause, nulliparity) increases the risk of breast cancer.

History

Patients can present with a **breast lump,** breast infection, or **nipple discharge.** Many are asymptomatic and present with a nonpalpable **mammographic abnormality.** Breast cancer most often presents in the **upper outer quadrant** of the breast.

PE

Firm, immobile, painless lump in the breast; **skin changes** (redness, ulceration, edema, nodularity) and axillary adenopathy indicate more advanced disease.

Differential

Mammary dysplasia, fibroadenoma, papilloma (OB.14), mastitis, fat necrosis.

Evaluation

Diagnosis is suggested by a palpable mass or by **mammographic abnormalities** (microcalcifications, hyperdense regions). **Ultrasound** may be used to examine a lump (if cystic, follow or biopsy; if solid, proceed to biopsy). **Biopsy** may be performed by multiple modalities: direct needle/core biopsy (of a palpable lump), stereotactic core biopsy (of a mammographic lesion), or open surgical biopsy (with needle localization if there is no palpable mass). Special variants include **inflammatory breast cancer** (lymphatic spread; poor prognosis), Paget's disease (ductal carcinoma in situ of the nipple), and **bilateral breast cancer** (more commonly seen with lobular carcinoma).

Treatment

Positive estrogen receptor status of the tumor is a good prognostic factor.

Treatment depends on the type and stage:

- **Carcinoma in situ** (CIS) is classified as lobular (LCIS) or ductal (DCIS). LCIS carries a risk of subsequent invasive carcinoma in both breasts, so patients should elect either close follow-up or bilateral mastectomy (especially if there is a positive family history). DCIS can be treated with surgical excision plus radiation (no node dissection is necessary) and follow-up.
- **Invasive cancer** can be either lobular or ductal. The tumor must be staged based on size, node status, and metastases (bone scan, CBC, serum calcium, and CXR). Localized disease can be treated either with lumpectomy + axillary node dissection + radiation or with mastectomy + axillary node dissection. The decision to use chemotherapy is based on the **number of positive nodes** or the presence of **metastases.**
- Positive **estrogen receptor status** makes tamoxifen therapy an option.
- Metastatic or recurrent disease is treated with chemotherapy +/− BMT.
- Metastatic sites include **bone marrow, chest wall, brain,** and **liver.**

Prevention

- **Monthly breast self-exam** for women ≥ 20 years old.
- **Clinical breast exam** every 2–3 years until age 40, then annually.
- **Screening mammography** should be performed yearly in all women > 40–50 years old and earlier in patients with a positive family history.
- New data suggest that prophylactic tamoxifen therapy may decrease the incidence of breast cancer in high-risk women (those with a positive family history). Tamoxifen increases the risk of uterine cancer, so this is an individual decision.
- Consider genetic testing in high-risk families.

PROSTATE CANCER   UC**V** *Surg-48*

Risk factors include advanced age (most men > 80 have a focus of prostate cancer) and a positive family history. Prostate cancer is the most common cancer in men and the second leading cause of cancer death in men.

History

Prostate cancer is usually **asymptomatic** but may present with **urinary retention,** a decrease in force of the urinary stream, lymphedema (metastases), weight loss, and **back pain** (spinal metastases and/or perineural invasion).

PE

Physical findings can include a **palpable nodule**/area of induration on **digital rectal exam.** Early carcinoma is usually not detectable on physical exam.

Differential

BPH (*Surg.46*), prostatitis (e.g., bacterial, TB), urethral stricture, neurogenic bladder.

Evaluation

Diagnosis is suggested by clinical findings and/or by a markedly **elevated PSA** (mild elevations in PSA may be seen with BPH). Diagnosis is made with **biopsy** (transrectal ultrasound guided); tumors are graded by the **Gleason histologic** system. Look for metastases with bone scan and CXR.

Treatment

- Although many cases of prostate cancer are latent and do not progress without treatment, a significant number do lead to metastases (local perineural invasion and bone metastases) and death. Appropriate treatment is controversial.
- **Radical prostatectomy** may result in **incontinence** and/or **impotence** (nerve-sparing surgery decreases the risk of side effects).
- Radiation therapy (brachytherapy) is used in some centers.
- Some patients, especially those of advanced age, choose follow-up with serial PSA/examination/ultrasound.
- Follow PSA in all patients post-treatment.
- Treat **metastatic disease** with **androgen ablation** (GnRH agonists + orchiectomy/flutamide) + chemotherapy (most cases recur).

Prevention

- Screening with PSA is common, although its utility is controversial.
- All males > age 40 should have an annual **digital rectal exam.**

Risk factors include **smoking** (all types except bronchoalveolar carcinoma) and exposure to secondhand smoke, **asbestos,** and other environmental agents.

History

Lung cancer is the leading cause of cancer death and the second most common cancer in men and women.

Patients can present with **hemoptysis, cough,** dyspnea, chest pain, systemic symptoms (fatigue, malaise, weight loss), or paraneoplastic syndromes (Table 2.8–1). Some patients are **asymptomatic** and present with a lung nodule noted on CXR/CT.

PE

Physical examination is usually unremarkable but may reveal abnormalities on respiratory exam (crackles, atelectasis). Other findings include **Horner's syndrome** (miosis, ptosis, anhidrosis) in patients with Pancoast's tumor and many **paraneoplastic syndromes** (Table 2.8–1).

TABLE 2.8–1. Paraneoplastic Syndromes in Lung Cancer.

Classification	Syndrome	Histologic Type of Cancer
Endocrine and metabolic	**Cushing's syndrome**	Small cell
	SIADH	Small cell
	Hypercalcemia	Squamous cell
	Gynecomastia	Large cell
Connective tissue and osseous	Hypertrophic pulmonary osteoarthropathy	Squamous cell, adenocarcinoma, large cell
Neuromuscular	Peripheral neuropathy (sensory, sensorimotor)	Small cell
	Subacute cerebellar degeneration	Small cell
	Myasthenia **(Eaton–Lambert syndrome)**	Small cell
	Dermatomyositis	All
Cardiovascular	Thrombophlebitis	Adenocarcinoma
	Nonbacterial verrucous (marantic) endocarditis	
Hematologic	Anemia	All
	DIC	
	Eosinophilia	
	Thrombocytosis	
Cutaneous	Acanthosis nigricans	All
	Erythema gyratum repens	

HIGH-YIELD FACTS

Oncology

Differential

TB/other granulomatous diseases, fungal disease (aspergillus, histoplasmosis), lung abscess, metastasis, benign tumor (bronchial adenoma), hamartoma.

Evaluation

Lung cancer is usually first noted as a nodule on CXR and is best seen with **lung CT. Bronchoscopy with biopsy** or brushing or **fine needle aspiration** under CT guidance can usually establish the diagnosis. Mediastinoscopy may be necessary for biopsy of hilar nodes. Thoracoscopic biopsy may be performed, with conversion to open thoracotomy if the lesion is found to be malignant.

Treatment

- Although there are multiple types of lung cancer (large cell, bronchoalveolar, adenocarcinoma, squamous, small cell), they can be grouped into **non-small cell** (NSCLC) and **small cell** (SCLC) for the purposes of treatment.
- **NSCLC** should be treated with **surgical resection** if possible. The decision is based on the size of the lesion, the presence of metastases (metastatic disease is usually not resected unless there is only a single brain met), and the patient's age, general health, and lung function. Follow surgery with radiation/chemotherapy (depends on stage). Unresectable disease should be treated with radiation and chemotherapy.
- SCLC is not considered resectable and often responds initially to **chemotherapy** but usually recurs, carrying a much **lower survival rate** than NSCLC.
- Treat oncologic emergencies (e.g., SVC syndrome) with radiation.
- Treat metastases (brain, liver, bone) palliatively.

> **Lung cancer—**
> **SPHERE of complications**
> **S**uperior vena caval syndrome
> **P**ancoast's tumor
> **H**orner's syndrome
> **E**ndocrine (paraneoplastic)
> **R**ecurrent laryngeal symptoms (hoarseness)
> **E**ffusions (pleural or pericardial)

Prevention

Smoking cessation (nothing else, including CXR screening, has been shown to help).

SOLITARY PULMONARY NODULE

An **asymptomatic** lung nodule < 5 cm in size that is discovered on CXR or CT. Solitary pulmonary nodules are most often benign, with a 5–10% likelihood of malignancy.

Five to ten percent of asymptomatic solitary pulmonary nodules are malignant.

Differential

Granuloma (e.g., old or active TB infection, fungal infection, foreign body reaction), carcinoma, **hamartoma,** metastasis (usually multiple), bronchial adenoma (95% carcinoid tumors), Pancoast's tumor (Horner's syndrome), **pneumonia.**

Evaluation

Older age of patient and larger size of nodule favor malignancy.

Obtain old x-rays if available and perform a CT scan to determine the nature, location, progression, and extent of the nodule. Proceed to biopsy or resection if diagnosis is still in doubt.

Benign lesions may be distinguished from malignant lesions by the following means:

- **Characteristics favoring carcinoma:** Age > 45–50 years; lesions new or larger in comparison to old films; absence of calcification or **irregular calcification;** size > 2 cm; irregular margins.
- **Characteristics favoring a benign lesion:** Age < 35 years; no change from old films; **central/uniform/laminated calcification;** smooth margins; size < 2 cm; regular margins.

Treatment

- A nodule in a patient > 35 years old should be **resected** unless there is radiologic proof that the lesion has not changed in size or appearance in at least two years.
- If the patient is young, if the lesion is unchanged, or if the patient objects, the lesion can be followed with a **second study in 3–6 months** (resect lesions that change in size or character).
- Surgical excision is preferred over biopsy. In some cases, surgeons opt for thoracoscopic biopsy with conversion to open resection if necessary.

COLORECTAL CANCER

Risk factors include a positive **family history,** IBD, colorectal polyps, and a **low-fiber, high-fat** diet. **Familial syndromes** include familial adenomatous polyposis (FAP) and hereditary nonpolyposis colorectal cancer (HNPCC). FAP is characterized by a colon full of polyps (Figure 2.8–2), any of which can progress to cancer, whereas HNPCC is characterized by an increased risk that a single polyp will progress to cancer.

History

Presenting symptoms can include a **change in bowel habits,** pencil-thin stools, **frank or occult blood in the stool,** abdominal obstruction, abdominal pain, symptoms of anemia, and **systemic symptoms** (malaise, fatigue, weight loss).

PE

Physical examination should include a **digital rectal exam,** a **stool guaiac test,** and palpation for an abdominal mass.

Differential

Diverticular disease, IBD, benign polyps of the colon, infectious colitis (amebiasis, C. *difficile* colitis), GI blood loss from the stomach/duodenum (peptic ulcer).

Evaluation

Colonoscopy or barium enema followed by colonoscopy (Figure 2.8–1). **Biopsy** suspicious areas. If a diagnosis of cancer is made, stage according to the TNM or the **Dukes system:** Dukes A (tumor within the muscularis propria), Dukes B (tumor invading the muscularis), Dukes C (positive lymph nodes), Dukes D (metastases).

Iron-deficiency anemia in an elderly male patient is colon cancer until proven otherwise.

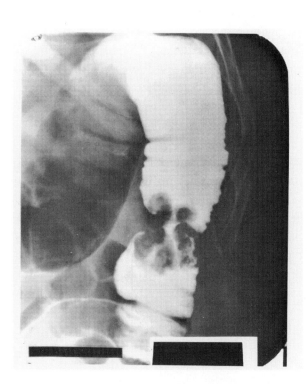

FIGURE 2.8–1. Colon carcinoma. The encircling carcinoma appears as an "apple core" filling defect in the descending colon on barium enema x-ray.

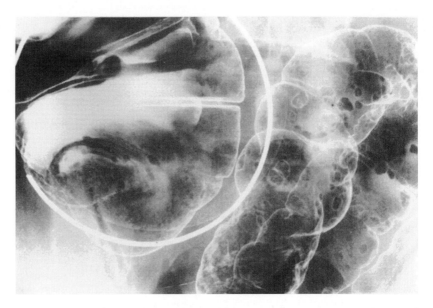

FIGURE 2.8–2. Familial adenomatous polyposis. Double-contrast barium enema x-ray reveals innumerable small polyps.

Treatment

Management of colon cancer depends on lymph node status.

- **Surgical resection** following the pattern of lymphatic and vascular drainage is the primary therapy. Rectal cancer is resected by abdominoperineal or low anterior resection.
- Node-negative disease is usually resected and followed.
- **Node-positive** disease is treated with **adjuvant chemotherapy** or radiotherapy following resection.
- Colon cancers are resected even if metastatic. Small to moderate liver mets are resected (with increased five-year survival and the possibility of cure) with subsequent chemotherapy.

Prevention

- **Annual digital rectal examination,** beginning at age 40.
- **Annual stool guaiac test** beginning at age 50. If stool guaiac is positive, perform a flexible sigmoidoscopy/colonoscopy.
- A **flexible sigmoidoscopy** should be performed **every 3–5 years** in patients > 50 years of age.
- Conduct more aggressive screening in patients with a positive family history.
- Consider prophylactic colectomy for patients with FAP or ulcerative colitis.
- CEA levels can help monitor for recurrence.

Risk factors include a family history of **breast or ovarian cancer, infertility, and nulliparity.** BRCA1 and BRCA2 syndromes are associated with an increased risk of breast and ovarian cancer.

History

Ovarian cancer is **usually asymptomatic until late in the course of the disease.** Patients may present with abdominal pain and bloating, early satiety, constipation, vaginal bleeding, and systemic symptoms (fatigue, malaise, weight loss).

PE

Physical findings can include a palpable abdominal/adnexal mass and ascites **(increasing abdominal girth).**

Differential

Uterine leiomyomas (should not increase in size after menopause), ectopic pregnancy, pelvic kidney, retroperitoneal fibrosis/tumor, colorectal cancer, PID, ovarian cyst, metastasis.

Evaluation

CA-125; transvaginal ultrasound and possibly CT/MRI; biopsy with **diagnostic laparoscopy or open resection.** Epithelial tumors are the most common histologic variant; other types include germ cell/functional tumors.

CA-125 levels may be elevated in ovarian cancer.

Treatment

- Primary therapy consists of **resection** as part of a **TAH/BSO.**
- Postsurgical **chemotherapy** is warranted for almost all patients.
- Ovarian cancer has a **poor prognosis;** most recur despite treatment.

Prevention

- Women with a strong family history (two or more affected first-degree relatives) can be screened annually with **CA-125** and **transvaginal ultrasound. Prophylactic oophorectomy** is sometimes recommended after childbearing is complete.
- **Oral contraceptive** use decreases the risk of ovarian cancer.

HIGH-YIELD FACTS

Oncology

- Note risk factors for malignancy (family history, nulliparity, infertility), previous malignancy, and previous ovarian cysts (e.g., polycystic ovarian syndrome). Feel for a palpable mass. Check for ascites, cervical motion tenderness, and abdominal tenderness.
- Perform a transvaginal ultrasound.
- CT/MRI may help delineate the lesion.
- Check CA-125 level.
- The mass should be **resected** if imaging suggests possible malignancy, if the patient has risk factors for ovarian cancer, and if CA-125 is elevated.

CERVICAL CANCER UCV OB.4

Risk factors include intercourse early in life, multiple sexual partners, **tobacco use,** and HPV infection.

History

Cervical cancer is usually diagnosed in asymptomatic patients by Pap smear, colposcopy, and biopsy, but patients may present with dysfunctional uterine bleeding, **postcoital bleeding,** pelvic pain, and vaginal discharge.

PE

Cervical discharge/ulceration, pelvic mass, or fistulas.

Differential

Cervicitis, vaginitis, STDs, actinomycosis.

Evaluation

Positive Pap smear/colposcopy must be followed with cone biopsy. The diagnosis may be invasive cervical carcinoma or cervical intraepithelial neoplasia (CIN), which is divided into low-grade squamous intraepithelial lesion (LSIL) and high-grade squamous intraepithelial lesion (HSIL).

Treatment

- CIN is usually treated with **cryosurgery** or **loop resection** (LSIL) or with **conization** of the cervix (HSIL/carcinoma in situ).

HIGH-YIELD FACTS

Oncology

- Invasive carcinoma is treated with **surgical resection**—simple **hysterectomy** for early disease, and radical hysterectomy +/– radiation for advanced/extracervical disease.

Prevention

- **Annual Pap smears** should be obtained beginning with the onset of sexual activity, with appropriate follow-up of indeterminate or positive results. After three consecutive normal Pap smears, screening every three years is recommended.

Screening with annual Pap smears has dramatically reduced the incidence of invasive cervical cancer.

THYROID NODULE UC**V** *Surg.8*

Thyroid nodules are found in 1% of individuals between the ages of 20 and 30 and in 5% of individuals > 60 years. The vast majority of thyroid nodules are benign. There is a higher risk of malignancy in patients with a **history of neck irradiation, "cold" nodules** (on radionuclide scan), firm and fixed solitary nodules, and **rapidly growing nodules** with **hoarseness or dysphagia.**

History

Usually **asymptomatic** on initial presentation. Note the presence of systemic symptoms (e.g., hypo/hyperthyroidism), local symptoms (dysphagia, dyspnea/respiratory difficulties, odynophagia, hoarse voice), family history (especially **medullary thyroid cancer**), and history of neck irradiation (for thyroid cancer, hyperthyroidism, or salivary gland tumors).

PE

Carcinoma will likely be palpable, **firm, fixed,** and **nontender.** Check for anterior cervical lymphadenopathy.

Differential

Lymphocytic thyroiditis, multinodular goiter, colloid nodule, benign follicular adenoma, papillary or follicular carcinoma.

Evaluation/Treatment

- TSH and **thyroid function tests.**
- **Ultrasound** can determine if the nodule is cystic; a radioactive scan can determine if it is cold or hot (cancers are usually cold and solid).
- The best method of assessing a nodule for malignancy is **fine needle aspiration** (high sensitivity and moderate specificity).

Malignant thyroid nodules are usually cold and solid.

HIGH-YIELD FACTS

Oncology

187

- If the FNA is benign, treat with **thyroxine** (suppresses TSH and shrinks nodule) and follow with ultrasound.
- If malignant, perform **surgical resection.**
- If the distinction between benign and malignant is not clear (this is often a difficult diagnosis), perform a lobectomy and wait for final pathology.
- Medullary thyroid cancer/anaplastic carcinomas are aggressive variants with a worse prognosis. Medullary thyroid carcinoma is associated with MEN IIA and IIB cancer syndromes.
- Look for metastases with radioactive iodine scans.

An **embryonal tumor of renal origin** that is the most common renal tumor in children (usually seen in 1- to 4-year-olds). Risk factors include a positive family history, Beckwith–Wiedemann syndrome, neurofibromatosis, aniridia, hemihypertrophy, and congenital GU anomalies.

History

Painless abdominal/flank mass, hematuria (usually microscopic), weight loss, nausea, emesis, bone pain, dysuria, and polyuria.

PE

Physical examination may reveal an **abdominal/flank mass,** abdominal tenderness, **fever,** and **hypertension.**

Differential

Neuroblastoma, abdominal neoplasms.

Evaluation

Abdominal CT/ultrasound will show an **intrarenal mass.** Assess extent of disease with CXR, chest CT, CBC, LFTs, and BUN/creatinine.

Treatment

- **Transabdominal nephrectomy.**
- Administer chemotherapy after surgery **(vincristine/dactinomycin).**
- Flank irradiation is used in some cases.

A tumor of **neural crest cell origin.** Risk factors include neurofibromatosis, tuberous sclerosis, Klippel–Feil syndrome, Waardenburg syndrome, pheochromocytoma, and Hirschsprung's disease. Children < 5 years of age are most commonly affected.

History

Lesions can appear anywhere in the body, so symptoms vary. May present as an **abdominal mass,** abdominal distention, anorexia, malaise, fever, diarrhea, or **neuromuscular symptoms** (if paraspinal).

PE

Abdominal mass, tenderness, distention, leg edema, hypertension, fever, pallor, and periorbital bruises.

Differential

Wilms' tumor, Ewing's sarcoma, rhabdomyosarcoma, peripheral neuroepithelioma, lymphoma.

Evaluation

Diagnose with abdominal CT plus 24-hour urinary catecholamines (look for **elevated VMA** and **HVA**). Assess extent of disease with CXR, bone scan, CBC, LFTs, BUN/creatinine, and coagulation screen.

Treatment

- Localized tumors are usually cured with **excision.**
- Localized but unresectable tumors also have a favorable prognosis.
- Chemotherapy includes **cyclophosphamide and doxorubicin.**
- Radiation is a useful adjunct.

Primary malignancy of **plasma cell origin.** Risk factors include monoclonal gammopathy of unknown significance (MGUS). Patients > 50 years of age are most commonly affected, and blacks are affected more frequently than whites.

HIGH-YIELD FACTS

Oncology

History

Patients can present with **back pain, hypercalcemic symptoms** (weakness, weight loss, altered mental status, constipation), **pathologic bone fractures,** and frequent infections (secondary to dysregulation of antibody production).

PE

Pallor, bone tenderness, bone deformities, and lethargy.

Differential

Metastatic carcinoma, lymphoma, MGUS, Waldenström's macroglobulinemia, primary amyloidosis, hyperparathyroidism.

Evaluation

Obtain CBC (anemia), peripheral smear (plasmacytosis; Figure 2.8–3), SPEP/UPEP **(monoclonal gammopathy, Bence Jones proteinuria),** electrolytes, BUN/creatinine (renal disease/hypercalcemia), a full-body **skeletal survey** ("punched-out" **osteolytic lesions** of the skull and long bones), **bone scan (negative),** and bone marrow biopsy **(plasma cell infiltration).**

Treatment

- Multiple-agent **chemotherapy** (alkylating agents), melphalan, and corticosteroids (prednisone).
- Bone marrow/stem cell transplant is an option.
- Patients with multiple osteolytic lesions in a single bone (e.g., femur) may require prophylactic **intramedullary fixation.**
- Pathologic fractures require open reduction–internal fixation.
- The disease usually recurs and carries a poor prognosis.
- Complications include infection, anemia, neurologic disease, and renal failure.

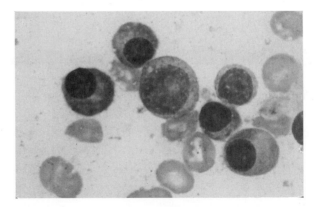

FIGURE 2.8–3. Multiple myeloma. Note the abundance of plasma cells on peripheral blood smear. RBCs will often be in rouleaux formation.

Table 2.8–2 summarizes features of non-Hodgkin's and Hodgkin's lymphoma.

TABLE 2.8–2. Non-Hodgkin's and Hodgkin's Lymphoma.		
	Non-Hodgkin's Lymphoma	**Hodgkin's Lymphoma**
Risk factors	EBV (Burkitt's), HIV infection.	15–45 years (women > men) or > 60 years
Histology	Varies.	**Reed–Sternberg cells.**
Variants	Many; separated into low, intermediate, and high grade.	Nodular sclerosis, mixed cellularity, lymphocyte predominance or lymphocyte depleted.
History	Painless adenopathy, fever, night sweats, other systemic symptoms (malaise, weight loss).	Fever, night sweats, weight loss, pruritus, systemic symptoms.
PE	**Systemic** adenopathy +/– hepatosplenomegaly.	**Regional** adenopathy +/– hepatosplenomegaly.
Differential	Hodgkin's lymphoma, mononucleosis, cat scratch disease, HIV, sarcoid.	Non-Hodgkin's lymphoma, HIV, sarcoid, lymphadenitis, drug reaction.
Evaluation	**Biopsy** for diagnosis followed by CXR, body CT scans, and possibly bone marrow biopsy/LP.	**Biopsy** largest, most central node (choose with neck → pelvis CT scan, physical exam), then CXR, possibly bone marrow biopsy/LP.
Treatment	Radiation + chemotherapy.	Radiation therapy for localized disease, plus chemo for advanced/widespread disease.

LEUKEMIAS

Leukemias result from the malignant proliferation of hematopoietic cells and are the most common type of cancer in **children.** Categorization is based on their cellular origin (e.g., promyeloid, myeloid, lymphoid) and level of differentiation of neoplastic cells. **Acute leukemias** are associated with the proliferation of minimally differentiated blast cells, while **chronic leukemias** are associated with the proliferation of more mature, differentiated cell forms. Tumor invasion of the bone marrow results in **pancytopenia** (thrombocytopenia, anemia). Thus, the major medical complications of end-stage leukemia are **bleeding** (from thrombocytopenia), **infection,** and anemia.

Leukemias are the most common type of cancer in children.

ACUTE LYMPHOCYTIC LEUKEMIA (ALL)   **UCV** *Ped.14*

ALL is most common in children, and whites are affected more frequently than blacks. **Most common cancer of childhood.**

History

Patients can present with limp, **bone pain,** refusal to walk, and **fever.**

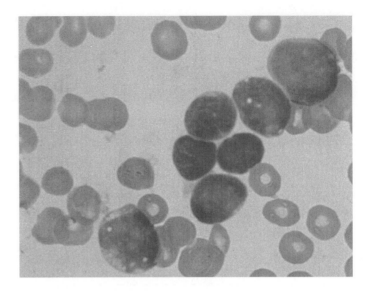

FIGURE 2.8–4. Acute lymphocytic leukemia. Peripheral blood smear reveals numerous large, uniform lymphoblasts with fine granular cytoplasm and faint nucleoli.

PE

Physical examination may reveal fever, pallor, widespread **petechiae/purpura,** adenopathy, **hepatosplenomegaly,** easy bruising, and bleeding.

Differential

Aplastic anemia, mononucleosis/other viral infections, rheumatic diseases, other neoplasms.

Evaluation

Look for depression of bone marrow elements (e.g., anemia, severe thrombocytopenia, leukopenia; see Figure 2.8–4), **elevated LDH/uric acid,** and cytogenetic changes. Diagnosis can be made with **bone marrow aspirate.** Obtain CXR (rule out mediastinal involvement), LP (rule out brain metastasis), and CT scan.

Treatment

Good prognosis with **chemotherapy,** with 85% of children achieving long-term survival (30% of adults).

Eighty-five percent of children achieve complete remission with chemotherapy.

ACUTE MYELOGENOUS LEUKEMIA (AML)

Affects children and adults. The adult form increases in incidence with age.

History

The adult form of AML presents as **fatigue, dyspnea, fever,** skin disease (leukemia cutis), CNS symptoms, and a history of **frequent infections.**

PE

Fever, lethargy, bleeding, **purpura/petechiae,** and variable hepatosplenomegaly.

Differential

CML, myelodysplastic syndromes, lymphoma, hairy cell leukemia, mononucleosis.

Evaluation

Bone marrow examination demonstrates depression of all blood cell elements except monocytes (anemia, thrombocytopenia, neutropenia). Blasts are often seen in peripheral blood (Figures 2.8–5 and 2.8–6), and **Auer rods** are pathognomonic. Cytogenic studies provide key prognostic information.

Treatment

Treat with intensive multiple-agent **chemotherapy,** transfusions, antibiotics as

WHAT'S "MY NE" IS AUERS

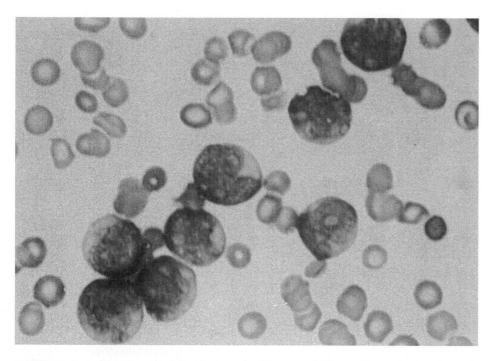

FIGURE 2.8–5. Acute myelogenous leukemia. Large, uniform myeloblasts with notched nuclei and prominent nucleoli are characteristic.

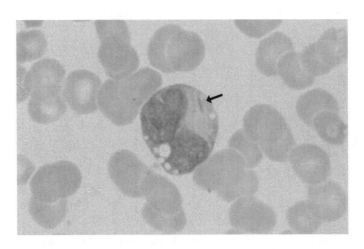

FIGURE 2.8–6. Auer rod in acute myelogenous leukemia. The red rod-shaped structure (arrow) in the cytoplasm of the myeloblast is pathognomonic.

needed, and allogenic/autologous **bone marrow transplants. Retinoic acid** may induce remission in the promyelocytic form. AML has a moderate prognosis, with 70–80% of adults < 60 years old achieving complete remission.

CHRONIC LYMPHOCYTIC LEUKEMIA (CLL)   UCV IM1.45

Primarily affects **patients > 65 years of age.** The disease is slowly progressive and is associated with good short-term and poor long-term survival.

History/PE

Lymphadenopathy, fatigue, and hepatosplenomegaly. This is usually an **indolent disease,** and many patients are diagnosed by incidental lymphocytosis.

Differential

Viral disease, other leukemias, myelodysplastic disorders.

Evaluation

Look for **isolated lymphocytosis** on CBC (hematocrit and platelet count are often normal at presentation; see Figure 2.8–7). Bone marrow will be infiltrated with lymphocytes.

Treatment

Most patients are **managed supportively.** Treatment is usually not instituted until patients develop increasing fatigue or lymphadenopathy, anemia, or thrombocytopenia. Start with chlorambucil or fludarabine; splenectomy and

CLL is slowly progressive, with good short-term but poor long-term survival.

CLL may be complicated by autoimmune hemolytic anemia.

0 PBCLPH LYMPHOCYTOSIS

1 LAD

2 SPLGNO MEG

3 ANEMIA

4 THROMBO CYTO

Call
me
Smear

194

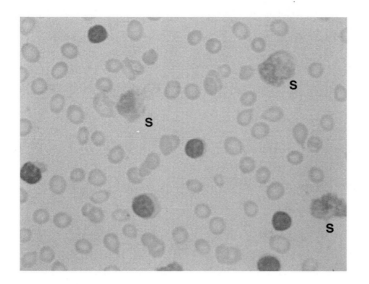

FIGURE 2.8–7. Chronic lymphocytic leukemia. The numerous small, mature lymphocytes and smudge cells (S; fragile malignant lymphocytes are disrupted during blood smear preparation) are characteristic.

steroids are appropriate for autoimmune hemolytic anemia and thrombocytopenia.

CHRONIC MYELOGENOUS LEUKEMIA (CML)   UCV IM1.46

Characterized by overproduction of myeloid cells, this disease is often stable for several years until it transforms into a more overtly malignant form. Associated with **prior radiation exposure.**

History/PE

In its early stages, CML is asymptomatic or presents with mild, nonspecific symptoms (e.g., **fatigue, fever, malaise,** decreased exercise tolerance, weight loss, night sweats). If detected at a later stage, patients present with early satiety, LUQ fullness/pain, splenomegaly, and bleeding. **Blast crisis** (associated with late presentation) presents as fever, bone pain, weight loss, and increasing **splenomegaly.** All patients eventually reach blast crisis with progressive pancytopenia and disseminated disease.

my
FRIEND
PHIL

Evaluation

Peripheral blood smear will demonstrate a significantly **elevated WBC** (median of 150,000 at time of diagnosis) and prominent myeloid cells. The leukocyte alkaline phosphatase score is low, and vitamin B_{12} levels are often markedly elevated. Bone marrow biopsy is performed as an adjunct. Definitive

The Philadelphia chromosome is the sine qua non of CML.

diagnosis can be made via cytogenics, which usually reveals the **Philadelphia chromosome** (9,22 translocation) or *bcr-abl* gene fusion product.

Treatment

CML often terminates in blast crises, which are rapidly fatal in most cases.

- CML is associated with a poor overall prognosis, with a median survival of 3–4 years.
- Treatment in the chronic phase is **palliative,** using myelosuppressive agents such as alpha-interferon and hydroxyurea.
- Allogenic **bone marrow transplant** is curative in about 60% of cases.
- Blast crisis is difficult to treat and is rapidly terminal in most cases.

Infectious Disease

SEPSIS

UCV EM.28

Systemic inflammatory response syndrome (SIRS) with a documented infection. Septic shock refers to sepsis-induced hypotension (systolic BP < 90). Gram-positive shock occurs secondary to fluid loss caused by the dissemination of exotoxins; common pathogens include staphylococci and streptococci. Gram-negative shock is caused by endotoxin (lipopolysaccharide) production by bacteria such as *E. coli, Klebsiella, Proteus,* and *Pseudomonas.* Other etiologies are as follows:

- **Neonates:** Group B streptococci, *E. coli, Klebsiella.*
- **Children:** *H. influenzae, Pneumococcus, Meningococcus.*
- **Adults:** Gram-positive cocci, aerobic bacilli, anaerobes.
- **IV drug users:** *S. aureus.*
- **Asplenic patients:** *Pneumococcus, H. influenzae, Meningococcus* (encapsulated organisms).

SIRS includes fever or hypothermia, chills, tachypnea, and tachycardia.

History

Abrupt onset of fever and chills, often associated with hyperventilation and altered mental status.

PE

Look for **fever** (15% present with hypothermia), **tachycardia,** and tachypnea. **Hypotension** and shock occur in severe cases. Septic shock may start with **warm skin and extremities** (warm shock; peripheral vasodilation) and may then progress to cold shock with **cool skin and extremities** (peripheral vasoconstriction). Petechiae or ecchymoses suggest DIC, which occurs in 2–3% of cases.

Evaluation

Findings include neutropenia or neutrophilia with increased bands. Thrombocytopenia occurs in 50% of cases. Blood, sputum, and urine cultures may be positive and CXR may show an infiltrate. Obtain coagulation studies and consider a DIC panel (fibrinogen, fibrin split products, D-dimers).

Septic shock requires empiric antibiotic therapy.

Treatment

Patients often require ICU admission. Treat aggressively with **IV fluids, pressors,** empiric **antibiotics** (Table 2.9–1), and **removal** of predisposing factors (take out Foley catheter, infected IV line, etc.).

TABLE 2.9–1. Examples of Empiric Antimicrobial Therapy for Acutely Ill Adults.

Suspected Diagnosis	Likely Etiology	Drugs of Choice
Meningitis, bacterial	Pneumococcus, meningococcus, *Listeria* (elderly, immuno-compromised)	Ceftriaxone or cefotaxime +/– vancomycin, ampicillin for *Listeria*
Brain abscess	Mixed anaerobes, pneumococci, streptococci	Penicillin G or metronidazole plus cefotaxime or ceftriaxone
Pneumonia, acute, community-acquired, severe	Pneumococci, *M. pneumoniae*, *Legionella*, *C. pneumoniae*	Erythromycin, doxycycline, cefotaxime, or ceftriaxone
Pneumonia, postoperative or nosocomial	*S. aureus*, anaerobes, gram-negative bacilli	Cefotaxime (or ceftriaxone) with gentamicin or tobramycin
Endocarditis, acute (including IV drug user)	*S. aureus*, *E. faecalis*, gram-negative aerobic bacteria, viridans streptococci	Antistaphylococcal penicillin (e.g., nafcillin, oxacillin) plus gentamicin or vancomycin plus gentamicin
Septic thrombophlebitis (e.g., IV tubing, IV shunts)	*S. aureus*, gram-negative aerobic bacteria	Nafcillin, gentamicin
Osteomyelitis	*S. aureus*, *Salmonella* in sickle cell patients	Nafcillin
Septic arthritis	*S. aureus*, *N. gonorrhoeae*	Ceftriaxone
Pyelonephritis with flank pain and fever (recurrent UTI)	*E. coli*, *Klebsiella*, *Enterobacter*, *Pseudomonas*, *Proteus*	Ciprofloxacin or levofloxacin
Intra-abdominal sepsis (e.g., postoperative, peritonitis, cholecystitis)	Gram-negative bacteria, *Bacteroides*, anaerobic bacteria, streptococci, clostridia, *Enterococcus*	Ampicillin plus gentamicin plus metronidazole

A retrovirus that targets and destroys CD4 lymphocytes, leading to AIDS. Risk factors include unprotected sexual intercourse, IV drug abuse, maternal HIV infection, needle sticks and mucocutaneous exposures, and receipt of blood products. Infection is characterized by a high rate of viral replication leading to a progressive decline in the CD4 count. Broadly stated, the **CD4 count** is a surrogate marker for the **extent** of disease progression, while the **viral load** is an indicator for the **rate** of disease progression.

CD4 count is a marker for the extent of disease, while viral load indicates rate of disease progression.

History/PE

Primary HIV infection is often **asymptomatic;** patients may present with **flu-like symptoms,** e.g., generalized malaise, fever, generalized lymphadenopathy, rash, or even viral meningitis. Later, HIV may present as night sweats, weight loss, and cachexia. Complications correlate with CD4 count, as indicated in Table 2.9–2.

Evaluation

The **ELISA test (high sensitivity, moderate specificity)** detects anti-HIV antibodies in the bloodstream (which can take up to six months to appear after exposure). Confirm a positive ELISA with a **Western blot (low sensitivity, high specificity).** If the patient is HIV positive, then check viral load, PPD with anergy panel, VDRL, and CMV and toxoplasmosis serologies.

A positive ELISA must be confirmed with a Western blot.

Treatment

Management is evolving rapidly. Currently, **antiretroviral therapy** is initiated for patients with CD4 counts < 500 or with a detectable viral load. Start patients on two **nucleoside analogs** (e.g., AZT, ddI, 3TC, D4T). **Protease in-**

TABLE 2.9–2. HIV Complications.

CD4 Count	Associated Complications
> 500	Lymphadenopathy, recurrent vaginal candidiasis.
200–500	Pneumococcal pneumonia, pulmonary TB, shingles, oral candidiasis, cervical intraepithelial neoplasia, anemia, Kaposi's sarcoma, non-Hodgkin's lymphoma, histoplasmosis, coccidioidomycosis.
100–200	*Pneumocystis carinii* pneumonia, AIDS dementia complex, wasting syndrome.
50–100	Toxoplasmosis, cryptococcosis.
< 50	CMV retinitis *(IM2.12)*, MAC, cryptosporidiosis, PML, primary CNS lymphoma.

HIGH-YIELD FACTS

Infectious Disease

hibitors (e.g., saquinavir, ritonavir, indinavir) are added depending on drug–drug interactions, drug tolerance, and patient compliance. **Prophylaxis** for *Pneumocystis carinii* pneumonia and toxoplasmosis (TMP-SMX) is started in patients with CD4 counts < 200. Prophylaxis for MAC (clarithromycin or azithromycin) is started in patients with CD4 counts < 100. Opportunistic infections are treated as they arise (Table 2.9–3).

TABLE 2.9–3. Opportunistic Infections in HIV.

Disease	Treatment
CMV	Ganciclovir, foscarnet
Esophageal candidiasis	Fluconazole, ketoconazole
Cryptococcal meningitis	Amphotericin B, fluconazole
HSV	Acyclovir, foscarnet
Herpes zoster	Acyclovir, foscarnet
Kaposi's sarcoma	Cutaneous—observation, intralesional vinblastine; severe cutaneous—systemic chemotherapy, alpha-interferon, radiation; visceral disease—combination chemotherapy
Lymphoma	Combination chemotherapy, radiation therapy with dexamethasone (if CNS lymphoma)
MAC	Clarithromycin, azithromycin, ethambutol, rifabutin
Mycobacterium tuberculosis	Multiagent therapy (INH, rifampin, pyrazinamide, ethambutol, streptomycin)
Pneumocystis carinii pneumonia	TMP-SMX ± steroids, atovaquone, pentamidine
Toxoplasmosis	Pyrimethamine, sulfadiazine, clindamycin

IM2.5

Syphilis is caused by *Treponema pallidum*, a spirochete.

History/PE

- **Primary** (10–60 days after infection): **Painless ulcer (chancre)** found on or near the area of contact (Figure 2.9–1). The lesion often goes unnoticed and heals spontaneously in 3–9 weeks.
- **Secondary** (4–8 weeks after appearance of chancre): Low-grade **fever,**

headache, malaise, anorexia, and generalized **lymphadenopathy; diffuse, symmetric, asymptomatic maculopapular rash on soles and palms.** Highly infective secondary eruptions (mucous patches) can coalesce, forming condylomata lata; lesions heal spontaneously in 2–6 weeks.

- **Early latent:** No symptoms, positive serology, first year of infection.
- **Late latent:** No symptoms, positive or negative serology, > 1 year of infection. One-third will progress to tertiary syphilis.
- **Tertiary** (1–20 years after initial infection): Destructive, granulomatous **gummas** can severely damage the CNS, heart, and great vessels (notably the aorta). Neurologic findings include **tabes dorsalis** (posterior column degeneration) and **Argyll–Robertson pupil** (small, irregular pupil that reacts to accommodation but not to light).

Evaluation

Evaluation (see Table 2.9–4) consists of **dark-field microscopy** (motile spirochetes) of primary or secondary lesions, **VDRL/RPR** (a rapid, nonspecific screening test), and **FTA-ABS/MHA-TP** (specific, diagnostic).

Treatment may induce a Jarisch–Herxheimer reaction with fever and flulike symptoms due to massive destruction of spirochetes.

TABLE 2.9–4. Diagnostic Test for Syphilis.

Test	Comments
Dark-field microscopy	Identifies motile spirochetes (only on primary or secondary lesions).
VDRL/RPR	Rapid, cheap, but sensitivity only 60–75% in primary disease; nonspecific. Reverts to negative with treatment.
FTA-ABS	Sensitive, specific. Used as a secondary, diagnostic test. Positive for life.

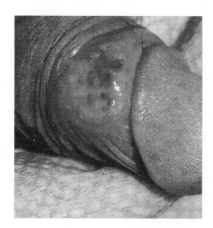

FIGURE 2.9–1. Primary syphilis. The chancre, which appears at the site of infection, is an ulcerated papule with a smooth, clean base; raised, indurated borders; and scant discharge.

HIGH-YIELD FACTS

Infectious Disease

Treatment

Treat with **penicillin.** Tetracycline or doxycycline can be used in patients with penicillin allergies.

A temperature that exceeds 38.3°C for at least three weeks' duration and remains undiagnosed after one week of intensive evaluation. In adults, **infections** and **cancer** account for > 60% of cases of FUO, while **autoimmune diseases** account for approximately 15%. Causes of FUO include:

- **Infectious: TB** and **endocarditis** (e.g., HACEK organisms) are the most common systemic infections causing FUO, while **occult abscess** is the most common localized infection.
- **Neoplastic: Leukemias** and **lymphomas** are the most common neoplasms causing FUO, while **hepatic and renal cell carcinomas** are the most common solid tumors.
- **Autoimmune:** Still's disease, SLE, temporal arteritis, and polyarteritis nodosa are the most common autoimmune disorders giving rise to FUO, but many rheumatologic/autoimmune diseases can cause FUO.
- **Miscellaneous**: This category includes sarcoidosis, Whipple's disease, recurrent pulmonary emboli, alcoholic hepatitis, drug fever, and factitious fever.
- **Undiagnosed** (10–15%).

Evaluation

Asymptomatic patients with FUO do not require empiric antibiotic therapy.

Evaluation should include serial physical exams, CBC with differential, ESR, and multiple blood cultures. CT and MRI scans should be done if malignancy or occult abscess is suspected. Specific tests (ANA, RF, viral cultures, viral/fungal antibody/antigen tests) can be obtained if an infectious or autoimmune etiology is suspected.

Treatment

Treat the underlying disorder. Severely ill patients are usually started empirically on broad-spectrum antibiotics until the precise etiology has been determined. However, antibiotics should be stopped if there is no response.

MENINGITIS

UCV *Neuro.4, 5, Ped.43*

Infection of the leptomeninges caused by viruses, bacteria, or fungi. Risk factors include recent ear infection, sinusitis, immune deficiencies, recent neurosurgical procedures, and sick contacts.

HIGH-YIELD FACTS

Infectious Disease

History/PE

Patients present with **fever,** malaise, **headache, neck stiffness, photophobia,** altered mental status, or seizures. Signs of meningeal irritation (Kernig and Brudzinski) are often absent in infants < 2 years of age.

Children < 2 years of age may not manifest meningeal signs.

Differential

Brain abscess, subdural empyema, mastoiditis, tumors, cysts, lead encephalopathy, trauma, vasculitis.

Evaluation

A high degree of clinical suspicion is required in children < 2 years of age owing to the possible absence of specific meningeal signs. Evaluation should include **LP** (if no papilledema or focal neurologic deficits) and possibly **CT or MRI** to rule out other diagnoses. CBC may reveal leukocytosis. CSF findings vary (see Table 2.9–5).

Check for papilledema or focal neurologic deficits before performing an LP!

Treatment

Treat with **antibiotics** (for bacterial infection) and **supportive care.** Viral disease can be treated with supportive care and close follow-up (except herpes meningoencephalitis; treat with acyclovir). The initial choice of antimicrobial agent is based on the most likely organisms involved given the patient's age (Table 2.9–6). Contacts of patients with meningococcal meningitis should receive rifampin prophylaxis.

Complications

- **Hyponatremia:** Administer fluids and monitor sodium concentration.
- **Seizures:** Treat with benzodiazepines and phenytoin.
- **Subdural effusions:** May be seen on CT scan. Occur in 50% of infants with *H. influenzae* meningitis. No treatment is necessary.
- **Cerebral edema:** Presents with loss of oculocephalic reflex. Treat with IV mannitol.
- **Subdural empyema:** Presents as intractable seizures. Requires surgical evacuation.

TABLE 2.9–5. CSF Findings in Meningitis.

Etiology	CSF Findings
Bacterial	Pressure↑, polys↑↑, protein↑, glucose ↓
Viral	Pressure normal/↑, lymphs↑, protein normal/↑, glucose normal
TB/fungal	Pressure↑, lymphs↑, protein↑, glucose ↓

TABLE 2.9–6. Treatment of Meningitis.

Age	Causative Organism	Treatment
< 1 month	Group B strep, *E. coli*, *Listeria*	Cefotaxime + ampicillin
1–3 months	Pneumococci, meningococci, *H. influenzae*	Cefotaxime + vancomycin ± steroids
3 months – 7 years	*H. influenzae*, meningococci	Ceftriaxone ± vancomycin ± steroids
7–50 years	Pneumococci, meningococci, *Listeria*	Ceftriaxone ± vancomycin ± steroids
> 50 years/alcoholism/chronic illness	Coliforms, *H. influenzae*, *Listeria*, *Pseudomonas*, meningococci	Ceftriaxone + ampicillin ± steroids

- **Brain abscess:** Requires surgical drainage.
- **Ventriculitis:** Presents as worsening clinical picture with improved CSF findings. Requires ventriculostomy and possibly intraventricular antibiotics.

OTITIS EXTERNA

UCV *EM.11*

Also known as "swimmer's ear," otitis externa is an inflammation of the skin lining the ear canal and surrounding soft tissue. *Pseudomonas* (from poorly chlorinated pools) and enterobacteriaceae are the most common etiologic agents. Both grow in the presence of excess moisture.

History

Pain, pruritus, and a **purulent discharge** from the ear canal.

PE

Pain with movement of the tragus/pinna, an edematous and erythematous ear canal, and purulent discharge.

Treatment

Eardrops with polymyxin B, neomycin, and hydrocortisone usually suffice. Use **dicloxacillin** for acute disease. **Diabetics** are at risk for malignant otitis externa and osteomyelitis of the skull base and thus require hospitalization and **IV antibiotics.**

Otitis media should not cause pain with movement of the tragus/pinna.

Includes cystitis, pyelonephritis, and urosepsis. UTIs affect women more frequently than men, and positive *E. coli* cultures are obtained in 80% of cases. Other pathogens include *Staphylococcus saprophyticus*, *Klebsiella*, *Proteus*, and *Enterococcus*. Risk factors include use of a **Foley catheter** or other urologic instrumentation, anatomic abnormalities (e.g., BPH, vesicoureteral reflux), a history of previous UTIs or acute pyelonephritis, **diabetes mellitus,** recent antibiotic use, immunosuppression, and **pregnancy.**

History/PE

Patients complain of **urinary frequency, dysuria,** and **urgency.** Acute pyelonephritis may present with nausea, vomiting, **fever,** and **back/flank pain.** Children often present with **bedwetting,** and infants can present with poor feeding, recurrent febrile episodes, and foul-smelling urine.

Urosepsis must be considered in any elderly patient with altered mental status.

Evaluation

Urine dipstick may reveal **increased leukocyte esterase** (75% sensitive for WBCs), **elevated nitrites** (low sensitivity; false positives with bacterial contamination), elevated urine pH (characteristic of *Proteus* infections), or hematuria (seen with cystitis). Microscopic analysis may show > **5 leukocytes/hpf** (indicative of GU infection) and a bacterial pathogen. WBC casts on UA indicate acute pyelonephritis. The gold standard is a clean-catch urine culture with > 10^5 **bacteria/mL** (diagnosis is often made on the basis of dipstick alone).

UTI bugs—

SEEKS PP
S. saprophyticus
E. coli
Enterobacter
Klebsiella
Serratia

Proteus
Pseudomonas

Treatment

Treat healthy young females on an outpatient basis with oral **TMP-SMX** or **ciprofloxacin** for three days. Elderly patients, those with comorbid diseases, or those with acute toxicity in the setting of acute pyelonephritis should be hospitalized and treated with **IV antibiotics** (ciprofloxacin or ampicillin and gentamicin to cover enterococcus). **Prophylactic antibiotics** may be given to those with recurrent UTIs.

LYME DISEASE   **UCV** *Ped.28*

A tick-borne disease caused by the spirochete *Borrelia burgdorferi*. Lyme disease is usually seen during the summer months and is carried by *Ixodes* ticks; it is endemic to the Northeast, northern Midwest, and Pacific coast. It is the most common vector-borne disease in North America.

HIGH-YIELD FACTS

Infectious Disease

History

Fever, malaise, and rash are characteristic of primary Lyme disease.

Lyme disease is the most common vector-borne disease in North America.

PE

Erythema migrans begins as a small erythematous macule or papule **found at the tick-feeding site** and expands slowly over days to weeks. The border may be macular or raised, and **central clearing** is often present ("bull's eye"). Median lesion width is 15 cm. Primary Lyme disease may be followed by secondary Lyme disease, which is characterized by **arthralgias, migratory polyarthropathies,** neurologic phenomena (e.g., **Bell's palsy**), meningitis, and/or **myocarditis** (presents as conduction abnormalities). Tertiary Lyme disease is characterized by arthritis and subacute encephalitis (memory loss and mood change).

Differential

- **Early:** Viral exanthem.
- **Later:** Collagen vascular disease, chronic fatigue syndrome, other causes of neuropathies, encephalitis, aseptic meningitis, myocarditis.

Evaluation

A positive ELISA indicates exposure but does not indicate active Lyme disease.

Diagnosis is based on clinical and laboratory findings (ELISA and Western blot). Use Western blot to confirm a positive or indeterminate ELISA. A positive ELISA denotes **exposure** and is not specific for active disease (culture/molecular tests are currently under development).

Treatment

Treat with **doxycycline** or **ceftriaxone.** Consider empiric therapy for patients with characteristic rash, arthralgias, or a tick bite acquired in an endemic area.

ROCKY MOUNTAIN SPOTTED FEVER   UCV *Ped.33*

The rash of Rocky Mountain spotted fever begins on the palms and soles and spreads centrally.

A tick-borne rickettsial disease caused by *Rickettsia rickettsii*, Rocky Mountain spotted fever is carried by the *Dermacentor* tick and is endemic to the **East Coast.** The organism invades the endothelial lining of capillaries and leads to **small vessel vasculitis.**

History

Patients present with **headache, fever,** malaise, and a **rash beginning on the palms and soles.**

PE

The rash characteristic of Rocky Mountain spotted fever is initially macular (beginning on the **palms** and **soles**) but becomes petechial/purpuric as it spreads centrally. Altered mental status or DIC may develop in severe cases.

Differential

Meningococcemia, Lyme disease, endocarditis, hemorrhagic fevers (Ebola, Hanta), vasculitis, other rickettsial diseases (e.g., ehrlichiosis).

Evaluation

This is a **clinical diagnosis** that is confirmed retrospectively with acute and convalescent antibody titers utilizing complement fixation or the Weil–Felix test (antigen cross-reactivity with *Proteus* antigens).

Treatment

Treat with **doxycycline;** use chloramphenicol in children and pregnant women. The condition can be rapidly fatal if left untreated.

CONGENITAL INFECTIONS

UCV OB.37, Ped.23, 24

Infections that may occur at any time during pregnancy, labor, and delivery and that can have severe consequences after birth. Common sequelae include premature delivery, CNS abnormalities, anemia, jaundice, hepatosplenomegaly, and growth retardation. The most common pathogens can be remembered by the mnemonic **TORCHeS:**

- **T**oxoplasmosis: Transplacental transmission from mom, with primary infection via consumption of **raw meat** or contact with **cat feces.** Specific findings include hydrocephalus, **intracranial calcifications,** and **ring-enhancing lesions** on head CT.
- **O**ther: **HIV,** parvovirus, varicella, *Listeria*, TB, malaria, fungi.
- **R**ubella: Transplacental transmission in the first trimester. Specific findings include a purpuric **"blueberry muffin" rash,** cataracts, hearing loss, and PDA.
- **C**MV (cytomegalovirus): The **most common congenital infection,** primarily transmitted transplacentally. Specific findings include petechial rash (similar to blueberry muffin rash) and **periventricular calcifications.**
- **H**erpes: Intrapartum transmission if mom has **active lesions.** Specific findings include skin, eye, and mouth **vesicles.** Can progress to life-threatening CNS/systemic infection.
- **S**yphilis: Primarily intrapartum transmission. Specific findings include **maculopapular skin rash,** lymphadenopathy, hepatomegaly, **"snuffles"**

The maternal-fetal transmission rate of HIV drops from 25% to 8% if the mother receives AZT during pregnancy.

(mucopurulent rhinitis), and osteitis. In childhood, late congenital syphilis is characterized by Hutchinson's triad: **peg-shaped upper central incisors, deafness,** and **interstitial keratitis** (photophobia, lacrimation).

Evaluation

Evaluation should include **serologic testing** for rubella, toxoplasmosis, and herpes. Perform urine culture for CMV and dark-field examination of skin lesions/maternal serology for syphilis. Other tests include viral isolation, amniocentesis, and antigen detection. All ill newborns require blood cultures and lumbar puncture.

Treatment

- **Toxoplasmosis:** Pyrimethamine, sulfadiazine, spiramycin.
- **Syphilis:** Penicillin.
- **HSV:** Acyclovir.
- **CMV:** Ganciclovir.

Prevention

- **Toxoplasmosis:** Avoid exposure to cats during pregnancy; treat women with primary infection with pyrimethamine and sulfadiazene.
- **Rubella:** Immunize before pregnancy; otherwise, consider abortion. Vaccinate the mother after delivery if titers remain negative.
- **Syphilis:** Penicillin in pregnant women.
- **CMV:** Avoid exposure.
- **HSV:** Perform a **C-section** if lesions are present at delivery.
- **HIV:** AZT in pregnant women with HIV.

Pregnant women should not change the cat's litterbox.

Musculoskeletal

OSTEOMYELITIS

UCV Surg.44

Bone infection secondary to **direct spread** from a soft tissue infection (80% of cases) or to **hematogenous seeding** (20% of cases). Osteomyelitis secondary to local soft tissue infection is seen in patients with peripheral vascular disease, diabetes (chronic foot ulcers), and penetrating soft tissue injuries. Hematogenous osteomyelitis is most commonly found in children (affecting the metaphyses of the long bones) and IV drug users (affecting the vertebral bodies). **Acute osteomyelitis** is osteomyelitis without a previous bone infection at that site. **Chronic osteomyelitis** occurs when acute osteomyelitis goes untreated or when treatment fails (recurrent infection). Common pathogens responsible for osteomyelitis are listed in Table 2.10–1.

Osteomyelitis is associated with IV drug use, diabetes, peripheral vascular disease, and penetrating soft tissue injuries.

History

Patients present with **fever** and **localized bone pain.**

PE

Localized warmth, tenderness, swelling, erythema, and limited motion of the adjacent joint.

TABLE 2.10–1. Pathogens in Osteomyelitis.	
If	**Think**
Most people	*S. aureus*
IV drug use	*S. aureus* or *E. coli*
Sickle cell disease	*Salmonella*
Hip replacement	*S. epidermidis*
Foot puncture wound	*Pseudomonas*
Chronic	*S. aureus, Pseudomonas,* Enterobacteriaceae

Differential

Cellulitis, soft tissue infection, septic arthritis, rheumatic fever, gout, Ewing's sarcoma, osteoarthritis.

Evaluation

Radiographs are often negative in early osteomyelitis.

WBC count, **ESR,** and **C-reactive protein** levels are **usually elevated.** Blood cultures may be positive. Radiographs are often negative on acute presentation; however, radiographic findings **(periosteal elevation)** may be seen 10–14 days later. **Bone scans** are sensitive for osteomyelitis but lack specificity; **indium-labeled leukocyte scanning** is more specific. MRI will show increased signal in the bone marrow consistent with bone marrow edema and may also reveal associated soft tissue infection. Definitive diagnosis is made by **bone aspiration** (Gram stain and culture).

Treatment

Treat with **IV antibiotics** for 4–6 weeks and **surgical debridement** of necrotic, infected bone. Empiric antibiotic selection is based on the suspected organism and Gram stain. Consider oxacillin, nafcillin, a cephalosporin, or vancomycin if *S. aureus* is suspected. Empiric gram-negative coverage includes a third-generation cephalosporin, gentamicin, or ciprofloxacin.

Complications

Chronic osteomyelitis, systemic sepsis, soft tissue infection, septic arthritis. Long-standing chronic osteomyelitis with a draining sinus tract may eventually lead to **squamous cell carcinoma.**

OSTEOPOROSIS

Obesity is protective against osteoporosis.

A common metabolic bone disease characterized by **osteopenia with normal bone mineralization.** Osteoporosis most often affects **thin, Caucasian, postmenopausal women.** Bone mass peaks at age 30–35 and then progressively declines. **Smoking** and long-term administration of heparin and glucocorticoids are associated with an increased risk of osteoporosis.

History/PE

Commonly asymptomatic. Patients often present with **hip fractures, vertebral compression fractures,** or **distal radius fractures** after minimal trauma. Loss of height may result from progressive thoracic kyphosis secondary to multiple vertebral compression fractures.

Differential

Osteomalacia, hyperparathyroidism, multiple myeloma, metastatic carcinoma (pathologic fracture).

Evaluation

Laboratory tests are normal; radiographs show global demineralization after > 30% of bone density is lost. Dual-energy x-ray absorptiometry (DEXA) scanning may show significant osteopenia, most commonly in the vertebral bodies, proximal femur, and distal radius.

Laboratory tests are all normal in osteoporosis, and radiographic changes are apparent only after significant osteopenia has developed.

Treatment

Prevention is key; **hormone replacement therapy (HRT)** is the most effective means of preventing bone loss in perimenopausal women. **Calcium supplementation with vitamin D** should be taken throughout adulthood to maintain bone density. **Smoking cessation** and weight-bearing exercises help maintain bone density, while **alendronate** and intranasal calcitonin can increase bone density.

Complications

Fractures of the proximal femur, distal radius, and vertebrae.

SYSTEMIC LUPUS ERYTHEMATOSUS (SLE)   UCV *IM2.56*

A multisystem autoimmune disorder that most frequently affects women (90%), especially **black women.** Its pathogenesis is related to antibody-mediated cellular attack and to the deposition of antigen-antibody complexes. Drugs, including hydralazine and procainamide, may produce a lupus-like syndrome that resolves when the drug is discontinued.

History

Fever, anorexia, weight loss, **joint pain, photosensitivity,** and oral ulcers.

PE

Malar rash, joint tenderness and inflammation, pericarditis, pleuritis, and neurologic, renal, and hematologic abnormalities (Figure 2.10–1).

Differential

RA and other vasculitic diseases.

Criteria for SLE—

4 RASHNIA
4 rashes
- Malar rash
- Discoid rash
- Photosensitivity
- Oral ulcers

Renal—proteinuria
Arthritis
Serositis
Hematologic—
  hemolytic anemia, leukopenia, thrombocytopenia
Neurologic—
  psychosis, seizures
Immunologic—anti-dsDNA, anti-SmAb, false positive VDRL
ANA

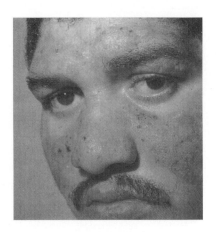

FIGURE 2.10–1. SLE. The malar rash is a red to purple continuous plaque extending across the bridge of the nose and to both cheeks.

Evaluation

A positive ANA is sensitive but not specific. **Anti-DNA** and **anti-SM antibodies** are very specific but not as sensitive.

Treatment

Treat with **NSAIDs** initially. **Steroids** are used for **acute exacerbations.** Steroids, hydroxychloroquine, cyclophosphamide, and azathioprine are used in progressive or refractory cases. Patients should **avoid sun exposure.**

Complications

Progressive impairment of the lung, heart, brain, or kidneys; opportunistic infections.

RHEUMATOID ARTHRITIS (RA)
UCV IM2.55

A chronic, destructive, systemic inflammatory arthritis characterized by **symmetric** involvement of both large and small joints. RA causes synovial hypertrophy and pannus formation with resultant erosion of adjacent cartilage, bone, and tendons. It is most common in **females 20–40 years old.** There is a high incidence in patients with the HLA-DR4 serotype.

History

Insidious onset of **morning stiffness, pain, warmth,** boggy swelling, and decreased mobility that affects numerous joints (polyarthropathy) and is associated with fatigue, **malaise,** anorexia, and weight loss.

PE

The most commonly involved joints are the **wrists, metacarpophalangeal (MCP)** and **proximal interphalangeal (PIP) joints,** ankles, knees, shoulders, hips, elbows, and cervical spine. Ulnar deviation of the fingers with MCP joint hypertrophy is a common finding in RA (Figure 2.10–2). Extra-articular manifestations include **subcutaneous nodules,** vasculitis, and carpal tunnel syndrome.

Distal interphalangeal (DIP) joints are spared in RA.

Differential

Seronegative spondyloarthropathies (e.g., ankylosing spondylitis, Reiter's syndrome) (IM2.48, 54), psoriatic arthritis (DIP joint involvement), SLE, osteoarthritis, gout, chronic Lyme disease, polymyalgia rheumatica.

Evaluation

Rheumatoid factor (anti-F_c IgG antibody) is elevated in > 75% of cases but is not specific for RA. ESR is also elevated. Synovial fluid aspiration reveals slightly turbid fluid with decreased viscosity and a WBC count of 3000–50,000. Early in the course of the disease, radiographs show soft tissue swelling and juxta-articular demineralization. Later findings include joint space narrowing and erosions.

Treatment

Treat with **NSAIDs.** Severe cases are treated with corticosteroids, methotrexate, hydroxychloroquine sulfate, gold, and azathioprine. Be aware of the potential complications associated with NSAIDs, corticosteroids, and other therapies for this disease. Operative therapy may be necessary in advanced cases.

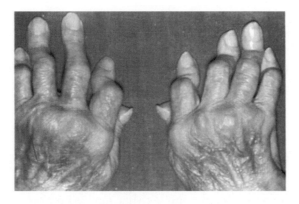

FIGURE 2.10–2. Rheumatoid arthritis. Note the swan-neck deformities of the digits, ulnar deviation of the fingers, MCP joint hypertrophy, and severe involvement of the proximal interphalangeal joints.

A chronic, noninflammatory arthritis of movable joints that is also known as degenerative joint disease (DJD). OA has **no systemic manifestations** and is characterized by deterioration of the articular cartilage and osteophyte formation at joint surfaces. Risk factors for OA include family history, **obesity,** and previous joint trauma (particularly previous intra-articular fractures).

History

OA typically has an asymmetric pattern.

Joint pain, crepitus, decreased range of motion of the affected joint, insidious onset of joint stiffness and pain that is **worsened by activity and weight bearing and relieved by rest.**

PE

Nodes in OA—

"HO DIP and BO PIP"
Heberden's nodes = **DIP**
Bouchard's nodes = **PIP**

OA most commonly involves the **weight-bearing joints** (hip, knee, and lumbar spine) but may also involve the DIP joints **(Heberden's nodes),** PIP joints **(Bouchard's nodes),** metatarsophalangeal joint of the big toe, and cervical spine. Physical examination usually reveals stiffness and marked **crepitus** of the affected joint.

Differential

RA, seronegative spondyloarthropathies, psoriatic arthritis (DIP joints), pseudogout, gouty arthritis, neuropathic joint.

Evaluation

The ESR is normal in osteoarthritis.

Laboratory values are normal. Radiographs show irregular **joint space narrowing,** osteophytes, and dense subchondral bone. ESR is normal. Synovial fluid aspiration reveals straw-colored, normal-viscosity fluid with a WBC count < 3000.

Treatment

Treat mild cases with **physical therapy, weight reduction,** and **NSAIDs.** Intra-articular corticosteroid injection may also provide temporary relief of symptoms. **Elective joint replacement** (e.g., total hip/knee arthroplasty) may be necessary when symptoms significantly interfere with activities of daily living.

An exceedingly common pain complex that may arise from paraspinous muscles, ligaments, facet joints, or disk or nerve roots. Strains refer to muscular injuries, whereas sprains refer to ligamentous injuries.

HIGH-YIELD FACTS

Musculoskeletal

History/PE

Low back pain is associated with the following manifestations and conditions:

- Paraspinous muscular pain/spasm suggest a back sprain.
- Pain radiating to the posterior thigh and exacerbated by coughing or straining implies a herniated disk with root impingement.
- **Positive straight leg raise** favors nerve **root impingement** most commonly due to a herniated disk (see Table 2.10–2).
- Pain with walking or prolonged standing (**pseudoclaudication**) and hyperextension suggests **spinal stenosis.**
- Pain that worsens with rest and improves with activity is typical of ankylosing spondylitis.
- Pain that worsens at night and is unrelieved by rest or positional changes suggests malignancy.
- Point tenderness over a particular vertebral body suggests vertebral osteomyelitis, fracture, or malignancy.
- **Bowel or bladder dysfunction** and **saddle area anesthesia** is consistent with **cauda equina syndrome.**

Differential

Herniation, strain, sprain, degenerative arthritis. Rule out infection, cancer, cauda equina syndrome, ankylosing spondylitis, and aortic aneurysm.

Cauda equina syndrome is a surgical emergency.

Evaluation

Diagnosis is primarily **clinical.** X-rays may reveal evidence of osteomyelitis, cancer (pathologic vertebral fractures, punched-out or sclerotic lesions), fractures, or ankylosing spondylitis. MRI/CT/bone scans are used to evaluate persistent radiculopathy or myelopathy (Figure 2.10–3).

TABLE 2.10–2. Motor and Sensory Deficit in Back Pain.

Root	Associated Deficits
L4	Motor: Foot dorsiflexion (tibialis anterior). Reflex: Patellar. Sensory: Medial aspect of the leg.
L5	Motor: Big toe dorsiflexion (extensor hallucis longus). Reflex: None. Sensory: Medial forefoot and lateral aspect of the leg.
S1	Motor: Foot eversion (peroneus longus/brevis). Reflex: Achilles. Sensory: Lateral foot.

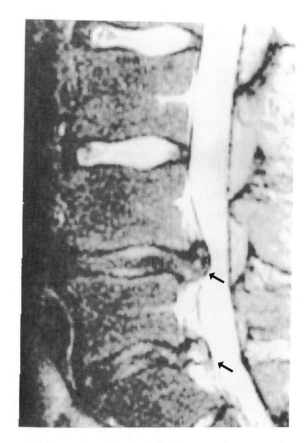

FIGURE 2.10–3. Disk herniation. MRI reveals herniations of L4–L5 and L5–S1 (arrows).

Treatment

The majority of patients with low back pain recover spontaneously in 3–4 weeks.

For sprains and strains, **NSAIDs** and continuation of ordinary activities as tolerated are recommended. **Rest for more than 1–3 days is considered unnecessary.** Ninety percent of patients recover spontaneously within 3–4 weeks. Surgery (laminectomy, discectomy) is indicated for patients with correctable spinal disease. Cauda equina syndrome is a surgical emergency requiring immediate decompression with laminectomy.

GOUT

UCV IM2.50

A metabolic condition causing recurrent attacks of **acute monoarticular arthritis.** Gout results from the intra-articular deposition of monosodium urate crystals and is especially common in **men** (90%) and Pacific Islanders. Most patients have hyperuricemia secondary to uric acid underexcretion. Other causes include Lesch–Nyhan syndrome, diuretic use, cyclosporin use, malignancies, and hemoglobinopathies.

History

The patient is typically awakened from sleep with excruciating joint pain.

PE

Gout most commonly affects the **first metatarsophalangeal joint** (podagra), midfoot, knees, ankles, and wrists and spares the hips and shoulders. Joints are erythematous, swollen, and exquisitely tender. Patients with long-standing disease may develop **tophi,** deposits of urate crystals that lead to deformed joints.

Differential

Pseudogout, cellulitis, septic joint, trauma, foreign body synovitis, avascular necrosis, malignancy.

Evaluation

Joint fluid aspiration may reveal **needle-shaped, negatively birefringent** (yellow when parallel to the condenser) **crystals** and elevated WBC. In many cases, serum uric acid > 7.5, but some patients have normal uric acid levels. Radiographs show no changes in early gout. Characteristic punched-out erosions with overhanging cortical bone ("rat bite") are seen in more advanced gout.

The presence of gout crystals on joint fluid aspiration confirms the diagnosis.

Treatment

Administer **NSAIDs** or **steroids** for **acute** attacks. **Colchicine, allopurinol,** and **probenecid** can be given for **maintenance** therapy. Avoid use of thiazide/loop diuretics (worsen hyperuricemia). The most frequent adverse effect of allopurinol is the precipitation of an acute gouty attack.

Allopurinol is contraindicated in acute attacks.

PSEUDOGOUT

A metabolic disease characterized by recurrent attacks of **acute monoarticular arthritis.** Pseudogout results from the deposition of calcium pyrophosphate crystals within the joint space and most commonly affects patients > 60 years of age. Risk factors include previous joint trauma, hemochromatosis, diabetes, hyperparathyroidism, hypothyroidism, and gout.

History

Joint tenderness, erythema, and warmth.

PE

The **knee** and **wrist** are most commonly involved. Pseudogout is often less severe than gout.

Differential

See "Gout."

Evaluation

Joint aspirate reveals **rhomboid-shaped crystals** that are **positively birefringent.** X-rays often show calcification of adjacent cartilaginous structures (chondrocalcinosis) as well as degenerative changes.

Treatment

Treat with **NSAIDs** or **intra-articular steroids** for acute attacks. **Colchicine** is used for prophylaxis.

PAGET'S DISEASE (OSTEITIS DEFORMANS)

A poorly characterized disease with excessive bone turnover. Paget's disease is frequently associated with paramyxovirus infection.

History/PE

The condition is often asymptomatic, although patients may complain of deep bone pain. Bone softening results in tibial bowing, kyphosis, and frequent fractures. It is also associated with an increase in cranial diameter (frontal bossing). Deafness may occur in advanced cases.

Differential

Osteogenic sarcoma, multiple myeloma, fibrous dysplasia, metastatic carcinoma.

Evaluation

Alkaline phosphatase and urinary hydroxyproline are elevated. Serum Ca^{2+} and phosphate are normal. X-rays show a **markedly expanded bony cortex** of increased density, thickened bony trabeculae, and bowing of the long bones (Figure 2.10–4).

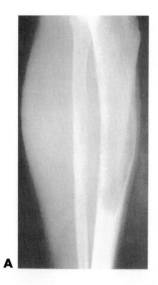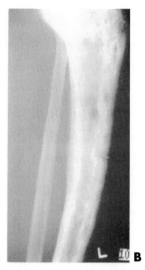

FIGURE 2.10–4. Pagets disease. (A) 45 years old. There are lytic changes in the proximal tibia associated with bulging of the anterior cortex. (B) 65 years old. There is increased cortical density of the tibia in this x-ray taken 20 years later.

Treatment

Treat symptomatic patients with **alendronate.** Calcitonin is used in some cases.

Complications

Fractures, vertebral collapse leading to spinal cord compression, high-output cardiac failure, arthritis, deafness, **osteosarcoma.**

POLYMYALGIA RHEUMATICA (PMR)

A rheumatologic disorder most commonly seen in **elderly females.** Polymyalgia rheumatica is considered to be part of the same spectrum of diseases as **temporal arteritis** (same HLA haplotypes), and the two frequently coexist.

PMR is rarely seen in patients < 55.

History

Pain and stiffness of the shoulder and pelvic girdle area, often associated with **fever,** malaise, weight loss, and minimal joint swelling. Patients classically have great difficulty getting out of a chair or lifting their arms above their heads.

PE

Although patients often complain of leg and shoulder weakness, weakness is not appreciated on physical exam.

Always rule out tempo-
ral arteritis in patients
with PMR.

Differential

Multiple myeloma, malignancy, chronic infection, temporal arteritis.

Evaluation

Evaluation is primarily clinical. **Anemia** and markedly **elevated ESR** are almost always present.

Treatment

Low-dose prednisone (5–20 mg/day) works in almost all cases.

COMMON ADULT ORTHOPEDIC INJURIES

Table 2.10–3 summarizes the major adult orthopedic injuries.

TABLE 2.10–3. Common Adult Orthopedic Injuries.

Injury	Mechanics	Treatment
Shoulder dislocation *Surg.45*	Most commonly anteriorly dislocated. Axillary artery and nerve are at risk for injury. Posterior shoulder dislocations are associated with seizures and electrical shocks.	Closed reduction followed by sling and swathe.
Hip dislocation *Surg.39*	Most commonly posteriorly dislocated, via a posteriorly directed force on **internally rotated, flexed,** adducted hip ("dashboard injury").	Closed reduction followed by abduction pillow/bracing.
Colles' fracture *Surg.37*	Most common wrist fracture. Involves the distal radius and commonly results from a **fall onto an outstretched hand,** resulting in a dorsally displaced, dorsally angulated fracture. Commonly seen in the **elderly** (osteoporosis) as well as in children.	Closed reduction followed by application of long arm cast.
Scaphoid (carpal navicular) fracture	**Most commonly fractured** carpal bone. May take 1–2 weeks for radiographs to show the fracture; thus, a high index of suspicion is necessary. Assume there is a fracture if there is **tenderness in the anatomical snuff box.**	Short arm thumb spica cast. With proximal third scaphoid fractures, **avascular necrosis** may result from disruption of blood flow (vessel enters at the distal portion of the bone).

..

TABLE 2.10–3 (continued). Common Adult Orthopedic Injuries.

Injury	Mechanics	Treatment
Boxer's fracture	Fracture of the fifth metacarpal neck. Often results from forward trauma of **closed fist** (e.g., punching a wall, an individual's jaw, or another fixed object).	Closed reduction and ulnar gutter splint. Percutaneous pinning if fracture angulation is excessive. If skin is broken, assume infection by human oral pathogens **("fight bite"),** and treat with surgical irrigation, debridement, and IV antibiotics.
Humerus fracture	Direct trauma, radial nerve at risk (travels in spiral groove of the humerus). Signs of radial nerve palsy include wrist drop and loss of thumb abduction.	Hanging arm cast vs. coaptation splint and sling. Functional bracing.
Monteggia's fracture	Dislocation of the radial head with diaphyseal fracture of the ulna. Also known as **"nightstick fracture"** (self-defense with arm against a blunt instrument).	Closed reduction of the radial head and open reduction/internal fixation (ORIF) of the ulna.
Galeazzi's fracture	Dislocation of the distal radioulnar joint with fracture of the diaphysis of the radius.	ORIF of the radius with casting of the forearm in supination to reduce the distal radioulnar joint.
Hip fracture	Falls, common in **osteoporotic women.** Patients are **at risk for subsequent DVT.** Patients present with the affected leg **shortened** and **externally rotated.** Displaced femoral neck fractures are associated with a high risk of avascular necrosis and fracture nonunion.	ORIF with parallel pinning of the femoral neck. Displaced fractures in elderly patients (> 80 years old) may require hemiarthroplasty. **Anticoagulate** to prevent DVT.
Femur fracture	Direct trauma (motor vehicle accident). Beware of fat emboli syndrome (presents with fever, scleral petechiae, confusion, dyspnea, and hypoxia).	Intramedullary nailing of the femur. Open fractures also require thorough irrigation and debridement.
Tibial fracture	Direct trauma (car + pedestrian bumper injury).	Casting vs. intramedullary nailing. Be aware of **compartment syndrome** (swelling in a confined space causes pain on passive extension of the toes, sensory/motor deficits, etc.).
Ankle fracture	Supination/external rotation injury resulting in fractures of medial and lateral malleoli.	ORIF.

Surg.41

HIGH-YIELD FACTS

Musculoskeletal

SALTER–Harris Classification:
I **S**ideways
II **A**bove
III **L**ower
IV **T**hrough (epiphyseal plate)
V **ER** (**E**verything's **R**uined!)

Growth plate injuries in children are commonly classified by the Salter–Harris system (see Figure 2.10–5).

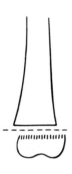 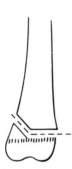 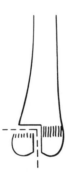 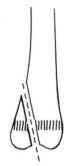 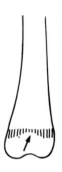

I. Through growth plate

II. Through metaphysis and growth plate

III. Through growth plate and epiphysis into joint

IV. Through metaphysis, growth plate, and epiphysis into joint

V. Crush of growth plate. May not be seen on x-ray

FIGURE 2.10–5. Salter–Harris classification of growth plate injuries.

Neurology

HEADACHE

Approach

- Note whether the headache is new or old. Recent-onset, severe headaches (such as headaches that awaken the patient in the middle of the night) warrant immediate workup (for SAH, tumor, temporal arteritis, meningitis, etc.).
- An old headache also requires prompt evaluation if there has been a change in character or intensity.

Note the **characteristics** of the headache (temporal relationship, location) and look for **associated symptoms** (jaw claudication, fever, nausea, vomiting, weight loss) and **neurologic symptoms** (paresthesias, numbness, ataxia, visual disturbances, photophobia, neck stiffness). Focal neurologic defects or papilledema warrants immediate workup.

"New" headaches warrant immediate workup.

Additional Studies

Obtain CBC, ESR, and CT/MRI in patients suspected of having SAH or elevated ICP, or if a patient has **focal neurologic findings.** CT without contrast is the preferred study for an acute hemorrhage.

CT without contrast is the preferred study for an acute hemorrhage.

Differential

- **Acute: SAH,** hemorrhagic stroke, meningitis, seizure, acutely elevated ICP, **hypertensive encephalopathy,** post-LP, ocular disease (glaucoma, iritis), new migraine headache.
- **Subacute: Temporal arteritis,** intracranial **tumor,** subdural hematoma, pseudotumor cerebri, trigeminal/glossopharyngeal neuralgia (Neuro.52), postherpetic neuralgia, hypertension.
- **Chronic/episodic:** Migraine, cluster headache, tension headache (Neuro.51), sinusitis, dental disease, neck pain.

A traumatic intracranial hemorrhage of arterial origin that is commonly due to a lateral skull fracture (blunt trauma), with resultant tear of the **middle meningeal artery.**

History/PE

With an epidural hematoma, mental status changes occur within minutes to hours.

Patients present with a **lucid interval** ranging from several minutes to hours followed by the onset of headache, progressive obtundation, and hemiparesis; ultimately it may lead to a "blown pupil" (fixed and dilated pupil; usually occurs secondary to uncal herniation).

Evaluation

CT shows a **lens-shaped, convex hyperdensity** (see Figure 2.11–1). Patients require close observation and serial neurologic examinations before surgery.

Treatment

Emergent neurosurgical evacuation.

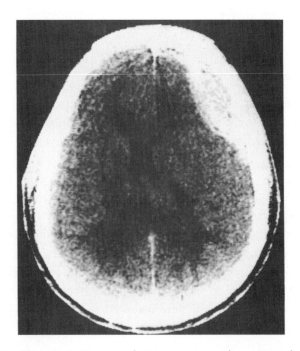

FIGURE 2.11–1. Epidural hematoma. CT scan without contrast reveals a convex, lens-shaped hyperdensity.

An intracranial hemorrhage that typically occurs after head trauma with resultant rupture of the **bridging veins** (especially in the **elderly** and **alcoholics**).

History/PE

Headache, changes in mental status, contralateral hemiparesis, or other focal changes. In contrast to epidural hematoma, changes can be **subacute** or **chronic** and may present as **dementia,** especially in the elderly. There may be a **remote history of a fall.**

With a subdural hematoma, mental status changes occur within days to weeks.

Evaluation

CT demonstrates a **crescent-shaped, concave hyperdensity** (see Figure 2.11–2).

Treatment

Surgical evacuation if symptomatic.

Commonly caused by a ruptured aneurysm (e.g., congenital berry), stroke, AVM, or trauma. Berry aneurysms are associated with polycystic kidney disease and coarctation of the aorta.

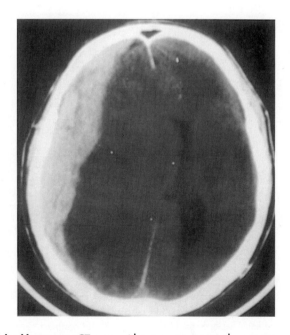

FIGURE 2.11–2. Subdural hematoma. CT scan without contrast reveals a concave, crescent-shaped hyperdensity with compression of the left lateral ventricle and midline shift of the cortex.

HIGH-YIELD FACTS

Neurology

History/PE

SAH will give the patient "the worst headache of my life."

A **sudden-onset, intensely painful** headache, often with **neck stiffness** (and other signs of meningeal irritation), fever, nausea/vomiting, and a fluctuating level of consciousness. SAH may be heralded by milder **sentinel headaches** in preceding weeks. Seizure may result from blood irritating the cerebral cortex.

Differential

Hemorrhagic stroke, trauma, meningitis, migraine headache.

Evaluation

Xanthochromia distinguishes SAH from traumatic LP.

Immediate **head CT** without contrast (Figure 2.11–3) to look for blood in the subarachnoid space (contrast can trigger a seizure if leaks occur beyond the blood-brain barrier). Obtain an immediate **LP if CT is negative** to look for red cells, **xanthochromia** (yellowish CSF due to breakdown of red blood cells), and elevated ICP. Four-vessel angiography should be performed once SAH is confirmed.

Treatment

Focus on **preventing elevation of ICP** by raising the head of the bed, limiting IV fluids, treating hypertension, and administering calcium channel blockers **(nimodipine)** and anti-seizure medications **(phenytoin).** Surgical treatment involves open or interventional radiologic clipping or coiling of an aneurysm or AVM.

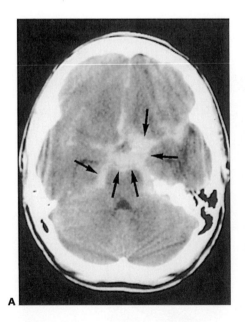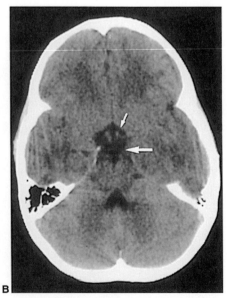

FIGURE 2.11–3. Subarachnoid hemorrhage. (A) CT scan without contrast reveals blood in the subarachnoid space at the base of the brain (arrows). (B) A normal CT scan without contrast shows no density in this region (arrows).

Complications

Rebleeding (more common with aneurysm than with AVM), extension into the brain parenchyma (more common with AVM), arterial vasospasm (occurs in one-third of aneurysmal SAHs).

A hemorrhage within the brain parenchyma. Etiologies include hypertension, tumor, and amyloid angiopathy (seen in the elderly).

History

Lethargy and **headache.**

PE

Focal motor and sensory deficits. Patients may have some degree of obtundation.

Evaluation

Immediate head CT reveals an intraparenchymal hemorrhage (Figure 2.11–4). Look for mass effect or edema that may predict herniation.

Treatment

Treatment is similar to that for SAH: raise the head of the bed and institute anti-seizure prophylaxis. Surgical evacuation may be necessary.

TEMPORAL ARTERITIS UCV Neuro.50

Generally not seen before age 50, temporal arteritis (or giant cell arteritis) affects twice as many women as men. It is often due to subacute granulomatous inflammation of the external carotid (especially the temporal branch) and vertebral arteries. The most feared complication of temporal arteritis is **blindness** secondary to occlusion of the central retinal artery (a branch of the internal carotid artery). Half of all patients will also have polymyalgia rheumatica (PMR).

Always assess for temporal arteritis in patients with PMR.

History/PE

A new headache that is unilateral or bilateral and associated with scalp pain, **temporal tenderness, jaw claudication,** and transient or permanent **monocular blindness.** It is also associated with weight loss, myalgia/arthralgia, and fever.

HIGH-YIELD FACTS

Neurology

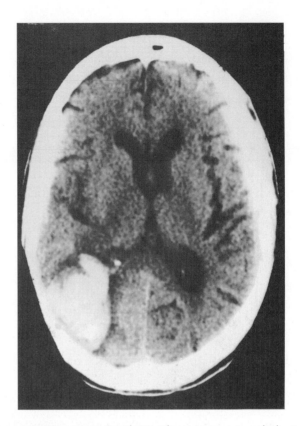

FIGURE 2.11–4. Intracerebral hematoma. Head CT without contrast reveals the irregularly shaped hyperdensity with midline shift of the choroid plexus.

Evaluation

Obtain **ESR** (> 50, usually > 100), ophthalmologic evaluation, and **temporal artery biopsy.** On biopsy, look for inflammation in the media and adventitia with lymphocytes, plasma cells, and giant cells.

Treatment

Don't wait for biopsy results before starting high-dose prednisone.

Treat immediately with **prednisone** 60 mg daily for 1–2 months before tapering. Since blindness may be permanent, do not wait for biopsy results to initiate treatment. Continue to follow eye exam for improvements or changes.

INTRACRANIAL TUMORS   UCV *Neuro.41, 43, 45*

Metastatic brain tumors are more common than primary brain tumors.

Intracranial tumors may be primary (including low-grade gliomas, anaplastic astrocytomas, and glioblastoma multiforme) or metastatic (most commonly from lung, melanoma, breast, colon, and kidney). Metastatic brain tumors are far more common than primary brain tumors. In children, primary brain tumors are most commonly **infratentorial,** while in adults primary brain tumors are most commonly **supratentorial.**

History

Thirty percent of patients present with **headache.** Headache is typically **dull and steady; worse in the morning; exacerbated by coughing,** Valsalva, changing position, and exertion; and **associated with nausea and vomiting.** Crescendo symptoms should raise suspicion of an intracranial mass.

PE

Focal findings on neurologic exam, seizures, and lethargy.

Evaluation

CT with contrast and **MRI with gadolinium.**

Treatment

Emergent radiation therapy or surgical excision may slow tumor progression. Virtually all anaplastic astrocytomas and glioblastomas recur. Otherwise, management is largely supportive.

MIGRAINE $\blacksquare$ Neuro. 49

Most commonly affects women < 30 years of age and those with a **family history.** Its etiology is not fully understood; **vascular abnormalities** (such as intracranial vasoconstriction and extracranial vasodilation) due to abnormalities in brain neurotransmitters (serotonin) may be responsible. Migraines are often precipitated by certain foods, fasting, stress, menses, OCPs, and bright light.

History/PE

Throbbing (or possibly dull) headache that is often **unilateral** (but can also be bilateral or occipital; Figure 2.11–5). Headaches are typically associated with **nausea and vomiting, photophobia,** and noise sensitivity. "Classic migraines" are commonly unilateral, associated with **aura,** and preceded by **visual symptoms** such as scintillating lights, scotomas, and field cuts. "Common migraines" present without these associated symptoms and are in fact more common. There is often a **prior history of migraines.**

Evaluation

Consider CT or MRI on first presentation, especially if there are focal neurologic findings (migraine itself can be associated with transient focal neurologic deficits). Rule out meningitis with an LP if symptoms are acute in onset.

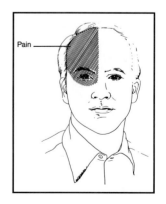

FIGURE 2.11–5. Distribution of pain in migraine headache. Pain is most commonly hemicranial but may be holocephalic, bifrontal, or unilateral frontal.

Treatment

Abortive therapy includes aspirin/NSAIDs, sumatriptan (a $5HT_1$ agonist), ergots (partial $5HT_1$ agonists), isometheptene, and opiates. **Prophylaxis** for patients with frequent/severe migraines includes NSAIDs, beta-blockers, ergots, tricyclic antidepressants, calcium channel blockers, and valproic acid. Narcotics should not be used prophylactically.

Affects **men** more often than women, with a mean age of onset of 25.

History

A **brief,** severe, **unilateral periorbital headache** (Figure 2.11–6). Attacks tend to occur in clusters, affecting the same part of the head and taking place at the same time of day (usually at night). Headaches may be precipitated by the use of alcohol or vasodilating drugs.

PE

Ipsilateral tearing of the eye and **conjunctival injection, Horner's syndrome,** and **nasal stuffiness.**

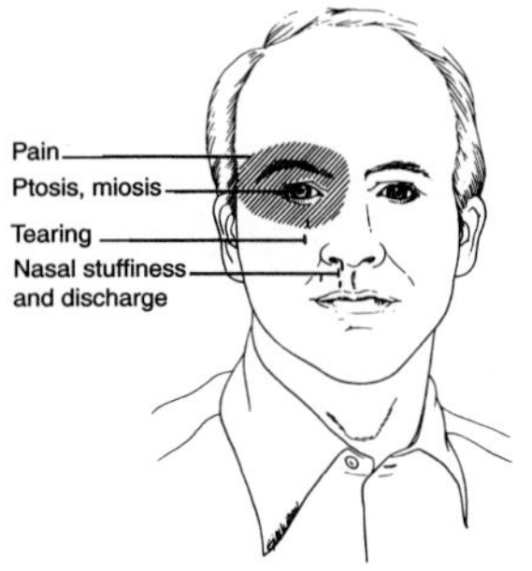

Evaluation

Classic presentations require no evaluation.

Treatment

Institute acute therapy with **high-flow oxygen** (100% nonrebreather oxygen), ergots, or sumatriptan. Prophylactic therapy includes ergots, calcium channel blockers, prednisone, and lithium.

FIGURE 2.11–6. Distribution of pain in cluster headache. Pain is commonly associated with ipsilateral conjunctival injection, tearing, nasal stuffiness, and Horner's syndrome.

Evaluate patients after their first seizure (for mass lesions, etc.) before initiating treatment for epilepsy.

Seizures involve excessive discharge by cortical neurons that results in focal and/or general neurologic symptoms. Epilepsy is the predisposition to recurrent, unprovoked seizures. Patients with a first seizure should be evaluated prior to the initiation of treatment. The type of medication used depends on the type of seizure. An **aura,** which is a subjective sensation/feeling preceding the onset of a seizure, is experienced by 50–60% of patients with epilepsy. The **EEG is the most important diagnostic test** used in the workup of seizures. Common etiologies of seizures according to age are listed in Table 2.11–1.

HIGH-YIELD FACTS

Neurology

TABLE 2.11–1. Causes of Seizures.

Infant	Child (2–10)	Adolescent	Adult (18–35)	Adult (35+)
Perinatal injury	Idiopathic	Idiopathic	Trauma	Trauma
Infection	Infection	Trauma	Alcoholism	Stroke
Metabolic	Trauma	Drug withdrawal	Brain tumor	Metabolic disorder
Congenital	Febrile seizure	AVM		Alcoholism

FOCAL (PARTIAL) SEIZURES

UCV Neuro.38

Focal (partial) seizures arise from a discrete region in one of the cerebral hemispheres and do **not** lead to loss of consciousness unless they evolve into generalized seizures. Focal seizures are broken down into simple partial and complex partial seizures (distinguished by the level of consciousness; see below).

History/PE

Manifestations of focal seizures depend on the region of the cortex that is affected. **Simple partial seizures** may involve motor (e.g., Jacksonian march, the progressive jerking of successive body regions), sensory (parietal lobe), or autonomic functions **without alteration of consciousness.** Postictally, there may be a focal neurologic deficit (**Todd's paralysis**) that resolves within 1–2 days.

Complex partial seizures typically involve the **temporal lobe** (70–80%) and are characterized by **impaired level of consciousness,** auditory or visual hallucinations, déjà vu, automatisms (e.g., lip smacking, chewing, or even walking), and **postictal confusion**/disorientation and amnesia. Symptoms may mimic schizophrenia or acute psychosis. Both types may secondarily generalize.

Evaluation

Rule out systemic causes with CBC, electrolytes, calcium, glucose, ABGs, LFTs, renal panel, RPR, ESR, and tox screen. Perform diagnostic tests, including EEG (to look for epileptiform waveforms) and CT or MRI (MRI is preferable).

Treatment

Treat the underlying cause if possible. Otherwise, phenytoin, carbamazepine, phenobarbital, valproate, lamotrigine, or gabapentin can be prescribed.

Generalized seizures involve both cerebral hemispheres and lead to a **sudden loss of consciousness** with a period of **postictal confusion.** The two most common types of generalized seizures are absence (petit mal) and tonic-clonic (grand mal).

ABSENCE (PETIT MAL) SEIZURES   UCV Neuro.37

Absence **(petit mal)** seizures typically begin in childhood, subside before adulthood, and are often familial.

History/PE

Children with absence seizures often get into trouble for daydreaming in class.

Brief, often unnoticeable episodes of impaired consciousness lasting only **5–10 seconds** and occurring up to hundreds of times per day. Patients are amnestic during and immediately after seizures. Classically, a teacher may observe a child "daydreaming" or "staring" in class.

Evaluation

EEG shows classic **three-per-second spike-and-wave** discharges.

Treatment

Ethosuximide or valproate.

TONIC-CLONIC SEIZURES   UCV Neuro.40

History/PE

In patients with loss of consciousness, always differentiate between seizure and syncope.

Tonic-clonic (grand mal) seizures begin with loss of consciousness and tonic extension of the back and extremities, followed by 1–2 minutes of repetitive, symmetric clonic movements. **Cyanosis** (secondary to limited respiratory function) and **incontinence** may occur during the seizure. Consciousness slowly returns in the postictal period. Patients may then complain of muscle aches and headache. Serum prolactin level is usually elevated during the postictal period. Generalized seizure must be differentiated from syncope (Table 2.11–2). Examine the patient for tongue lacerations, head injuries, and shoulder dislocations (typically posterior).

Treatment

Treat the underlying cause, if possible. Otherwise use valproate, phenytoin, or carbamazepine.

TABLE 2.11—2. Seizure Versus Syncope.

	Seizure	Syncope
Onset	Sudden onset without prodrome. Focal sensory or motor phenomena. Sensation of fear, smell, memory.	Progressive lightheadedness. Dimming of vision, faintness.
Course	Sudden LOC with tonic-clonic activity. May last 1–2 minutes. May see tongue laceration, head trauma, and bowel/urinary incontinence.	Gradual LOC, limp or with jerking. Rarely lasts longer than 15 seconds. Less commonly injured.
Recovery	Postictal confusion and disorientation.	Typically immediate return to lucidity.

STATUS EPILEPTICUS

Status epilepticus, a medical emergency, consists of prolonged (**> 30 minutes**) or repetitive seizures without a return to baseline consciousness between them. Common causes include anticonvulsant withdrawal/noncompliance, EtOH/sedative **withdrawal** or other drug intoxication, **metabolic disturbances** (e.g., hyponatremia), trauma, and infection. Status epilepticus is associated with a 20% mortality rate.

Status epilepticus is a medical emergency associated with a 20% mortality rate.

History/PE

Continuous seizure activity or multiple episodes of seizure activity occur without return to consciousness.

Evaluation

Determine cause with pulse oximetry, CBC, electrolytes, calcium, glucose, ABGs, LFTs, BUN/creatinine, ESR, and toxicology screen. Defer EEG and brain imaging until the patient is stabilized.

Treatment

Maintain airway, breathing, and circulation (**ABCs**). Consider rapid intubation for airway protection. Administer an IV **benzodiazepine** such as lorazepam or diazepam and a loading dose of **phenytoin.** If seizures continue, intubate and load with phenobarbital. Consider an IV sedative such as midazolam or pentobarbital if seizures continue.

233

Acute onset of **focal neurologic deficits** resulting from diminished blood flow **(ischemic stroke)** or hemorrhage **(hemorrhagic stroke).** Risk factors include diabetes, hypertension, smoking, atrial fibrillation, and cocaine. Incidence increases with advancing age and occurs more frequently in males than in females. The most common etiology is atherosclerosis of the extracranial vessels (internal and common carotids, basilar, and vertebral arteries). **Lacunar infarcts** occur in regions supplied by small perforating vessels and result from atherosclerosis, hypertension, or diabetes.

History/PE

- **Middle cerebral artery (MCA):** Aphasia, neglect, hemiparesis, gaze preference, and homonymous hemianopsia (Figure 2.11–7).
- **Anterior cerebral artery:** Leg paresis.
- **Posterior cerebral artery:** Homonymous hemianopsia.
- **Basilar artery:** Coma, cranial nerve palsies, apnea.
- **Lacunar stroke:** Pure motor or sensory stroke, dysarthria–clumsy hand syndrome, ataxic hemiparesis.
- **TIA:** Transient neurologic deficit that lasts < 24 hours (EM.34).

Differential

Brain tumor, subdural or epidural hematoma, brain abscess, endocarditis, multiple sclerosis, metabolic abnormalities (hypoglycemia), neurosyphilis.

Evaluation

Evaluation should include:

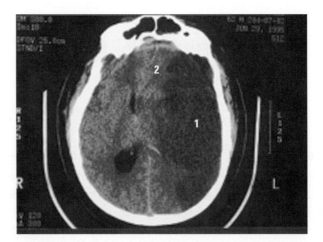

FIGURE 2.11–7. Left MCA stroke. Note the ischemic brain parenchyma (1) subtle midline shift to the right (2), and left lateral ventricles obliterated by edema. There is no visible hemorrhage.

- CT without contrast (to differentiate ischemic from hemorrhagic stroke).
- MRI (to identify early ischemic changes and neoplasms and to adequately image the brainstem/posterior fossa).
- CBC, glucose, coagulation panel, lipid evaluation, ESR, and a treponemal assay.
- EKG and an echocardiogram if embolic stroke is suspected (transesophageal echo is most sensitive for mural thrombus).
- **Vascular studies** for extracranial disease (carotid ultrasound, MRA or traditional angiography) and for intracranial disease (transcranial doppler or MRA).
- Screen for hypercoagulable states (if history of bleeding, first stroke, or < 50 years of age).

Treatment

- **Heparin** and **aspirin** should be used for embolic strokes and those due to a hypercoagulable state after hemorrhagic stroke has been ruled out by CT or MRI.
- Maintain vigilance for signs and symptoms of brain swelling, increased ICP, and herniation.
- **Thrombolysis** and **neuroprotective agents** are investigational medical interventions.
- **Do not overtreat hypertension** (may diminish cerebral perfusion).

Allow BP to rise up to 200/100 to maintain cerebral perfusion.

Prevention

Preventive and long-term treatment should consist of the following:

- **Aspirin** or clopidogrel if stroke is secondary to small vessel disease or thrombosis or if anticoagulation is contraindicated.
- Carotid endarterectomy if stenosis is > 60% (endarterectomy is contraindicated in vessels that are 100% occluded).
- **Anticoagulation** (heparin initially, then warfarin) in cases of cardiac emboli, new atrial fibrillation, or hypercoagulable states.
- Management of hypertension (including isolated systolic hypertension).

WERNICKE'S APHASIA

UCV *Neuro.22*

A disorder in the comprehension of language—an expressive (fluent) aphasia. Features are as follows:

Wernicke's is **W**ordy but makes no sense.

- Etiology is usually embolic.
- **Fluent, expressive speech** that is empty of meaning.
- **Comprehension and repetition of language are impaired;** marked paraphasic errors.
- Hemiparesis is mild or absent.
- No dysarthria.

- The patient is often not aware of his deficit.
- The lesion is frequently in the left posterior superior temporal lobe (Sylvian fissure) secondary to a **left inferior MCA** stroke.

Treatment

Institute speech therapy. Patients have a wide range of outcomes, and prognosis is intermediate.

A disorder in the production of language—a nonfluent aphasia. Features are as follows:

- **Speech is nonfluent** with decreased rate and short phrase length, and **impaired speech articulation.**
- **Comprehension is intact.**
- Associated with a hemiparesis, hemisensory loss, and apraxia of oral muscles.
- The patient is often frustrated by the deficit.
- The lesion is frequently in the left superior temporal gyrus in the inferior frontal lobe secondary to a **superior MCA stroke.**

Broca's is Broken speech.

Treatment

Institute speech therapy. Patients have a wide range of outcomes, and prognosis is intermediate.

A slowly progressive degenerative brain disease that is the **most common cause of dementia.** Age is the most important risk factor. Other risk factors include female gender, family history, Down's syndrome, and low educational level. Pathology includes neurofibrillary tangles, neuritic plaques with amyloid deposition, amyloid angiopathy, and neuronal loss.

5 A's of dementia:
Aphasia
Apraxia
Agnosia
Amnesia
Abstract thought

History/PE

Memory impairment is usually the first presenting sign, followed by language deficits, acalculia, depression, agitation, and apraxia (inability to perform skilled movements).

Differential

A useful mnemonic is **DEMENTIAS:**

- **D**egenerative diseases (Parkinson's, Huntington's)
- **E**ndocrine (thyroid, parathyroid, pituitary, adrenal)
- **M**etabolic (alcohol, fluid electrolytes, B_{12} deficiency, glucose, hepatic, renal, Wilson's disease)
- **E**xogenous (heavy metals, carbon monoxide, drugs)
- **N**eoplasia
- **T**rauma (subdural hematoma)
- **I**nfection (meningitis, encephalitis, abscess, endocarditis, HIV, syphilis, prion diseases, Lyme disease)
- **A**ffective disorders (depression)
- **S**troke/Structure (multi-infarct dementia *(Neuro.25)*, ischemia, vasculitis, normal pressure hydrocephalus)

The three most common causes of dementia are Alzheimer's disease, multi-infarct dementia, and depression (pseudodementia).

Evaluation

AD is a **diagnosis of exclusion.** MRI or CT may show atrophy and can rule out multi-infarct dementia, normal pressure hydrocephalus, subdural hemorrhage, abscess, or tumor. Other tests include CBC, B_{12}, glucose, electrolytes, calcium, TSH, ESR, and RPR. Neuropsychologic testing helps distinguish between dementia and depression.

Treatment

Institute supportive therapy. Tetrahydroaminoacridine, donepezil, or tacrine may temporarily slow disease progression.

AMYOTROPHIC LATERAL SCLEROSIS (ALS)

UCV *Neuro.12*

A chronic, progressive degenerative disease of unknown origin characterized by loss of motor neurons within the spinal cord, brainstem, and motor cortex. ALS almost always progresses to respiratory failure and death.

History

Asymmetric, slowly progressive weakness affecting the arms, legs, and cranial nerves. Some patients initially complain of fasciculations.

PE

Upper motor neuron signs (spasticity, increased DTRs, upward-going toes) and/or **lower motor neuron signs** (flaccid paralysis, loss of DTRs, fasciculations, downward-going toes).

A combination of upper and lower motor neuron signs in three or more extremities is diagnostic of ALS.

Differential

Spondylitic cervical myopathy, syringomyelia, neoplasms, demyelinating diseases, benign fasciculations, polio, hypothyroidism, hyperparathyroidism, dysproteinemia, lymphoma, heavy metal poisoning, post-radiation effects, Guillain–Barré syndrome.

Evaluation

EMG/nerve conduction studies reveal **widespread denervation and fibrillation potentials.** Obtain CT/MRI of the cervical spine to exclude structural lesions. Rule out systemic causes with CBC, TSH, SPEP, UPEP, Ca^{2+}, PTH, urine for heavy metals (if history of exposure), and PFTs.

Treatment

Supportive measures, patient education, and aggressive pulmonary toilet. Riluzole, which reduces presynaptic glutamate release, may slow disease progression.

MULTIPLE SCLEROSIS (MS)

An acquired demyelinating disease of the CNS that may have a T-cell-mediated **autoimmune pathogenesis** (involving both environmental and genetic components). MS is twice as common in **women** as in men and has a peak incidence at **20–40 years of age.** It is generally a disorder of **temperate climates.**

History/PE

MS is classically defined as **two distinct episodes of focal neurologic deficits.** Patients present with neurologic complaints that frequently cannot be explained by a single lesion. The most common presenting complaints include **limb weakness, optic neuritis, paresthesias, diplopia, urinary retention,** and **vertigo.** Neurologic symptoms can wax and wane or be progressive. Exacerbating factors include heat, trauma, pregnancy, and vigorous activity.

Differential

CNS tumors or trauma, vasculitis, vitamin B_{12} deficiency, CNS infections (Lyme disease, neurosyphilis), sarcoidosis.

Evaluation

MRI reveals **multiple, asymmetric, often periventricular lesions.** Active lesions enhance with gadolinium on MRI. CSF analysis may show **mononuclear** pleocytosis (> 5 cells/μL) in 25% of cases, elevated CSF IgG in 80% of cases, and/or **oligoclonal bands** (nonspecific).

Treatment

Steroids should be given during acute exacerbations. **Prophylactic immunosuppressants or beta-interferon** may decrease the number and severity of relapses.

An **acute, acquired demyelinating autoimmune disorder** of the peripheral nerves resulting in weakness. GBS is associated with recent *Campylobacter jejuni* infection, preceding viral infection, and recent vaccination.

History

Rapidly progressive weakness that begins distally and progresses proximally to involve the trunk, diaphragm, and cranial nerves **(ascending paralysis).** It is often accompanied by a history of **recent viral infection, diarrhea,** or **immunization.**

PE

Weakness with areflexia. Dysesthesias may also be present.

Differential

Myasthenia gravis, multiple sclerosis, chronic inflammatory demyelinating polyneuropathy, ALS, poliomyelitis, porphyria, heavy metal poisoning, botulism, transverse myelitis, diphtheric neuropathy, tick paralysis.

Evaluation

Findings include evidence of **diffuse demyelination** on EMG and nerve conduction studies. Diagnosis is supported by a **CSF protein level > 55 mg/dL** with little or no pleocytosis.

Treatment

Plasmapheresis or **IV immunoglobulin** with close monitoring of respiratory function (intubation may be necessary). Most cases improve as long as proper supportive therapy (e.g., ventilatory support) is administered.

Closely monitor respiratory function in patients with GBS.

HIGH-YIELD FACTS

Neurology

A common form of **peripheral** (i.e., end-organ) vertigo. BPPV results from a dislodged piece of otolith that causes disturbances in the semicircular canals.

History/PE

Transient, episodic vertigo (lasting less than one minute) and nystagmus with specific head postures (classically **while turning in bed or getting up in the morning**), together with **nausea and vomiting.** Dizziness is usually exacerbated by changes in position. Fatigable nystagmus is present on physical examination when the patient lies on his side. BPPV is also characterized by **habituation,** which is decreased vertigo/nystagmus with repetitive testing. Table 2.11–3 summarizes the different signs and symptoms of central and peripheral vertigo.

Differential

Hypothyroidism, aminoglycoside or furosemide toxicity, stroke, trauma, Ménière's syndrome, labyrinthitis, acoustic neuroma.

Evaluation

Evaluation should include the Nylen–Bárány maneuver, i.e., having the patient go from a sitting to a supine position while quickly turning the head to the side. If vertigo and/or nystagmus is reproduced, BPPV is the likely diagnosis. Other studies can include CT/MRI (with attention to the posterior fossa and temporal bone to rule out cerebellopontine-angle lesions), an audiogram to rule out Ménière's disease, and TSH.

Peripheral causes of vertigo always produce horizontal nystagmus, whereas vertical nystagmus indicates a central lesion.

TABLE 2.11–3. Etiologies of Peripheral and Central Dysequilibrium.

Peripheral Vestibular Disorders	Acute Central Ataxias	Chronic Central Ataxias
Benign positional vertigo	Drug intoxication	Multiple sclerosis
Ménière's disease	Wernicke's encephalopathy	Cerebellar degeneration
Acute peripheral vestibulopathy	Vertebrobasilar ischemia	Hypothyroidism
Otosclerosis	Vertebrobasilar infarction	Wilson's disease, CJD
Cerebellopontine-angle tumor	Inflammatory disorders	Posterior fossa masses
Vestibulopathy/acoustic neuropathy	Cerebellar hemorrhage	Ataxia–telangiectasia

Treatment

Treat with **repositioning exercises.** Vestibular suppressant medications (antihistamines, antiemetics, benzodiazepines) generally are not effective and should be used only for acute vertiginous states.

LABYRINTHITIS

A form of **peripheral** vertigo that arises spontaneously and may be caused by **viral or bacterial infection.**

History

Acute onset of **severe, continuous vertigo** associated with nausea and vomiting as well as with **tinnitus** and **hearing loss.** Symptoms often last for days. A recent history of viral infection is common.

PE

Physical exam may reveal spontaneous nystagmus toward the unaffected ear, and the patient may fall to the side of the lesion on Romberg test.

Differential

Other causes of peripheral vertigo.

Evaluation

Diagnosis is primarily **clinical.** Studies may include CT/MRI (with attention to the posterior fossa and temporal bone), an audiogram to rule out Ménière's disease, and TSH.

Treatment

Bed rest and **avoidance of rapid head movements.** Consider amoxicillin-clavulanic acid or TMP-SMX if bacterial infection is suspected.

Patients with labyrinthitis should avoid rapid head movements.

A form of **peripheral vertigo** that results from distention of the endolymphatic compartment of the inner ear. Causes include head trauma and syphilis.

History/PE

Episodic vertigo associated with nausea and vomiting, **ear fullness, hearing loss,** and **tinnitus.** Episodes resolve within hours to days.

Differential

Other causes of peripheral vertigo.

Evaluation

Audiometry shows **low-frequency pure-tone hearing loss** that fluctuates in severity.

Treatment

Treat with a **low-salt diet** and **acetazolamide.** Antihistamines, antiemetics, and benzodiazepines may be given for acute attacks. Surgical decompression may be necessary in refractory cases.

Obstetrics

PRENATAL CARE

Prenatal care is critical to the delivery of a healthy baby. The pregnant patient's prenatal labs should be scheduled as described in Table 2.12–1.

TABLE 2.12–1. Standard Prenatal Labs and Studies.

Gestation	Labs to Be Obtained
Initial visit	CBC Type, Rh, and antibody screen Rubella antibody titer Cervical gonorrhea and chlamydia cultures VDRL for syphilis screening Hepatitis B surface antigen test Pap smear Urinalysis PPD Sickle prep in high-risk groups HIV testing (with consent), counseling in high-risk groups Glucose test if patient has risk factors for diabetes
15–20 weeks	**Maternal serum alpha-fetoprotein level** should be measured to screen for any neural tube defect (very high level) and trisomy 21 (low level). Perform triple screen (AFP, HCG, estriol) at 16 weeks to screen for trisomy 18, trisomy 21, and neural tube defects. If abnormal, perform ultrasound or amniocentesis.
18–20 weeks	Ultrasound for dating if unknown or uncertain. This is the best time during fetal development to assess the age of the fetus if there is only one chance of obtaining an ultrasound.
24–28 weeks	**Glucose test** for everyone (risk factors or not).
28–30 weeks	RhoGAM administered to patients initially determined to be Rh antibody negative.
34–38 weeks	CBC
36–40 weeks	Cervical chlamydia and gonorrhea cultures in high-risk patients.

ALPHA-FETOPROTEIN (AFP) IN PRENATAL TESTING

High levels of MSAFP suggest open neural tube defects.

AFP is produced by the fetus and found primarily in amniotic fluid. Small amounts of AFP cross the placenta and enter the maternal circulation. **Maternal serum alpha-fetoprotein (MSAFP) should be measured at 16–18 weeks' gestation.** The results of AFP testing depend on accurate gestational dating. Causes of elevated MSAFP include open neural tube defects (anencephaly or spina bifida), abdominal wall defects, multiple gestation, incorrect gestational dating, fetal death, and placental abnormalities (e.g., placental abruption). An abnormally low MSAFP level warrants amniocentesis and karyotyping to rule out chromosomal abnormalities (such as trisomy 21).

GESTATIONAL DIABETES   UCV *OB.38*

Gestational diabetes occurs in 3–5% of all pregnancies. Risk factors include past history of gestational diabetes, prior abortions, stillbirths, obesity, a previous history of macrosomic baby, maternal age > 30, and a family history of diabetes. A prior history of polyuria, recurrent UTIs, as well as a fetus that is large for gestational age, may indicate occult diabetes.

History/PE

A fetus that is large for gestational age may indicate occult diabetes.

Typically **asymptomatic.**

Differential

Diabetes mellitus, volume overload, sugar overload, urinary tract abnormalities.

Evaluation

UA reveals **glycosuria.** Other findings include **fasting hyperglycemia** (serum glucose > 105 mg/dL) and an **abnormal glucose tolerance test** (routinely performed between 24 and 28 weeks' gestation). One-hour (50 g) glucose tolerance testing with postprandial serum glucose > 140 mg/dL suggests the diagnosis and should be followed by a three-hour (100 g) glucose tolerance test (GTT).

Treatment

Treatment consists of strict adherence to **ADA diet.** Administer **insulin** if the diabetes cannot be controlled by diet alone. **Avoid oral hypoglycemics** (can cause fetal hypoglycemia).

Complications

Complications of gestational diabetes are listed in Table 2.12–2.

TABLE 2.12–2. Complications of Gestational Diabetes.

Maternal Complications	Fetal Complications
Preterm labor	Macrosomia
Polyhydramnios	Shoulder dystocia
Cesarean section for macrosomia	Perinatal mortality 2–5%
Preeclampsia/eclampsia	Congenital defects
Glucose intolerance or diabetes mellitus type II later on (50% of gestational diabetes patients have impaired glucose tolerance later in life)	Hypoglycemia

PREECLAMPSIA AND ECLAMPSIA

Pregnancy-induced hypertension (PIH) is defined by two blood pressure measurements of 140/90 (without a history of hypertension) at least six hours apart at > 20 weeks' gestation. **Preeclampsia** is defined as **PIH, proteinuria** (> 300 mg/24 hours), and/or **nondependent (hand and face) edema. Eclampsia** is defined as **seizures** in a patient with preeclampsia. Risk factors include nulliparity, black race, extremes of age (< 15 or > 35), multiple gestations, vascular disease (secondary to SLE or diabetes), a family history of preeclampsia, and chronic hypertension. **HELLP syndrome** is a variant of preeclampsia that has a poor prognosis (see sidebar).

> **HELLP syndrome**
>
> **H**emolysis,
> **E**levated **L**FTs,
> **L**ow **P**latelets (thrombocytopenia)

History/PE

Mild and severe preeclampsia share the same spectrum of signs and symptoms (Table 2.12–3).

Differential

Molar pregnancy, essential hypertension, renal disease, renovascular hypertension, primary aldosteronism, Cushing's syndrome, pheochromocytoma, primary seizure disorder, TTP, and SLE.

Evaluation

CBC, electrolytes, serum BUN/creatinine, uric acid, UA, 24-hour urine protein, **amniocentesis** (to **check** for **fetal lung maturity**), LFTs, PT/PTT, fibrinogen, fibrin split products, urine tox screen, ultrasound, and non-stress tests/biophysical profiles (as indicated).

TABLE 2.12–3. Signs and Symptoms of Preeclampsia and Eclampsia.

Mild Preeclampsia	Severe Preeclampsia	Eclampsia
Blood pressure greater than **140/90** measured two times six hours apart	Signs and symptoms of mild preeclampsia plus:	The three most common symptoms preceding an eclamptic attack are **headache, visual changes,** and **right upper quadrant/ epigastric pain**
Cerebral changes (headaches, somnolence)	Blood pressure greater than **160/110** measured two times six hours apart	**Seizures;** severe if not controlled with anticonvulsant therapy
Visual changes (blurred vision, scotomata)	Proteinuria (> 5 g over 24 hours, or > 3+ on urine dipstick)	
GI symptoms (epigastric pain)	Oliguria	
Rapid weight gain, **edema**	Right upper quadrant/epigastric pain	
Jugular venous distention	Pulmonary edema/cyanosis	
Hyperactive reflexes, clonus	HELLP syndrome	
Proteinuria (> 300 mg/24 h)	Oligohydramnios	
	IUGR	

Seizures require magnesium ± benzodiazepines.

Treatment

The only cure for preeclampsia/eclampsia is delivery. Use IV **magnesium sulfate** for seizure prophylaxis in severe preeclampsia (continue 12–24 hours after delivery) and for seizure management. Management should also include fetal monitoring until delivery and control of hypertension (e.g., hydralazine, methyldopa). Table 2.12–4 further details the management of preeclampsia and eclampsia.

Complications

Prematurity, fetal distress, intrauterine growth retardation (IUGR), placental abruption, seizure, DIC, cerebral hemorrhage, acute renal failure, fetal/maternal death.

ECTOPIC PREGNANCY   **UCV** *OB.41*

Any pregnancy outside the uterine cavity (Figure 2.12–1). It most commonly occurs in the ampulla of the oviduct. Risk factors include history of **PID** (most common), prior ectopic pregnancy, tubal/pelvic surgery, DES exposure in utero, and IUD use.

History/PE

Symptoms of **pregnancy** (amenorrhea, nausea, vomiting) as well as **abdominal/pelvic pain** and tenderness, **abnormal vaginal bleeding,** and/or **pelvic**

TABLE 2.12–4. Management of Preeclampsia and Eclampsia.

Preeclampsia

If term or fetal lung mature, deliver.

If severe, expedite delivery regardless of lung maturity.

Modified bed rest, check blood pressure, reflexes, daily weight and urine protein output, labs, fetal surveillance, patient education.

Control blood pressure with antihypertensives (hydralazine, methyldopa, labetalol, diazoxide) if diastolic blood pressure is higher than 110 mmHg. The goal is to maintain a blood pressure lower than 160/110, preferably with a diastolic blood pressure of 90–100 mmHg.

If severe, immediately hospitalize, check urine output, check for pulmonary edema, keep diastolic blood pressure 90–105 with antihypertensives, give magnesium sulfate for seizure prophylaxis, deliver as soon as possible by labor induction and/or cesarean section.

Postpartum: **continue magnesium sulfate** for the first 12–24 hours; check blood pressure, pulmonary status, and fluid retention. Follow heme, renal, and liver labs.

General course of disease: 30% of preeclampsia cases occurs before 30 weeks' gestational age, with the highest number of cases occurring at 34 weeks' gestational age.

Eclampsia

Supplemental oxygen. Place in left lateral decubitus position.

Prevent maternal trauma.

Control seizure with **magnesium sulfate** and consider benzodiazepines if seizures are poorly controlled.

Control blood pressure if severe hypertension (blood pressure > 160/110, or diastolic blood pressure > 110).

General measures: limit fluid intake, Foley catheter, monitor inputs and outputs, monitor magnesium blood level, carefully monitor fetal status, **initiate steps to delivery!**

Postpartum: same as preeclampsia.

General course of disease: 50% of seizures occur antepartum, 25% occur intrapartum, 25% occur within 24 hours postpartum.

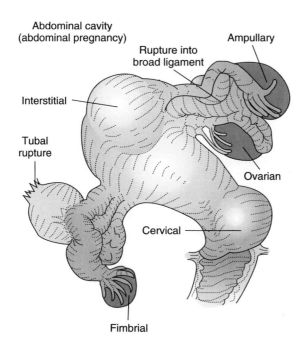

FIGURE 2.12–1. Sites of ectopic pregnancy.

mass. Ruptured ectopic pregnancy may present with orthostatic hypotension, tachycardia, generalized abdominal and adnexal tenderness with rebound, shoulder pain, and shock.

Differential

Intrauterine pregnancy, threatened abortion, PID, ruptured ovarian cyst, corpus luteum cyst, endometriosis, appendicitis, ovarian torsion, nephrolithiasis, diverticulitis.

Evaluation

Quantitative β-HCG levels are lower than expected for normal pregnancies of the same duration (usually < 6500) with **prolonged doubling times** (normal doubling time is two days). Serum progesterone is also below normal (usually < 15 ng/mL). An **elevated β-HCG in the absence of an intrauterine pregnancy on ultrasound** is highly suspicious. Evidence of an ectopic pregnancy can be found on ultrasound or by the return of > 5 cc of nonclotting blood on culdocentesis. Definitive diagnosis is made by laparoscopy or laparotomy.

Treatment

Patients with an ectopic pregnancy or suspicion of having one should be closely followed with serial β-HCG and ultrasound studies. Medical treatment for stable unruptured ectopic pregnancies < 3 cm with a β-HCG < 1000 is with **methotrexate.** All other ectopic pregnancies require surgery. Surgical options include salpingostomy, salpingectomy, and salpingo-oophorectomy. Give a **RhoGAM** shot if appropriate.

Complications

Inevitable loss of fetus, hemorrhagic shock, **future ectopic pregnancy,** infertility, maternal death, Rh sensitization.

SPONTANEOUS ABORTION UCV *EM.35, OB.31*

Spontaneous abortion is defined as a nonelective termination of a pregnancy at **< 20 weeks' gestational age** or at an estimated fetal weight of < 500 g. It is a common cause of first-trimester bleeding. Causes of habitual abortion include cervical incompetence, infections, uterine abnormalities, hormonal dysfunction, and chromosomal abnormalities.

History/PE

Vaginal bleeding and tissue passage. Closed vs. open cervical os on pelvic examination (see Table 2.12–5).

Any woman with abdominal pain needs a urine pregnancy test.

TABLE 2.12–5. Types of Spontaneous Abortion.

Abortion	Definition	Treatment
Complete abortion	Less than 20 weeks' gestation **All products of conception expelled** Internal **cervical os closed** Uterine bleeding	RhoGAM if appropriate
Incomplete abortion	Less than 20 weeks' gestation **Some products of conception expelled** Internal **cervical os open** Uterine bleeding	D&C RhoGAM if appropriate
Threatened abortion	Less than 20 weeks' gestation **No products of conception expelled** Membranes remain intact Internal **cervical os closed** Uterine bleeding Abdominal pain may be present Fetus still viable	Avoid heavy activity Pelvic rest Bed rest RhoGAM if appropriate
Inevitable abortion	Less than 20 weeks' gestation **No products of conception expelled** Membranes ruptured Internal **cervical os open** Uterine bleeding and cramps	Emergent D&C RhoGAM if appropriate
Missed abortion	No cardiac activity No products of conception expelled Retained fetal tissue Uterus not growing Internal cervical os closed No uterine bleeding Nonviable tissue not expelled in 4 weeks	Evacuate uterus D&C RhoGAM if appropriate
Septic abortion	Infection associated with abortion Endometritis leading to septicemia Maternal mortality 10–50%	Complete uterine evacuation D&C Intravenous antibiotics RhoGAM if appropriate
Intrauterine fetal death	No cardiac activity (fetal heart tones) Greater than 8 weeks' gestation, with 15 mm or larger crown–rump length	Evacuate uterus D&C RhoGAM if appropriate

Differential

Ectopic pregnancy, molar pregnancy, complete abortion, incomplete abortion, missed abortion, threatened abortion, septic abortion, intrauterine fetal death, local causes (e.g., cervicitis, genital tract trauma, infection).

Evaluation

Evaluation includes qualitative/quantitative β-HCG, transvaginal ultrasound, and possibly culdocentesis. Consider dilatation and curettage.

Treatment

Ensure hemodynamic stability if there has been significant bleeding. Management generally consists of **uterine evacuation,** prevention of infection, and **RhoGAM if appropriate** (Table 2.12–5).

Complications

Sepsis, hemorrhage.

RH DISEASE

Rh incompatibility can result when an Rh-negative mother gives birth to an Rh-positive baby. Rh factor is an antigenic protein located on RBCs in Rh-positive individuals and is transmitted in an autosomal-dominant fashion. Thus, an Rh-negative mother may have an Rh-positive fetus (if the father is Rh-positive) against which she can form antibodies. Since maternal anti-Rh IgG antibodies are able to cross the placenta, these maternal antibodies can react with the infant's RBCs, resulting in fetal RBC hemolysis (see Figure 2.12–2). Hemolytic disease usually occurs during the second pregnancy due to the rapid production of anti-Rh IgG antibodies by memory plasma cells.

History/PE

Severe fetal anemia can lead to heart failure, edema, ascites, and pericardial effusion **(erythroblastosis fetalis).** Fetal tissue hypoxia and acidosis may also be present.

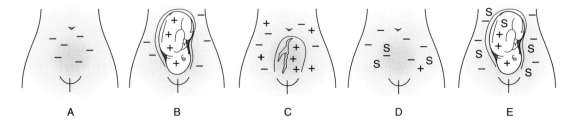

A   B   C   D   E

FIGURE 2.12–2.   Rh disease. (A) Rh-negative woman before pregnancy. (B) Pregnancy occurs. The fetus is Rh-positive. (C) Separation of the placenta. (D) Following delivery, Rh-isoimmunization occurs in the mother, and she develops antibodies (S=antibodies). (E) The next pregnancy with an Rh-positive fetus. Maternal antibodies cross the placenta, enter the bloodstream, and attach to Rh-positive cells, causing hemolysis. RhoGAM (Rh IgG) is given to the Rh-negative mother to prevent sensitization.

Evaluation

Findings include Rh-negative maternal RBCs, a positive indirect Coombs' test, high titers of maternal anti-Rh IgG, postnatal fetal cord blood that is Rh positive, and fetal Hgb < 10 g.

Treatment

- Prevention consists of **maternal indirect Coombs' testing and blood type testing at 28 weeks' gestation.** If the Coombs' test is negative, **give RhoGAM** (anti-IgG Rh). RhoGAM should also be given postpartum if the baby is Rh positive. RhoGAM should also be given to Rh-negative mothers who undergo spontaneous abortion, miscarriage, ectopic pregnancy, amniocentesis, vaginal bleeding, or placenta previa/placental abruption.
- Sensitized Rh-negative mothers should be closely monitored with serial ultrasound and amniocentesis.
- Fetal bilirubin levels are closely monitored to measure the amount of hemolysis. Enhance pulmonary maturity with betamethasone if fetal lungs are not mature; in severe cases, preterm delivery should be initiated when fetal lungs are mature.

Complications

Fetal kernicterus, fetal heart failure, fetal prematurity, fetal death.

PLACENTAL ABRUPTION AND PLACENTA PREVIA   UCV   EM.36, OB.44, 45

Placenta previa (Figure 2.12–3) and placental abruption are the two most common causes of **third-trimester bleeding.** Other causes include placenta accreta, bloody show, ruptured vasa previa, early labor, ruptured uterus, marginal placental separation, and genital tract lesions and trauma.

Table 2.12–6 describes the management of the two most common causes of third-trimester bleeding.

HYDATIDIFORM MOLE   UCV   OB.12

Gestational trophoblastic disease (GTD) can be benign or malignant. Benign GTD (molar pregnancy) accounts for approximately 80% of cases of GTD. **Complete molar pregnancies,** which result from sperm fertilization of an empty ovum, most commonly have a chromosomal pattern of **46, XX** and are completely derived from the father. **Incomplete molar pregnancies,** which result when a normal ovum is fertilized by two sperm, most commonly have a chromosomal pattern of **69, XXY.** Malignant GTD consists of invasive moles (10–15% of GTD) and choriocarcinoma (2–5% of GTD). Risk factors for

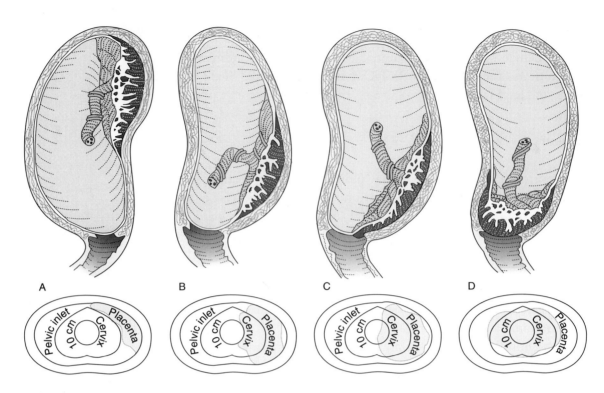

FIGURE 2.12–3. Placental implantation. (A) Normal placenta. (B) Low implantation. (C) Partial placenta previa. (D) Complete placenta previa.

GTD include extremes of age (< 20 or > 40), patients with **inadequate folate** or beta-carotene in their diet, and low socioeconomic status.

History/PE

Preeclampsia in the first trimester is pathognomonic for hydatidiform mole.

First-trimester **painless uterine bleeding, uterine size/date discrepancy,** preeclampsia, passage of molar vesicles, **hyperemesis gravidarum** (intractable nausea and vomiting), and hyperthyroidism. Pelvic examination may reveal bilaterally enlarged ovaries with bilateral theca lutein cysts.

Differential

Normal pregnancy, spontaneous abortion, threatened abortion, ectopic pregnancy, preeclampsia, placenta previa, placental abruption, multiple-gestation pregnancy.

Evaluation

Findings include **markedly elevated serum β-HCG** (usually > 100,000 mIU/mL) and **"snowstorm" appearance on pelvic ultrasound** with no fetus present.

TABLE 2.12–6. Abruptio Placentae Versus Placenta Previa.

	Abruptio Placentae	**Placenta Previa**
Pathophysiology	**Premature** (before the onset of labor) **separation** of normally implanted placenta.	**Abnormal implantation** of placenta **near or at the cervical os,** classified as: • Total: placenta covers cervical os • Partial: placenta partially covers os • Marginal: edge of placenta extends to margin of os • Low-lying: placenta within reach of the examining finger reached through the cervix
Incidence	1/100	1/200
Risk factors	**Hypertension, abdominal/pelvic trauma, tobacco or cocaine use.**	**Prior cesarean sections, grand multiparous.**
Symptoms	**Painful** vaginal bleeding (although in 10% of cases there is no bleeding); bleeding usually does not spontaneously cease. Abdominal pain, uterine hypertonicity. Fetal distress.	**Painless,** bright red bleeding (bleeding source is mom), with the first bleeding episode at 29–30 weeks' gestation. Bleeding often ceases in 1–2 hours with or without uterine contractions. Usually no fetal distress.
Diagnosis	Transabdominal/transvaginal ultrasound: look for retroplacental clot; can rule in diagnosis but cannot rule out.	**Transabdominal/transvaginal ultrasound:** look for abnormally positioned placenta; this test is very sensitive for the diagnosis.
Management	Stabilize patient with premature fetus; **expectant management** with continuous or frequent monitoring. **Moderate to severe abruption: immediate delivery** (vaginal delivery with amniotomy if fetal heart rate is stable; cesarean section if mom or fetus is in distress).	**NO vaginal exam!** **Stabilize patient with premature fetus;** bed rest. Tocolytics (magnesium sulfate). Serial ultrasound to assess fetal growth, resolution of partial previa. Amniocentesis to check fetal lung maturity; administer betamethasone to augment fetal lung maturity. Delivery by cesarean section or vaginal route depending on the lie of the placenta. **Delivery if persistent labor, blood loss of more than 500 mL, unstable bleeding requiring multiple transfusion, coagulation defects, documented fetal lung maturity, 36 weeks' gestational age.**
Complications	Hemorrhagic shock. Coagulopathy: DIC in 10% of all abruptions. Ischemic necrosis of distal organs. Recurrence risk is 5–16%; this risk increases to 25% after two previous abruptions. Fetal anemia.	Placenta accreta (up to 25% with one previous cesarean section). Vasa previa. Twofold increase in congenital abnormalities. Increased risk of postpartum hemorrhage. Fetal anemia.

HIGH-YIELD FACTS

Obstetrics

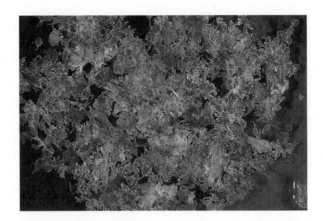

FIGURE 2.12–4. Hydatidiform mole. Note the characteristic "bunch of grapes" appearance on this gross specimen.

Treatment

Dilatation and curettage revealing "**cluster-of-grapes**" tissue (Figure 2.12–4); **chemotherapy** (methotrexate) with subsequent monitoring of β-HCG levels for malignant lesions; and **hysterectomy for invasive disease.**

Complications

Pulmonary metastases, trophoblastic pulmonary emboli, acute respiratory insufficiency.

LABOR STAGES

Table 2.12–7 and Figure 2.12–5 depict the normal stages of labor.

INDICATIONS FOR CESAREAN SECTION

Indications for performing cesarean section are as follows:

- Previous cesarean section (most common indication, but many women elect a trial of labor even if they have had a previous C-section)
- Cephalopelvic disproportion
- Placenta previa
- Placental abruption
- Fetal malposition (e.g., posterior chin position, transverse lie, brow presentation, shoulder presentation, compound presentation)
- Fetal distress
- Erythroblastosis fetalis (Rh incompatibility)
- Cord prolapse

TABLE 2.12–7. The Stages of Labor.

Stage	Starts/End	Events	Duration (hours)	
First			Nulli*	Multi**
Latent	Regular uterine contractions/cervix dilated to 4 cm	Highly variable duration, cervix effaces and slowly dilates	6–11	4–8
Active	4-cm cervical dilation/ complete cervical dilation (10 cm)	Regular and intense uterine contractions, cervix effaces and dilates more quickly, fetal head progressively descends into pelvis	4–6	2–3
Second	Complete cervical dilation/delivery of the baby	Baby undergoes all stages of cardinal movements	1–2	0.5–1
Third	Delivery of baby/ delivery of placenta	Placenta separates and uterus contracts to establish hemostasis	0–0.5	0–0.5

*Nulli = nulliparous (first-time mother)

**Multi = multiparous (pregnant and delivered before)

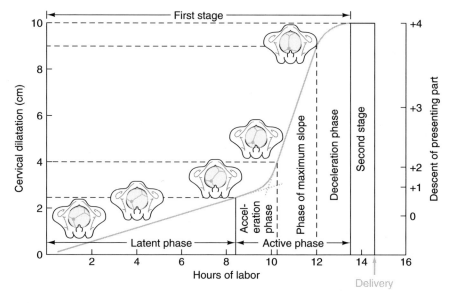

FIGURE 2.12–5. Stages of labor. Cervical dilatation, level of descent, and orientation of occipitoanterior presentation during various stages of labor.

- Carcinoma of the cervix
- Post-term pregnancy (relative indication)
- Cervical dystocia
- Failed operative vaginal delivery
- Active genital herpes infection
- Maternal trauma/demise

FETAL DISTRESS

During labor, the fetus can be monitored with an external fetal monitor, fetal scalp electrode, fetal scalp pH, and ultrasound. Normal fetal heart rate is 120–160 beats per minute. **Long-term variability** (external monitor), **beat-to-beat variability** (scalp monitor), and **transient accelerations** of the heart rate **are reassuring findings.** Decelerations are transient declines in the fetal heart rate in relation to a uterine contraction and may indicate fetal distress. They can be classified as indicated in Table 2.12–8.

TABLE 2.12–8. Fetal Heart Decelerations.

Fetal Deceleration	Description	Most Common Cause
Early deceleration	Decelerations begin and end at approximately the same time as the maternal contraction.	Cephalic compression (**no fetal distress**).
Variable deceleration	Decelerations occur at any time during the maternal contraction.	Umbilical cord compression. Change mother's position (e.g., back to side).
Late deceleration	Decelerations begin at the peak of the contraction and persist until the contraction has finished. Precipitated by hypoxemia.	Uteroplacental insufficiency, possibly due to abruption or hypotension. Further testing for fetal reassurance is necessary. If late decelerations are repetitious and severe, deliver the baby ASAP.

Table 2.12–9 summarizes the effects of some common teratogens.

TABLE 2.12–9. Birth Defects.

Teratogen	Effect
DES	Clear cell adenocarcinoma of the vagina/cervix; genital tract abnormalities
Thalidomide	Limb abnormalities (**phocomelia**) as well as auricle, eye, and visceral malformations
Amphetamines	Transposition of the great vessels, cleft palate
Ethanol	Fetal alcohol syndrome (microcephaly, mental retardation, facial abnormalities, limb dislocation, heart/lung fistulas)
Iodide	Congenital goiter, hypothyroidism, mental retardation
Tetracycline	Inhibition of bone growth, small limbs, syndactyly, discoloration of teeth
Fluoroquinolones	Cartilage damage
Aminoglycosides	Eighth-nerve damage, macromelia, multiple skeletal abnormalities
Sulfonamides	Kernicterus
Griseofulvin	Multiple anomalies
Isotretinoin	Multiple anomalies
Warfarin	Skeletal and facial abnormalities, mental retardation, stillbirth, IUGR
Phenytoin, carbamazepine	Multiple anomalies, including cleft lip/palate, hypoplasia of distal phalanges, and sacral teratomas (fetal anticonvulsive syndrome)
Valproic acid	Fetal anticonvulsive syndrome, neural tube defects
ACE inhibitors	Fetal renal damage

HIGH-YIELD FACTS

Obstetrics

Defined as a loss of > 500 mL of blood within the first 24 hours of delivery. Table 2.12–10 summarizes the management of postpartum hemorrhage. Complications include excessive blood loss and transfusion-related risks.

TABLE 2.12–10. Common Causes of Postpartum Hemorrhage.

	Uterine Atony	Genital Tract Trauma	Retained Placental Tissue
Risk factors	Overdistention of the uterus (multiple gestations, macrosomia) Abnormal labor (prolonged labor, precipitous labor) Conditions interfering with uterine contractions (uterine myomas, magnesium sulfate, general anesthesia) Uterine infection	Precipitous labor Operative vaginal delivery (forceps, vacuum extraction) Large infant Inadequate episiotomy repair	Placenta accreta/increta/pecreta Preterm delivery Placenta previa Previous cesarean section/ curettage Uterine leiomyomas
Diagnosis	Palpation of a softer, flaccid, "boggy" uterus without a firm fundus	Careful visualization of the lower genital tract looking for any laceration > 2 cm in length	Careful inspection of the placenta for missing cotyledons. Ultrasound may also be used to examine the uterus.
Treatment	**Most common cause of postpartum hemorrhage** (90%) Bimanual **uterine massage,** which is usually successful **Oxytocin** infusion Methylergonovine maleate (Methergine) if not hypertensive and/or prostaglandin F2-alpha if patient is not asthmatic or hypertensive	Surgical repair of the physical defect	Manual removal of the remaining placental tissue. Curettage with suctioning may also be used with care taken to avoid perforating the uterine fundus. In cases of true placenta accreta/increta/pecreta where the placental villi invade into the uterine tissue, hysterectomy is often required as a life-preserving therapy.

Gynecology

VAGINITIS

UCV *OB.1, 2, 27*

The vagina normally contains mixed bacterial flora in an acidic environment (pH 3.3–4.2) maintained by lactic acid–producing lactobacilli. A change in this acidic environment can lead to overgrowth of other bacterial species and hence to clinical infection. Bacterial vaginosis is a common vaginal infection that is most commonly caused by ***Gardnerella vaginalis***.

History/PE

Vulvovaginal pruritus with or without a burning sensation, odor, and increased vaginal discharge.

Differential

UTIs, STDs.

Workup

Obtain vaginal discharge slide smears with saline and KOH. A Gram stain of the vaginal discharge and chlamydia antigen tests should also be performed to rule out STDs. Also obtain a clean-catch urine culture and a UA to rule out UTI. Findings are noted in Table 2.13–1.

Treatment

See Table 2.13–1.

TABLE 2.13–1. Causes of Vaginitis.

Variable	Bacterial Vaginosis (usually *Gardnerella*)	*Trichomonas*	Yeast (usually *Candida*)
Relative frequency	50%	25%	25%
Discharge	Homogenous, grayish-white, watery, fishy and stale odor	Profuse, malodorous, yellow-green, frothy.	Thick, white, cottage cheese texture
Vaginal pH	> 4.5	> 4.5	Normal vaginal pH
Saline smear*	**Clue cells** (epithelial cells coated with bacteria; see Figure 2.13–1B)	**Motile trichomonads**	Nothing
KOH smear	Positive whiff test (**fishy smell**)	Positive whiff test	**Pseudohyphae** (See Figure 2.13–1A)
Treatment	Metronidazole**	Metronidazole** (**treat partner**; this is considered an STD)	Nystatin

*On saline smear, if you see lots of WBCs and no organism, suspect chlamydia.
**Patients taking metronidazole should not drink alcohol, which would lead to an Antabuse-like effect.

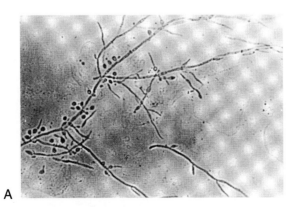

A

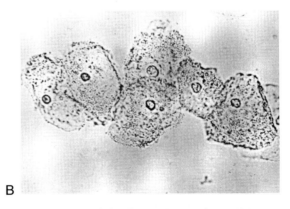

B

FIGURE 2.13–1. Causes of vaginitis. (A) Candidal vaginitis. Branched and budding *Candida albicans* are evident on KOH preparation of vaginal discharge. **(B)** *Gardnerella vaginalis*. Saline wet mount of vaginal fluid reveals granulations on vaginal epithelial cells ("clue cells") due to adherence of *G vaginalis* organisms to the cell surface.

STDs are among the most common outpatient/ER gynecologic complaints. All sexually active patients should be screened for STDs. Risk factors include multiple sexual partners, unprotected sexual intercourse, high frequency of sexual intercourse, high-risk behavior, young age at first intercourse, and unusual sexual practices. Twenty-five to fifty percent of patients with STDs have multiple genital tract infections.

Up to 50% of patients with STDs have multiple genital tract infections.

History/PE

Patients may be asymptomatic or may present with lesions or ulcerations in the vulvovaginal region, abnormal vaginal discharge, inguinal rashes, inguinal lymphadenopathy, or abdominal pain.

- **Syphilis:**
    - **Primary:** Painless genital ulceration **(chancre).**
    - **Secondary: Maculopapular rash on palms and soles;** fever, headache, and generalized lymphadenopathy; condylomata lata (mucous membrane lesions).
    - **Tertiary: Aortic aneurysms and aortic regurgitation;** granulomatous **gummas** of the CNS, heart, or great vessels.
- **Condylomata acuminata (venereal warts):** Painless, soft, fleshy, **"cauliflower-like"** lesions.
- **Gonorrhea:** Dysuria, urinary frequency, purulent yellow-green discharge. May progress to PID; high rate of coinfection with chlamydia.
- **Chlamydia:** Often asymptomatic, but may cause dysuria, cervicitis, PID, lymphogranuloma venereum, or infertility.
- **Herpes:** Paresthesias and burning followed by painful vesicles and ulcerations. In primary infections, patients may present with fever, malaise, and adenopathy. *IM2.19*

Differential

Candidiasis, UTIs.

Evaluation

Evaluation should include **cervical and urethral cultures** for chlamydia and gonorrhea, a **Tzanck smear** of suspicious lesions (for HSV), dark-field microscopy of suspicious lesions (for syphilis), VDRL/RPR (a rapid screening test for syphilis; nonspecific), and/or FTA-ABS (specific; diagnostic for syphilis), a chlamydia antigen test, and a **saline/KOH/Gram stain** of vaginal discharge. A UA and a clean-catch **urine culture** should also be obtained to rule out UTI. **Biopsy** suspicious lesions with 5% acetic acid staining (to detect condylomata acuminata).

FTA-ABS = Find **T**he **A**ntibody-**ABS**olutely.

1. Most specific
2. Earliest positive
3. Remains positive the longest

HIGH-YIELD FACTS

Gynecology

Treatment

Always treat patients for both gonorrhea and chlamydia (presume coinfection).

- **Primary/secondary/tertiary syphilis:** Penicillin.
- **Condylomata acuminata:** Podofilox, cryotherapy, biopsy.
- **Gonorrhea:** Ceftriaxone. Also treat for presumptive chlamydia coinfection.
- **Chlamydia:** Tetracycline/doxycycline. Azithromycin for cervicitis. Also treat for presumptive gonorrhea coinfection.
- **Herpes:** Acyclovir ointment during flare-up; oral acyclovir to decrease severity and rate of recurrence.

Complications

PID, coexisting STDs, recurrence, infertility, increased risk of **ectopic pregnancy,** chronic pelvic pain, **HIV,** systemic infection (e.g., gonococcal arthritis, tabes dorsalis), cervical cancer (associated with HPV subtypes 16, 18, 31, and 33).

PELVIC INFLAMMATORY DISEASE (PID)   UCV OB.18

Use of OCPs and barrier contraception decreases the incidence of PID.

Ascending genital tract infection secondary to cervical and/or vaginal infection. Causes of PID include *Neisseria gonorrhoeae, Chlamydia trachomatis,* and aerobic/anaerobic bacteria. Risk factors include multiple sexual partners, unprotected sexual intercourse, high frequency of sexual intercourse, high-risk behavior, young age at first intercourse, unusual sexual practices, and IUD use. Use of OCPs and barrier contraception decreases the incidence of PID.

History

One- to three-day history of **lower abdominal pain** with or without fever, **vaginal discharge, recent menses,** history of sexual exposure, or a past history of PID. Patients often believe they have appendicitis (especially if pain is right-sided).

PE

"Chandelier sign": severe CMT on exam that makes the patient "jump for the chandelier."

Lower **abdominal tenderness, cervical motion tenderness (CMT), adnexal tenderness,** and/or purulent cervical discharge.

Differential

Ectopic pregnancy, endometriosis, ovarian tumors, hemorrhagic ovarian cyst, appendicitis, UTI, diverticulitis.

Evaluation

The diagnosis of PID requires the presence of the above clinical findings along with **leukocytosis** (WBC > 10,000). Obtain β-**HCG** (to check pregnancy status) and Gram stain/cultures of the cervical discharge. Consider RPR/VDRL, HIV serology, and hepatitis serology. For definitive diagnosis, consider ultrasound, culdocentesis, and/or laparoscopy.

Treatment

Antibiotic treatment should address the most common pathogens (e.g., *N. gonorrhoeae*, *C. trachomatis*, and anaerobes).

- **Inpatient IV antibiotic regimen:** Cefoxitin and doxycycline.
- **Outpatient antibiotic regimen:** Ceftriaxone and doxycycline for 2–4 weeks.

Complications

Tubo-ovarian abscess, which requires hospitalization for IV antibiotics and possible surgical intervention. Ectopic pregnancy, chronic pelvic pain, infertility, recurrence, perihepatitis (inflammation of the liver capsule; Fitz–Hugh–Curtis syndrome).

CONTRACEPTIVES

Table 2.13–2 describes various methods of contraception.

AMENORRHEA UCV *OB.22, 23, 24, 25*

Amenorrhea is defined as the absence of menstruation. **Primary amenorrhea** is the absence of menses and the lack of secondary sexual characteristics by age 14 or the absence of menses by age 16 with or without secondary sexual characteristics. **Secondary amenorrhea** is the absence of menses for three cycles or for six months with prior normal menses.

History/PE

Absence of menstruation (see above).

Differential

The causes of primary amenorrhea include gonadal failure/agenesis (e.g., Turner's syndrome), müllerian duct abnormality, androgen insensitivity syndrome, hypopituitary failure, and constitutional developmental delay. The causes of secondary amenorrhea include pregnancy (most common), hyper- or hypothyroidism, polycystic ovarian syndrome, premature menopause, hypothalamic/pituitary failure (e.g., Sheehan's syndrome, Kallmann's syndrome), hyperprolactinemia (galactorrhea), and anorexia nervosa.

TABLE 2.13–2. Contraceptive Methods.

Method	Description	Side Effects
Rhythm	Uses body temperature and cervical mucus consistency to predict the time of fertility.	None, but method not very effective.
OCPs	Suppress ovulation by inhibiting FSH/LH; changing the consistency of cervical mucus makes the endometrium unsuitable for implantation.	Nausea, weight gain, breast tenderness, headache, acne, mood changes, hypertension, hepatic adenoma, post-pill amenorrhea, and increased incidence of DVT (but protective effects against PID and ovarian and endometrial cancer).
Levonorgestrel (Norplant)	Progestin-only subdermal implant that inhibits ovulation by suppressing LH peak. Contraceptive effects last for five years.	Irregular vaginal bleeding, weight gain, galactorrhea, acne, breast tenderness.
Medroxyprogesterone (Depo-Provera)	Intramuscular injection of medroxyprogesterone acetate given every three months, which suppresses ovulation by suppressing LH.	Irregular vaginal bleeding, weight gain, galactorrhea, acne, breast tenderness, mood changes, hair loss.
IUD	Causes local sterile inflammatory reaction within the wall of the uterus that prevents implantation.	Increased vaginal bleeding, uterine perforation, infection, increased risk of PID and ectopic pregnancy, IUD migration.
Barrier methods (e.g., condoms, diaphragms, spermicides, sponges)	Physically block entrance of sperm into the uterine cavity. Protective effects against PID, STDs, and cervical cancer.	Very few (possible allergic reactions to latex or spermicides).
Surgical sterilization (e.g., tubal ligation, vasectomy) OB.50	Tubes are ligated, cauterized, or mechanically occluded.	Essentially irreversible; bleeding, infection, failure, ectopic pregnancy.

Evaluation

Always rule out pregnancy in a patient with amenorrhea.

Evaluation begins with β-HCG (to rule out pregnancy) and prolactin; TSH in cases of hyperprolactinemia; gynecologic examination and imaging studies (to rule out genital tract outflow obstruction); and serum LH/FSH, baseline and with progestin challenge to localize ovarian–pituitary–hypothalamic axis dysfunction (see Figures 2.13–2 to 2.13–4).

Treatment

Treat the underlying cause.

HIGH-YIELD FACTS

Gynecology

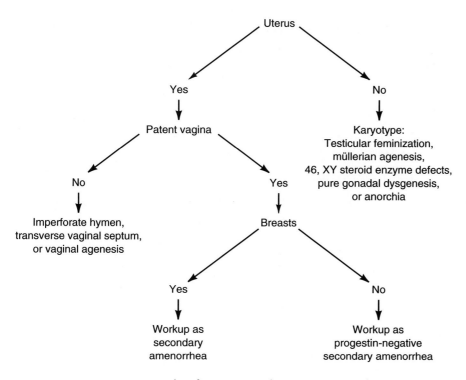

FIGURE 2.13–2. Workup for patients with primary amenorrhea.

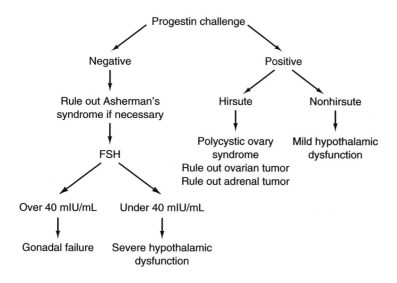

FIGURE 2.13–3. Workup for patients with secondary amenorrhea without hyperprolactine-mia.

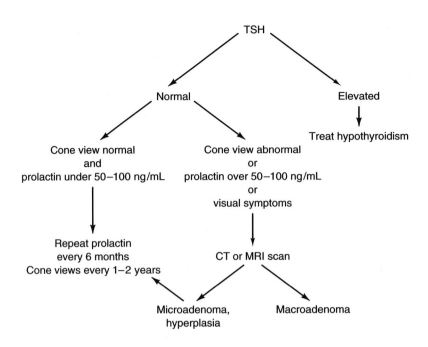

FIGURE 2.13–4. Workup for patients with secondary amenorrhea with hyperprolactinemia.

Abnormal uterine bleeding can be of many types, including menorrhagia (excessive or prolonged menses), metrorrhagia (irregularity), menometrorrhagia (irregular, prolonged, heavy menstrual bleeding), polymenorrhea (increased frequency of menstruation), or oligomenorrhea (scanty menstruation). The most common cause of postmenopausal vaginal bleeding is **atrophic vaginitis.**

History/PE

Uterine bleeding is considered abnormal if any of the following are present:

- Menstrual flow lasting > 8 days.
- A menstrual interval of < 21 days.
- Total blood loss/menstrual cycle > 80 mL.

Differential

Any postmenopausal woman with uterine bleeding requires an endometrial biopsy to rule out endometrial cancer.

Threatened abortion, ectopic pregnancy, endometriosis, trauma, **endometrial cancer,** atrophic vaginitis, ruptured ovarian cyst, blood dyscrasias.

Evaluation

Laboratory tests include β-HCG (to rule out pregnancy), CBC, coagulation studies, and endocrine tests (serum TSH/prolactin/FSH/LH). Perform endometrial biopsy on postmenopausal women.

Treatment

Anovulatory bleeding can be treated with hormone replacement therapy. **Women with regular menses are ovulating.** Dysfunctional uterine bleeding can be treated with **OCPs.** Patients with severe, uncontrollable uterine bleeding may require dilatation and curettage with **endometrial ablation.** Vaginal packing and uterine artery ligation may be necessary. **Hysterectomy** may be performed as a last resort.

ENDOMETRIOSIS

Defined as the presence of endometrial glands and stroma outside the uterus. The most common sites of endometriosis are the ovaries, broad ligament, and cul de sac. Proposed etiologies include direct implantation of endometrial cells by retrograde menstruation, vascular and lymphatic dissemination of endometrial cells, and metaplasia within the peritoneal cavity. Risk factors include positive family history, nulliparity, and infertility.

History/PE

Dysmenorrhea, **dyschezia** (painful defecation), **chronic pelvic pain, dyspareunia** (painful intercourse), abnormal bleeding, and/or **infertility.** Pelvic examination may reveal nodular thickening along the uterosacral ligament, a fixed, retroverted uterus, and/or tender, fixed adnexal masses.

Endometriosis is the most common cause of infertility.

Differential

PID, pelvic adhesions, ectopic pregnancy, appendicitis, adnexal torsion, ruptured corpus luteal cyst, primary/secondary amenorrhea, endometrioma.

Evaluation

Definitive diagnosis can be made by **laparoscopic examination**/biopsy, which will reveal functioning endometrial glands or **"chocolate cysts."** Laboratory tests include β-HCG, UA, and ultrasound (may reveal endometriomas).

Treatment

Medical options include OCPs, progestin, danazol, and GnRH agonists. Surgical options include **laparoscopic ablation** or **total abdominal hysterectomy** with lysis of adhesions in patients with severe, recurrent disease.

The most **common** benign gynecologic lesion, also known as uterine fibroids. More common in black women and those > 35 years of age. Leiomyomas can change in size with the menstrual cycle but usually regress after menopause.

History

Asymptomatic or may present with dysmenorrhea, abdominal pain, menorrhagia (excessive uterine bleeding), metrorrhagia (irregular uterine bleeding), anemia, infertility, or urinary frequency.

PE

Firm, irregular, palpable uterine mass on pelvic examination.

Differential

Cervical or endometrial carcinoma, leiomyosarcoma, pregnancy, ovarian carcinoma, endometriosis, adenomyosis.

If a uterine mass continues to grow after menopause, it is not a leiomyoma.

Evaluation

The condition can usually be diagnosed by **ultrasound.**

Treatment

- Can be followed with **ultrasound.**
- If symptoms worsen, the lesion can be **resected.**
- Rarely, a myoma resected for symptomatic relief turns out to be a leiomyosarcoma, an aggressive tumor that is usually not responsive to therapy.
- Leiomyomas stop growing after menopause.

Also known as Stein–Leventhal syndrome, polycystic ovarian syndrome affects **women aged 15–30,** resulting in amenorrhea and infertility. Its exact etiology is unknown, but it is thought to involve a disorder of the hypothalamic–pituitary axis.

History

Hirsutism, amenorrhea/oligomenorrhea, **obesity,** and **infertility.**

PE

Bilaterally enlarged ovaries are found on bimanual exam.

Differential

Androgen-secreting ovarian tumor, endometriosis, adrenal tumor, Cushing's syndrome, congenital adrenal hyperplasia.

Evaluation

Findings include a **serum LH:FSH ratio > 3** and **increased serum androstenedione and DHEA.** Ultrasound shows bilaterally enlarged ovaries with numerous large subcapsular cysts.

Treatment

Treatment consists of **weight reduction, clomiphene citrate** (induces ovulation and may result in multiple pregnancies), and **OCPs.**

Complications

Infertility, increased risk of endometrial cancer (secondary to unopposed estrogen stimulation).

MENOPAUSE   **UCV** OB.15

The permanent cessation of menstruation secondary to end-organ ovarian resistance to gonadotropins. The mean age of onset of menopause in U.S. women is 50–51 years. Premature menopause is the cessation of menstruation before **age 40** and is often secondary to idiopathic premature ovarian failure. Early menopause is frequently associated with **cigarette smoking.** Postmenopausal women lose the protective effects of estrogen and are thus at increased risk of developing **osteoporosis** and **heart disease.**

History/PE

Menstrual symptoms (e.g., menorrhagia, polymenorrhea, oligomenorrhea, amenorrhea), **hot flashes** (secondary to vasomotor instability), **sweats,** sleep disturbances, **mood changes,** depression, dyspareunia (secondary to vaginal wall atrophy), cystocele, urinary frequency/incontinence, and **dysuria.**

Differential

Premature ovarian failure.

> Menopause causes
> **HAVOC:**
> **H**ot flashes
> **A**trophy of the
> **V**agina
> **O**steoporosis
> **C**oronary artery
>   disease

Evaluation

Elevated serum FSH is diagnostic.

Treatment

Treatment consists of **hormone replacement therapy** with opposed (if the patient still has her uterus) or unopposed (if the patient has undergone TAH/BSO) estrogen therapy.

Complications

Osteoporosis, atrophic vaginitis, **heart disease.**

Endometriosis is the most common cause of female infertility followed by PID.

Failure on the part of a couple to achieve pregnancy after **repeated attempts over a 12-month period.** Infertility can be classified into four etiologies: male dysfunction (30–40%), ovulatory problems (15–20%), pelvic factor (30%), and cervical factor (5%). In approximately 5–20% of cases, the cause of infertility is unknown.

History/PE

Look for signs of endocrine dysfunction (e.g., hirsutism, acne, galactorrhea). Look for varicoceles in males.

Differential

Ovulatory dysfunction (e.g., ovarian failure, prolactinoma), genital tract damage/scarring (endometriosis, PID, Asherman's syndrome), defects in spermatogenesis, varicoceles (interfere with normal sperm development).

Evaluation

Evaluation includes semen analysis, postcoital test (assess cervical mucus), daily basal body temperature measurements (verify ovulation), endometrial biopsy, serum FSH/LH/midcycle progesterone/prolactin (to rule out endocrine dysfunction) and hysterosalpingogram (to rule out tubal disease and uterine cavity abnormalities). Assess cervical mucus for antisperm antibodies.

Treatment

Treat the underlying cause. **In vitro fertilization** may be the best option if other treatments fail.

Pediatrics

VENTRICULAR SEPTAL DEFECT (VSD) UCV Ped.3

A congenital "hole" in the ventricular septum that causes symptoms which depend on the degree of **left-to-right** shunting. VSD can be membranous, perimembranous, or muscular (the last two often close spontaneously). VSDs are seen in tetralogy of Fallot, Apert's syndrome, Down's syndrome, cri-du-chat syndrome, and trisomy 13/18. VSD is the most common congenital heart defect.

VSD is the most common congenital heart defect.

History

Usually **asymptomatic** at birth if the "hole" is small. Frequent respiratory infections, failure to thrive, dyspnea, exercise intolerance, shortness of breath from pulmonary edema, and other symptoms of cardiac failure may be seen in severe cases.

PE

Pansystolic murmur at the lower left sternal border, loud pulmonic S_2, systolic thrill (if severe), cardiomegaly (if severe), and crackles (if severe).

Distinguish VSD from ASD by ASD's fixed, split S_2.

Differential

Mitral regurgitation, aortic stenosis, cardiomyopathy, other congenital heart defects (including VSD as part of tetralogy of Fallot).

Evaluation

Diagnosis is made by clinical presentation and **echocardiogram.** EKG may show RVH or LVH. EKG is normal in patients with small VSDs.

Treatment

- Follow small VSDs, since most will close spontaneously.
- Surgically repair large VSDs (or VSDs in patients with Down's syndrome) as soon as possible to prevent pulmonary vascular disease and heart failure.
- If a VSD remains open, Eisenmenger's syndrome may develop. Eisenmenger's syndrome is characterized by pulmonary vascular hyperplasia and consequent pulmonary hypertension that leads to right heart failure (cor pulmonale) and shunt reversal. Eisenmenger's syndrome presents as cyanosis, is often **irreversible,** and renders the patient inoperable.
- Patients with patent VSDs are at increased risk for **endocarditis** and septic emboli.
- Treat post-MI VSD in adults with nitroprusside (reduces afterload) and intra-aortic balloon pump as a bridge to surgical repair.

Eisenmenger's syndrome: L → R shunt causes pulmonary hypertension and shunt reversal.

PATENT DUCTUS ARTERIOSUS (PDA) · UCV *Ped.1*

Failure of the ductus arteriosus to close within the first few days of life. Risk factors include prematurity, high altitude (low O_2 tension), and maternal first trimester rubella infection. It is more common in females and preterm infants.

History

Asymptomatic or may present with symptoms of heart failure, lower extremity clubbing, and dyspnea.

**L → R shunts—
The 3 D's:**
VS**D**
AS**D**
P**D**A

PE

Wide pulse pressure, a continuous **"machinery" murmur** at the second intercostal space on the left upper sternal border, loud S_2, and bounding peripheral pulses.

Differential

Aortopulmonary window, truncus arteriosus, mitral regurgitation, VSD, aortic stenosis, Eisenmenger's syndrome.

Evaluation

Diagnosis is made by echocardiography. EKG may show LVH.

Treatment

- Treat with **indomethacin** unless the PDA is necessary for survival (transposition of the great vessels).
- If indomethacin fails or if a child is > 6–8 months old, surgical closure is preferred.

274

A condition in which the pulmonary and systemic circulations exist in **parallel:** the aorta is connected to the right ventricle and the pulmonary artery to the left ventricle. Risk factors include Apert's syndrome, Down's syndrome, cri-du-chat syndrome, and trisomy 13/18.

History

Patients present with **cyanosis** and are **critically ill.** The condition is fatal without correction unless the patient has a PDA or VSD.

PE

Cyanosis, tachypnea, and progressive respiratory failure.

Differential

Large VSD, aortic coarctation, tetralogy of Fallot, hypoplastic left ventricle.

Evaluation

Echocardiography.

Treatment

- Keep the ductus open with **prostaglandin E_1 (PGE_1).**
- **Balloon atrial septostomy** if immediate surgery is not feasible.
- **Surgical correction** (arterial or atrial switch).

In transposition of the great vessels, a PDA or VSD is required for mixing of pulmonary and systemic blood flow (required for survival).

R → L Shunts—

The 5 T's:
Tetralogy
Transposition
Truncus arteriosus
Tricuspid atresia
Total anomalous pulmonary venous return

HIGH-YIELD FACTS

Pediatrics

VSD, right ventricular outflow obstruction, RVH, and anteriorly overriding aorta. Early cyanosis results from right-to-left shunting across the VSD. Risk factors include Down's syndrome, cri-du-chat syndrome, and trisomy 13/18.

History

Patients present during infancy with **cyanosis** and **dyspnea.** Children often **squat for relief ("tet spells").** They may have dyspnea on exertion, failure to thrive, fatigue, and mental status changes.

PE

Systolic ejection murmur at the left sternal border, **RV lift,** and single second heart sound.

Tetralogy of Fallot—

PROVe
Pulmonary stenosis
RVH
Overriding aorta
VSD

275

Differential

Tricuspid or pulmonary atresia, transposition of the great vessels, hypoplastic left heart syndrome, PDA.

Evaluation

Echocardiography and catheterization. CXR shows a **"boot-shaped" heart.** EKG shows right-axis deviation and RVH.

Treatment

- Administer **PGE$_1$** to keep the ductus arteriosus patent.
- Treat cyanotic spells with oxygen, propranolol, knee-chest position, fluids, and morphine.
- **Surgical correction.** Temporary palliation can be achieved through the creation of an artificial shunt (e.g., balloon atrial septostomy).
- There is an increased risk of arrhythmia even after correction.
- Prognosis depends on the degree of pulmonary stenosis.

COARCTATION OF THE AORTA
UCV *Surg.2*

Constriction of the aorta leading to decreased flow below the coarctation and increased flow above it (to the upper extremities). **Turner's syndrome** is a risk factor, and males are affected more frequently than females.

History

Patients often present during childhood with asymptomatic hypertension. Dyspnea on exertion, syncope, claudication, epistaxis, and headache may be present.

PE

Higher systolic BP in the upper extremities than in the lower extremities, decreased femoral and distal pulses, a late systolic murmur (heard in the left axilla), and forceful apical impulses. BP in the right arm may be greater than that in the left arm depending on the location of the coarctation.

Differential

Primary hypertension, pheochromocytoma, aortic stenosis, renal artery stenosis, renal disease, Cushing's syndrome, hyperaldosteronism.

Coarctation of the aorta is a cause of secondary hypertension.

In advanced cases of coarctation, patients may have a well-developed upper body and lower-extremity wasting.

Pediatrics

Evaluation

Perform EKG (LVH), echocardiography, and possibly MRI. Diagnosis can be made by cardiac catheterization (aortography). CXR may reveal a **"reverse 3 sign"** due to pre- and post-dilatation of the coarct segment as well as **"rib notching"** due to collateral circulation through the intercostal arteries.

Treatment

- **Surgical correction** is often only partially successful and does not correct the intercostal aneurysms that result from long-standing coarctation.
- **Balloon angioplasty** is an alternative to surgical repair.
- Continue **endocarditis prophylaxis** even after treatment.
- **Initiate repair** as **early** as possible given the risks of heart failure, premature CAD, and intracerebral hemorrhage.
- Twenty-five percent of patients continue to have hypertension after repair.

FAILURE TO THRIVE (FTT)

There is no standard definition for failure to thrive; it refers to an infant or child whose weight or weight gain is significantly below that of children of similar age and the same sex (Table 2.14–1). Risk factors include chronic illness, low socioeconomic status, low maternal age, chaotic family situation, CF and other genetic diseases, and inborn errors of metabolism. Infants born with HIV comprise an increasing number of cases of FTT.

TABLE 2.14–1. Definitions of Failure to Thrive.

Attained growth
- Weight < 3rd percentile on NCHS* growth chart
- Weight for height < 5th percentile on NCHS growth chart
- Weight 20% or more below ideal weight for height
- Triceps skin-fold thickness ≤ 5 mm

Rate of growth
- Depressed rate of weight gain
    - < 20 g/day from 0–3 months of age
    - < 15 g/day from 3–6 months of age
- Falloff from previously established growth curve:
    - downward crossing of ≥ 2 major percentiles on NCHS growth charts
- Documented weight loss

*NCHS = National Center for Health Statistics.

History

Patients are of **low weight for their age and height** and exhibit little or no weight gain or even weight loss. Note caloric intake and parent-child interaction.

PE

Plot height and weight on a standardized chart and compare the values to the population norms; look for signs of systemic disease.

Differential

The differential is vast **(often no organic cause is identified)** and includes poverty, inadequate breast feeding, improper feeding, mechanical GI dysfunction, structural abnormalities (e.g., pyloric stenosis, intestinal atresia), infection, endocrine disease, congenital heart disease, lung disease, and neurologic disorders.

Evaluation

Evaluation should include CBC, electrolytes, creatinine, albumin, total protein, sweat test, UA/culture, stool ova and parasites, and assessment of bone age. Take a careful diet history including calorie count.

Treatment

Treatment depends on cause.

- **Reassure and educate** parents if no cause is found.
- Encourage **nutritional supplementation** if breast feeding is inadequate (a common cause of early FTT is poorly managed mammary engorgement). Keep a calorie count.
- **Hospitalize** the patient if there is evidence of neglect or severe malnourishment.

Hospitalize children if there is evidence of neglect or severe malnourishment.

INTUSSUSCEPTION   UCV *EM.16*

The telescoping of a segment of bowel into itself, usually proximal to the ileocecal valve (Figure 2.14–1). Intussusception is the **most common cause of bowel obstruction in the first two years of life** and affects males more than females. Risk factors include Meckel's diverticulum, intestinal lymphoma, Henoch–Schönlein purpura, and adenovirus infection.

Intussusception is the most common cause of bowel obstruction in the first two years of life.

History

Abrupt-onset abdominal pain in apparently healthy children. The pain is often **colicky** in nature and is accompanied by emesis and bloody mucus in the stool (**"currant jelly" stool**).

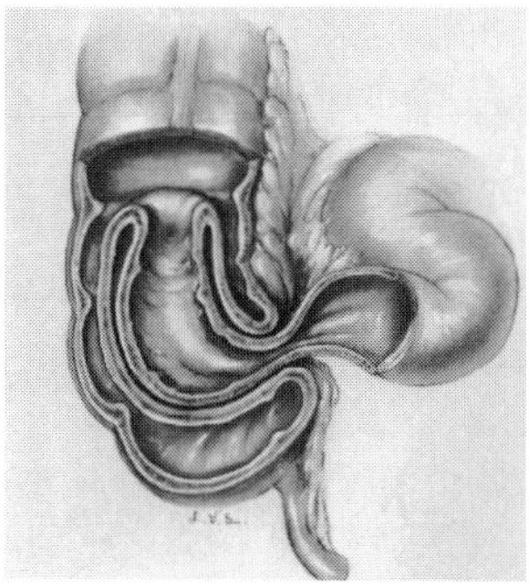

PE

Abdominal tenderness, positive stool guaiac, and pallor/diaphoresis. A **"sausage-shaped" abdominal mass** may be palpated.

Differential

Meckel's diverticulum, constipation, lymphoma (children > 6 years), GI infection, and meconium ileus (neonates).

Evaluation

CBC (leukocytosis), air contrast enema (if clinically stable), abdominal plain films, and ultrasound.

Treatment

- Correct volume/electrolyte abnormalities.
- **Air contrast enema** is diagnostic and often curative. If the child is not stable or if enema reduction is unsuccessful, proceed to **surgical reduction** and resection of gangrenous bowel.
- The appendix is usually removed during surgery to prevent future confusion.

FIGURE 2.14–1. Intussusception. A segment of bowel telescopes into an adjacent segment, causing obstruction.

Air contrast enema is both diagnostic and curative for intussusception.

NEONATAL JAUNDICE

Jaundice in the first day of life is not physiologic. "Physiologic" jaundice is jaundice after the first day of life and within 3–5 days of birth; bilirubin commonly rises to 9 mg/dL and then slowly falls. If bilirubin levels rise more quickly or to a higher level, infants need treatment and a search for a cause. **Kernicterus** results from the irreversible deposition of bilirubin in the basal ganglia, pons, and cerebellum; it occurs with bilirubin levels of > 20 mg/dL and is potentially fatal.

Direct hyperbilirubinemia is never physiologic.

History/PE

Neonates may be jaundiced with bilirubin levels > 5 mg/dL. Search for signs of infection, congenital malformations, cephalohematomas, and hepatomegaly. Note history of maternal-fetal ABO or Rh incompatibilities.

Differential

Physiologic jaundice, breast milk jaundice, breast-feeding jaundice, Crigler–Najjar syndrome, Gilbert's syndrome, hemolysis, neonatal hepatitis, biliary atresia, alpha-1-antitrypsin deficiency, infections, metabolic disorders, and hypothyroidism.

Evaluation

A jaundiced neonate with abnormal vital signs requires a full septic workup.

Assess direct (conjugated) and indirect (unconjugated) bilirubin levels. If indirect (but not direct) bilirubin is elevated, check blood smear **(hemolysis).** Coombs' test distinguishes between immune-mediated disorders (ABO incompatibility) and non-immune-mediated hemolytic disorders (G6PD deficiency, hereditary spherocytosis). If direct bilirubin is elevated, check liver enzymes, alkaline phosphatase, bile acids, sweat test, and tests for aminoacidopathies and alpha-1-antitrypsin deficiency. Blood cultures are warranted, and a jaundiced neonate who is febrile, hypotensive, and/or tachypneic needs a full septic workup and ICU monitoring.

Treatment

- Treat infectious causes (e.g., TORCHES) with appropriate therapy.
- If bilirubin rises above 15–20 mg/dL (regardless of cause), initiate **phototherapy.** In severe cases, **exchange transfusion** may be used.

MECKEL'S DIVERTICULUM
UCV Ped.7

Meckel's diverticulum—

Rule of 2's:
- Males are affected **2** times as often as females
- Symptomatic before **2** years of age
- **2** cm long
- **2** feet proximal to ileocecal valve
- **2** types of ectopic tissue (gastric or pancreatic)
- **2**% of the population

A remnant of the omphalomesenteric duct that can contain ectopic (usually gastric or pancreatic) mucosa. Meckel's diverticulum affects 1–3% of the population and conforms to the **"rule of 2's"** (see sidebar).

History

Often asymptomatic and noted incidentally during surgery. Patients may present with **painless rectal bleeding,** intussusception, peptic perforation, diverticulitis, fistula, obstruction, or abscess.

PE

Usually **unremarkable.** Possible physical findings include rectal bleeding, abdominal pain secondary to obstruction from intussusception, purulent or other discharge from the umbilicus, and umbilical cellulitis.

Differential

Omphalomesenteric fistula, enterocystoma, umbilical sinus, other GI structural abnormalities.

Evaluation

Evaluation should include a **technetium radionuclide scan** (detects ectopic gastric mucosa). The condition is rarely seen on barium studies.

Meckel's diverticulum is rarely seen on barium studies.

Treatment

- Hydrate/transfuse as needed.
- Perform **surgical exploration if symptomatic. Resection** of bowel may be required depending on the location and complexity of the lesion.

PYLORIC STENOSIS
UC**V** *Ped.41*

Hypertrophy of the pyloric sphincter causing gastric outlet obstruction. Males are most often affected. Incidence is 1 in 500 births.

History

Nonbilious emesis progressing to **projectile emesis** in the **first two weeks to four months of life.** Babies feed well initially but eventually suffer from malnutrition and dehydration.

PE

Palpable **epigastric olive-shaped mass** or visible gastric peristaltic waves.

Differential

Hiatal hernia, duodenal atresia ("double bubble sign"), malrotation/volvulus, meconium ileus, GERD, gastroenteritis.

Evaluation

Obtain plain abdominal films and electrolytes (look for hypokalemia and metabolic alkalosis secondary to emesis). Barium studies may reveal a narrow pyloric channel **("string sign")** or a **pyloric beak.** Abdominal ultrasound may reveal the hypertrophic pylorus.

Treatment

- Correct dehydration and electrolyte abnormalities.
- **Surgical correction** (pyloromyotomy).

HIGH-YIELD FACTS

Pediatrics

A spectrum of conditions characterized by varying displacement of the proximal femur from the acetabulum. Congenital hip dislocations are seen more often in **females, firstborn children,** and **breech presentations.** The hip may be subluxed, dislocatable, or dislocated. Dislocations typically result from poor development of the acetabulum and hip due to **excessive uterine packing** (e.g., breech presentation), which causes excessive stretching of the posterior hip capsule and adductor muscle contracture. The deformity will progress if it is not corrected.

History/PE

Perform Ortolani's and Barlow's maneuvers on all newborns.

- **Barlow's maneuver:** Pressure is placed on the inner aspect of the thigh while the hip is abducted, causing posterior dislocation.
- **Ortolani's maneuver:** The thighs are gently abducted from the midline with anterior pressure on the greater trochanter. The greater trochanter is displaced anteriorly and produces a **soft click.**
- **Trendelenburg's sign:** A dip of the pelvis to the opposite side when the patient stands on the affected leg. With bilateral involvement, the patient may have a waddling gait.
- **Allis' (Galeazzi's) sign:** The knees are at unequal heights when the hips and knees are flexed (the dislocated side is lower).

Additional signs include asymmetric skin folds and limited abduction of the affected hip secondary to adductor contracture.

Evaluation

Evaluation is clinical, although ultrasound may help. X-rays are unreliable until the patient is at least four months old.

Treatment

Treat congenital hip dislocation early for the best results.

Splint with a **Pavlik harness** (maintains hip flexed and abducted) within the first four months of life. Delayed treatment is possible before two years of age by closed or open reduction of the hip, but the benefits of treatment diminish with time.

Complications

Joint contractures, dysplasia of the femoral head and acetabulum.

SLIPPED CAPITAL FEMORAL EPIPHYSIS (SCFE)

Separation of the proximal femoral epiphysis through the growth plate such that the femoral head is displaced medially and posteriorly to the femoral neck.

HIGH-YIELD FACTS

Pediatrics

SCFE occurs most commonly in **adolescent** (11- to 13-year-old), **obese African-American males.** Its etiology is not known. The condition is bilateral in about 30% of cases.

History

Thigh or **knee pain** and a **limp.**

PE

Limitation of internal rotation and abduction of the hip along with hip tenderness. Flexion of the hip leads to an **obligatory external rotation** secondary to physical displacement.

Evaluation

Radiographs of both hips in anteroposterior and frog-leg lateral views show **posterior and medial displacement** of the femoral head (Figure 2.14–2).

Patients may complain of knee and thigh pain instead of hip pain.

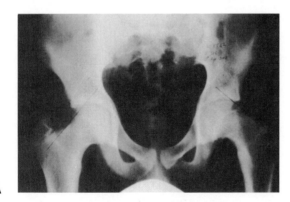

A

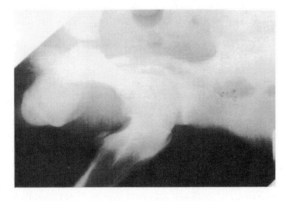

B

FIGURE 2.14–2. Slipped capital femoral epiphysis. (A) Anteroposterior x-ray. The medial displacement of the left femoral epiphysis is best seen with a line drawn up the lateral femoral neck. The abnormal epiphysis does not protrude beyond this line. (B) Frog-leg lateral x-ray. Posterior displacement of the femoral epiphysis is characteristic.

Treatment

- Prompt **surgical treatment** is warranted with fixing of the slip into the correct anatomic position (in situ screw fixation).
- **Gentle closed reduction** is warranted only in acute slips.
- Avascular necrosis results in 30% of uncorrected cases.
- Patients are at risk of developing premature degenerative arthritis.

Nonmigratory mono/polyarthropathy that occurs during childhood and lasts for at least three months. In 95% of cases, the disease resolves by puberty.

History/PE

- **Acute febrile:** Fevers, an **evanescent salmon-colored rash,** arthritis, and hepatosplenomegaly.
- **Polyarticular:** Multiple, inflamed, symmetrically involved joints (resembles adult RA). Systemic features are less prominent; patients may develop iridocyclitis.
- **Pauciarticular:** Chronic arthritis frequently involving weight-bearing joints. Up to 30% will develop insidious **iridocyclitis,** which may cause blindness if untreated.
- All three patterns may be accompanied by **fever, nodules, erythematous rashes, pericarditis,** and **fatigue.**

Differential

Trauma, reactive arthritis, septic arthritis.

Evaluation

There is no diagnostic test for JRA. Rheumatoid factor is positive in 15% of cases. A normal ESR does not exclude the diagnosis. Imaging may show soft tissue swelling and regional osteoporosis.

Treatment

Treat with **NSAIDs** and range-of-motion and **strengthening exercises.** Methotrexate is used as a second-line agent. Monitor for iridocyclitis with routine ophthalmologic examinations.

Complications

Iridocyclitis (most commonly seen in pauciarticular JRA) may lead to blindness if left untreated.

Table 2.14–2 describes common pediatric orthopedic injuries.

TABLE 2.14–2. Orthopedic Injuries in Children.

Fracture	Characteristics	Treatment
Clavicular fracture	The most frequently fractured long bone in children. Often occurs during athletic activity. May be birth related (especially in large infants) and can be associated with brachial nerve palsies. Fractures usually involve the **middle third of the clavicle,** with the proximal fracture end displaced superiorly due to pull of the sterno-cleidomastoid muscle.	Figure-of-eight sling vs. arm sling.
Greenstick fracture	Incomplete fracture involving the cortex of only one side of a bone.	Reduction with casting. Films should be obtained at 7–10 days to assess for adequate reduction.
Nursemaid's elbow	Radial head subluxation. Typically occurs as a result of being **pulled or lifted by the hand.** The child complains of pain and **will not bend the elbow.**	**Manual reduction by gentle supination of the elbow at 90 degrees of flexion.** No immobilization is necessary.
Torus fracture	Buckling of the cortex of a long bone secondary to trauma. Usually occurs in the distal radius or ulna.	Cast immobilization for 3–5 weeks.
Supracondylar humeral fracture	Tends to occur between the ages of 5 and 8. Dangerous because of proximity to **brachial artery.**	Closed reduction with percutaneous pinning. Beware of **Volkmann's ischemic contracture.**

CHILD ABUSE

UCV *Ped.53, Psych.10*

Includes physical abuse, sexual abuse, emotional abuse, neglect, and, rarely, Münchausen's syndrome by proxy. The diagnosis of physical abuse is based on a **discordant history and physical findings.** Red flags should go off if the mechanism of injury described by a caretaker does not correlate with physical findings.

Red flags should rise if the caretaker's story does not match the child's injury.

History

Pain, swelling, and multiple ecchymoses. Infants may present with irritability and failure to thrive. Evidence of neglect (poor hygiene) may be noted.

PE

Physical findings may include the following:

- **Cutaneous findings:** Oddly situated (e.g., head/face, back, thighs) **bruises of varying ages** (note: bruises on the shins, elbows, and knees occur with normal childhood activity) as well as **pattern injuries** such as wire-loop marks (electrical cords), burns (cigarettes, etc.), and belt marks. Ophthalmologic examination may reveal **retinal hemorrhages** (shaken baby syndrome; see Figure 2.14–3).
- **Skeletal trauma: Spiral fractures** of the humerus and femur in patients < 3 years of age indicate abuse until proven otherwise; **epiphyseal/ metaphyseal injuries** in infants are suggestive as well (they result from pulling, twisting, or shaking of the limbs). Look for **rib injuries** in infants < 2 years (ribs are extremely pliant).
- **Sexual abuse:** Symptoms of **STDs, genital trauma,** or behavioral abnormalities.

Evaluation

Skeletal survey shows multiple fractures in various stages of healing. Perform coagulation studies if there are multiple bruises. Gonorrhea and chlamydia cultures and HIV testing if sexual abuse is suspected. Ophthalmic exam may reveal retinal hemorrhages. In a shaken baby, CT may reveal bilateral subdural hemorrhages, and MRI will show white matter changes.

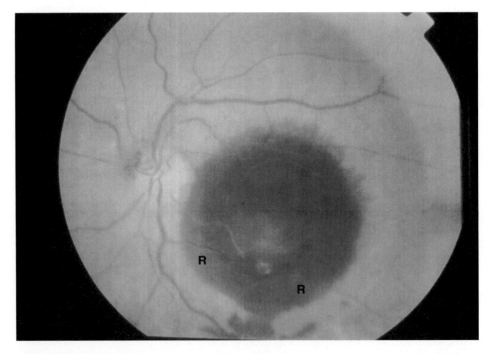

FIGURE 2.14–3. Subretinal hemorrhage. Note the preretinal blood and overlying retinal vessels (R). Subretinal hemorrhages may be seen in any condition with abnormal vessel proliferation (e.g., diabetes, hypertension) or from trauma.

Treatment

Notify child protective services for appropriate evaluation and possible removal from the home environment.

Fever-associated seizures that occur in children six months to six years of age.

History/PE

Febrile seizures may be classified as simple or complex.

- **Simple:** High fever (> 39°C), short duration (< 15 minutes), **generalized,** one per 24-hour period, fever onset within hours of the seizure.
- **Complex:** Low-grade fever, duration > 15 minutes, **focal** seizure, > 1 seizure per 24-hour period, fever for several days before seizure onset.

Differential

Meningitis, sepsis, dehydration, electrolyte imbalance, CNS malformations, tumors, intoxication.

Evaluation

None indicated if the presentation is consistent with febrile seizures. Electrolytes, serum glucose, blood cultures, UA, and CBC with differential if presentation is atypical. Perform an LP if CNS infection is suspected. Obtain an **EEG and MRI** of the brain for **complex febrile seizures.**

Treatment

Administer **antipyretics** (acetaminophen; avoid aspirin in children due to the risk of Reye's syndrome) and treat underlying illness. Children with febrile seizures should receive aggressive antipyretic therapy, even with low-grade fevers. Children with complex febrile seizures should have a thorough neurologic evaluation and may require chronic anticonvulsant therapy.

Complications

For simple febrile seizures there is **no increased risk** of epilepsy or of developmental, intellectual, or growth abnormalities. With complex seizures, the risk of epilepsy is 10%.

Perform LP if CNS infection is suspected in a patient with a febrile seizure.

Patients with complex febrile seizures may require chronic anticonvulsant therapy.

HIGH-YIELD FACTS

Pediatrics

287

Hereditary, progressive degenerative myopathies that include the following:

- **Duchenne muscular dystrophy:** See below.
- **Becker muscular dystrophy: X-linked;** similar to Duchenne muscular dystrophy but less severe and with onset after age 5.
- **Facioscapulohumeral dystrophy:** Autosomal dominant; onset between 10 and 20 years; characterized by facial muscle and shoulder girdle weakness.
- **Myotonic dystrophy:** Autosomal dominant; onset in adolescence; presents with characteristic facies, cataracts, testicular atrophy, and muscular weakness/wasting.

An **X-linked disorder** that results from a deficiency of **dystrophin** (Becker muscular dystrophy results from abnormal-sized dystrophin), a subsarcolemmal cytoskeletal protein. DMD is the most common and most lethal muscular dystrophy. Its usual onset is between two and six years of age and death occurs by age 20 secondary to respiratory complications.

History

Progressive **clumsiness, fatigability,** difficulty standing or walking, difficulty walking on toes (due to calf muscle shortening), and waddling gait. **Gowers' maneuver**—pushing off with the hands when rising from the floor—indicates proximal muscle weakness. Patients are usually wheelchair-bound by age 13 from proximal muscle weakness.

PE

Pseudohypertrophy of the calf muscles and possibly mental retardation. DMD affects the axial and proximal muscles before the distal muscles.

Differential

Other muscular dystrophies (facioscapulohumeral, limb-girdle, myotonic, Becker), myasthenia gravis, metabolic myopathies.

Evaluation

CK is consistently elevated. EMG shows polyphasic potentials and increased recruitment. **Muscle biopsy** shows degeneration and variation in fiber size with fibrosis and basophilic fibers. Immunostaining for dystrophin expression (absent) is diagnostic. DNA analysis may reveal the dystrophin mutation (but does not rule out Becker dystrophy).

Treatment

Institute **physical therapy** to maintain ambulation and prevent contractures. Perform Achilles tendon release as necessary.

A **nonprogressive,** nonhereditary disorder of impaired motor functioning and posture. CP most commonly results from a perinatal neurologic insult. Risk factors include prematurity, mental retardation, low birth weight, fetal malformation, neonatal seizures, neonatal cerebral hemorrhage, and perinatal asphyxia. Categories of CP include:

- **Pyramidal (spastic):** About 75% of cases are pyramidal; such cases involve spastic paresis of any or all limbs. Approximately 90% of patients are mentally retarded.
- **Extrapyramidal (nonspastic):** Extrapyramidal CP results from damage to extrapyramidal tracts. This category includes choreoathetoid, ataxic, rigid, hypotonic, and dystonic types.
- **Mixed:** Marked by spasticity and extrapyramidal symptoms.

History/PE

Patients may have an associated **seizure** disorder, **mental retardation,** or sensory and speech deficits. **Contractures** of the upper and lower extremities are common. Hip dysplasia/dislocation and scoliosis may develop.

Differential

Metabolic disorders, cerebellar dysgenesis, spinocerebellar degeneration.

Evaluation

EEG may be useful in patients with seizures; otherwise CP is largely a **clinical diagnosis.**

Treatment

Administer diazepam, dantrolene, or baclofen for spasticity. Special education, physical therapy, bracing, and surgical release/lengthening of contractures are often helpful. Baclofen pumps and posterior rhizotomy may alleviate contractures in severe cases.

HIGH-YIELD FACTS

Pediatrics

ADHD affects ~ 3% of children. Boys are affected more frequently than girls.

History/PE

Children must exhibit ADHD symptoms in more than one setting (i.e., home and school).

- **Inattention:** Patients exhibit **poor attention span** for schoolwork or play; do not listen when spoken to; have **difficulty following instructions;** lose items necessary for completion of school tasks; and are forgetful and **easily distracted.**
- **Hyperactivity/impulsivity:** Patients are **fidgety** and unexpectedly leave their desks; run around inappropriately; cannot play quietly; are often "on the go"; talk excessively; blurt out answers before questions have been completed; **do not wait for their turn;** and **interrupt others.**

Differential

Normal active child, medication side effects, head trauma, learning disabilities, major depression, bipolar disorder, anxiety disorder, cyclothymic disorder, conduct disorder, oppositional-defiant disorder.

Evaluation

To be diagnosed with ADHD, a child must exhibit six inattention symptoms and six hyperactivity symptoms before the age of 7, and these symptoms must cause **significant social and academic impairment.**

Treatment

Initial treatment involves reducing caffeine intake. Sugar and food additives are not etiologic factors.

Initial treatment should be conservative and nonpharmacologic. Reduce caffeine intake (sugar and food additives are not considered etiologic factors). Treatment for refractory/severe cases includes:

- **Psychostimulants: Methylphenidate,** dextroamphetamine, and pemoline. Adverse effects include stunted growth, tics, insomnia, irritability, and decreased appetite.
- **Antidepressants:** Nortriptyline, imipramine, bupropion.

A repetitive and persistent pattern of inappropriate conduct that lasts at least **six months** in which patients < 18 years of age ignore or violate the rights of others.

History/PE

Conduct disorder may be **aggressive** (e.g., **violence, destruction,** or **theft**) or **nonaggressive** (e.g., violation of rules, **lying**). The **undersocialized variant** affects individuals who cannot form social bonds with others. The **socialized** variant shows bonding, often with loyal groups that support deviant behavior (e.g., **urban gangs**).

Oppositional-defiant disorder is associated with loss of temper and defiance but not theft or lying.

Treatment

Address emotional conflicts and sociocultural factors.

CROUP   UCV *Ped.25*

An acute inflammatory disease of the larynx, primarily within the subglottic space; also known as **laryngotracheobronchitis.** Croup affects children from three months to five years of age. **Parainfluenza type 1** is the most common pathogen; others include parainfluenza type 2 and 3, RSV, influenza, rubeola, adenovirus, and *Mycoplasma pneumoniae.*

History/PE

Low-grade fever, mild dyspnea, inspiratory stridor that worsens with agitation, characteristic **barking cough** (usually at night), and a hoarse voice. Symptoms typically follow a URI.

Differential

Epiglottitis, foreign body aspiration, bacterial tracheitis, angioedema, retropharyngeal abscess.

Evaluation

Diagnosis is primarily **clinical.** Lateral neck film will show subglottic narrowing (**"steeple sign"**; Figure 2.14–4).

Treatment

- Manage mild cases **supportively** on an outpatient basis.
- **Mist therapy,** oxygen, **racemic epinephrine,** and **corticosteroids** may be useful.
- Hospitalize patients with stridor at rest.

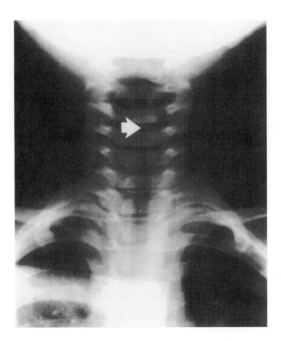

FIGURE 2.14–4. Croup. The x-ray shows marked subglottic narrowing of the airway (arrow).

EPIGLOTTITIS

UCV EM.26

Epiglottitis may cause life-threatening airway obstruction.

A serious and rapidly progressive infection of the epiglottis and contiguous structures that can cause life-threatening airway obstruction. Epiglottitis affects **children aged 2–7** and is most commonly caused by *Haemophilus influenzae* **type B** infection. Other pathogenic organisms include *Streptococcus* species. The incidence of epiglottitis has decreased with the widespread use of the *H. flu* vaccine.

History/PE

Sudden-onset high **fever** (39–40°C), **dysphagia, drooling, muffled voice,** inspiratory retractions, cyanosis, and **soft stridor.** Patients sit with the neck hyperextended and the chin protruding (**"sniffing dog"** position). If untreated, may progress to total airway obstruction and respiratory arrest.

Differential

Croup, tracheitis, foreign body aspiration, angioedema, retropharyngeal abscess.

Evaluation

Throat examination may precipitate laryngospasm and airway obstruction.

Diagnosis is primarily clinical (Table 2.14–3). **Do not examine the patient's throat** unless an anesthesiologist is present. Definitive diagnosis is made by direct fiberoptic visualization of cherry-red and swollen epiglottis and arytenoids. Lateral x-ray demonstrates a swollen epiglottis obliterating the valleculae (the classic **"thumbprint sign"**; see Figure 2.14–5).

TABLE 2.14–3. Characteristics of Croup, Epiglottitis, and Tracheitis.

Croup	Epiglottitis	Tracheitis
Age: 3 months to 5 years	Age: 2–7 years	Age: older child, but may affect any age
Usually viral etiology, commonly parainfluenza	Usually *Haemophilus influenzae* type B	Often *Staphylococcus aureus*
Develops over **2–3 days**	**Rapid onset** over hours	**Gradual onset** over 2–3 days followed by acute decompensation
Low-grade fever	High fever	High fever
Usually only mild to moderate respiratory distress	Commonly severe respiratory distress	Commonly severe respiratory distress
Prefers sitting up, leaning against parent's chest	Prefers perched position with neck extended	May have position preference
Stridor improves with aerosolized racemic epinephrine	No response to racemic epinephrine	No response to racemic epinephrine
"Steeple sign" on AP neck films	"Thumbprint sign" on lateral neck films	Subglottic narrowing

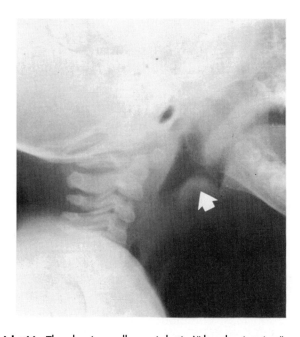

FIGURE 2.14–5. Epiglottitis. The classic swollen epiglottis ("thumbprint sign"; arrow) and obstructed airway are seen on lateral neck x-ray.

Treatment

This disease is a true emergency.

- Keep the patient (and his or her parents) calm, call anesthesia immediately, and **transfer the patient to the OR.**
- Treat with **endotracheal intubation** and **IV antibiotics** (ceftriaxone, chloramphenicol, ampicillin).

CYSTIC FIBROSIS (CF)

An **autosomal-recessive** disorder caused by mutations in the CFTR gene (chloride channel) and characterized by widespread exocrine gland dysfunction. CF is the most common severe genetic disease in the US (and is most common in **caucasians**).

History/PE

- **Respiratory:** Recurrent pulmonary infections (especially with **Pseudomonas**), cyanosis, cough, dyspnea, **bronchiectasis,** hemoptysis, chronic sinusitis.
- **Gastrointestinal:** Fifteen percent of infants present with **meconium ileus.** Patients usually have greasy stools and flatulence. **Malabsorption syndromes, failure to thrive,** pancreatitis, rectal prolapse, esophageal varices, and biliary cirrhosis may be seen.
- **Other: Abnormal glucose tolerance,** type II diabetes, "salty taste," unexplained hyponatremia. Ninety-five percent of males are **infertile.** Fifty percent of patients present with failure to thrive or respiratory compromise.

Evaluation

Sweat chloride test > 60 mEq/L; genetic testing.

Treatment

Pulmonary manifestations are managed by **DNase,** chest physical therapy, **bronchodilators, anti-inflammatory agents,** and **antibiotics.** Administer pancreatic enzymes and fat-soluble vitamins A, D, E, and K for malabsorption.

OTITIS MEDIA

Middle ear infection most commonly caused by **S. pneumoniae, H. flu,** or **Moraxella catarrhalis.** Predisposing conditions include URIs, trisomy 21, CF, immune deficiencies, passive smoke exposure, day care, and previous ear infections.

History/PE

Parents may report **fever, ear tugging,** crying, **hearing loss, irritability,** feeding difficulties, and vomiting. Otoscopic examination may reveal a **bulging or hyperemic tympanic membrane (TM), decreased movement of the TM with insufflation, loss of the TM light reflex,** or TM perforation (Figure 2.14–6).

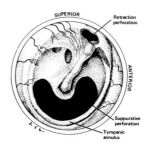

FIGURE 2.14–6. Perforated TM. Common sites of TM perforation.

Differential

Otitis externa, toothache, foreign body in the ear, ear canal furuncle, ear canal trauma, hard cerumen.

Evaluation

Diagnosis is clinical.

Treatment

Treat with **amoxicillin for 10 days;** amoxicillin–clavulanic acid or trimethoprim–sulfamethoxazole may be required in recurrent otitis media to cover *H. flu.*

Complications

Mastoiditis, sigmoid sinus thrombosis, meningitis, brain abscess, hearing loss.

RESPIRATORY DISTRESS SYNDROME   UCV *Ped.40*

The most common form of respiratory failure in **preterm infants;** results from **surfactant deficiency,** causing poor lung compliance and atelectasis. Respiratory distress syndrome is seen in 65% of infants born at 29–30 weeks' gestation.

History/PE

Patients present in the **first 48–72 hours of life** with a **respiratory rate > 60/min** and progressive **hypoxemia,** cyanosis, **nasal flaring, intercostal retractions,** and **expiratory grunting.**

Differential

Transient tachypnea of the newborn (TTN), meconium aspiration syndrome, congenital pneumonia, spontaneous pneumothorax, diaphragmatic hernia, cyanotic heart disease.

Evaluation

Evaluation depends primarily on characteristic CXR. Check ABGs, CBC, and blood cultures to rule out infection. Classic CXR findings include:

- **Respiratory distress syndrome:** Bilateral atelectasis causes a **"ground-glass"** appearance.
- **TTN:** Retained amniotic fluid causes prominent perihilar streaking in the interlobular fissures.
- **Meconium aspiration:** Coarse, irregular infiltrates and hyperexpansion.
- **Congenital pneumonia:** CXR is not helpful; neutropenia, tracheal aspirate, and Gram stain suggest the diagnosis.

Treatment

- **Intubation** is often required to maintain adequate oxygenation.
- **Surfactant replacement therapy** decreases mortality.
- Supportive care in a neonatal ICU is required.
- Prevent by administering **corticosteroids** to mothers at high risk for premature delivery and monitor fetal lung maturity with amniotic-fluid **lecithin-to-sphingomyelin ratio.**

Preventive Medicine

LEADING CAUSES OF DEATH

Table 2.15–1 presents the leading causes of death in different age groups.

TABLE 2.15–1. Leading Causes of Death by Age.*	
Age	**Most Common Causes of Death**
Birth to 18 months	Perinatal conditions, congenital abnormalities, injuries, pneumonia
2–6	Injuries, motor vehicle accidents (MVAs), congenital abnormalities, homicide, heart disease
7–12	MVAs, injuries, congenital abnormalities, leukemia, homicide, heart disease
13–39	MVAs, homicide, suicide, injuries, heart disease
40–60	Heart disease, lung cancer, CVA, breast cancer, COPD
Over age 60	Heart disease, cerebrovascular disease, COPD, pneumonia, lung cancer, colorectal cancer

*From U.S. Preventative Services Task Force, 1996.

Table 2.15–2 summarizes recommended screening measures by age.

TABLE 2.15–2. Health Care Screening.

Age	Screening Measure
Birth to 10 years	Height and weight, BP, vision screen, hemoglobinopathy screen (in high-risk populations*), phenylalanine level (at birth), TSH and/or T_4 (at birth).
11–24	Height and weight, BP, Pap smear (beginning when sexually active or at 18 years), chlamydia screen (sexually active), rubella serology or vaccination (women only), screen for alcohol abuse.
25–64	BP (< 140/90), height and weight, cholesterol, Pap smear, fecal occult blood test (FOBT) and/or sigmoidoscopy (> 50 years), mammography/clinical breast exam (50–69 years), screen for alcohol abuse, rubella serology or vaccination (women).
65 and older	BP, height and weight, FOBT and/or sigmoidoscopy, mammography/breast exam, Pap smear (sexually active), vision screening, hearing screening, screen for alcohol abuse.

* Individuals of African, Caribbean, Latin American, Mediterranean, Middle Eastern, or Southeast Asian descent.

Table 2.15–3 summarizes recommended screening measures.

TABLE 2.15–3. Recommended Cancer Screening Measures.*

Screening Measure	Ages and Intervals
Flexible sigmoidoscopy**	Q 3–5 years after 50
Fecal occult blood test	Q year after 50
Digital rectal examination**	Q year after 40
Prostate examination**	Q year after 50
Pap smear	Sexually active or 18, Q 1 year; after three normal smears, Q 3 years
Pelvic exam	20–40, Q 1–3 years; after 40, Q year
Endometrial tissue sample**	At menopause
Breast self-exam**	Q month after 20
Breast exam by clinician	20–40, Q 3 years; after 40, Q year
Mammography	Q year after 40–50 (exact timing controversial)
CXR	Not recommended as a screening test

*From U.S. Preventative Services Task Force, 1996.
**Additional recommendations from the American Cancer Society.

CXR is not effective in lung cancer screening.

COLORECTAL CANCER SCREENING

- Patients with **large/multiple adenomas** on sigmoidoscopy or colonoscopy should have a follow-up colonoscopy within three years.
- Patients with one or more **first-degree relatives** (parent, child, sibling) with a history of colorectal cancer should be screened beginning at age 40.
- Patients with **IBD of eight years' duration** should consider surveillance colonoscopy.
- Patients with **FAP** should be screened by genetic analysis and followed with serial colonoscopy/sigmoidoscopy.
- Patients with **FAP** or with long-standing **ulcerative colitis (10+ years)** should consider prophylactic colectomy to eliminate the risk of colon cancer.
- Patients with a first-degree relative with adenomatous polyps before age 60 should consider early screening.

Table 2.15–4 summarizes the recommended timetable for childhood immunizations.

TABLE 2.15–4. Timetable for Childhood Vaccinations.

Vaccine	Age
Diphtheria-tetanus-pertussis (DTP)	2, 4, 6, 15 months/4–6 years/15 years/Q 10 years
Polio	2, 4, 15 months/4–6 years
Measles-mumps-rubella	> 12 months/4–6 years
H. influenzae type B (Hib)	2, 4, 6, 12 months
Varicella	> 12 months
Hepatitis B	Birth/1, 6 months

- Avoid live vaccines in immune-compromised patients (oral polio, chicken pox, MMR). However, MMR may be administered to HIV-positive patients without immune compromise.
- For previously unvaccinated patients, Hib is not necessary for patients > 5 years of age and pertussis is not necessary for patients > 6 years of age.
- Avoid DTP in children with progressive neurologic disorders.
- Avoid influenza vaccine and MMR in patients with egg allergies.
- Asplenic patients should receive pneumococcal, meningococcal, and Hib vaccines.

HEPATITIS B VACCINE

Give the hepatitis B vaccine to Alaskan natives, Pacific Islanders, Native Americans, homosexual men, IV drug users, military personnel, and health care/lab workers.

PNEUMOCOCCAL VACCINE

Give the pneumococcal vaccine to patients with cardiopulmonary disease, diabetes, or asplenia (including patients with sickle cell disease), to Native American/Alaskan native populations, and to all people > 65.

HIGH-YIELD FACTS

Preventive Medicine

INFLUENZA A VACCINE

Give the influenza A vaccine to patients with cardiopulmonary disease, diabetics, elderly patients (especially in **chronic care facilities**), patients with hemoglobinopathies, immune-compromised individuals, patients with renal dysfunction, health care workers (to reduce nosocomial transmission), and to all people > 65.

CHOLESTEROL

Elevated cholesterol levels are a strong risk factor for cardiovascular disease. Screening should be done for men once between 20–39 years and then every five years; for women, screening should be conducted once between the ages of 40 and 49 years and then every five years. Additional risk factors for CAD include a family history of premature CAD, hypertension, smoking, HDL < 35, and diabetes. Males > 45 years of age and women > 55 are at greatest risk. Guidelines are as follows:

- **Total cholesterol** < 200 (mg/dL): Retest in five years.
- **Total cholesterol** > 200: Test lipid fractions; treat on basis of LDL.
- **LDL 130–159:** Borderline risk. Treat with dietary modification and exercise.
- **LDL** > 130 + CAD, LDL > 160 with two risk factors, or LDL > 190: High risk. Begin drug therapy.
- **Triglycerides** < 200 mg/dL: Considered normal.

Management is as follows:

- **Diet:** Modest (10–15%) reduction in cholesterol results in 15–30% reduction in cardiovascular events.
- **HMG-CoA reductase inhibitors:** Most effective cholesterol-lowering drugs. Can cause LFT abnormalities, warfarin potentiation, and/or myositis.
- **Bile acid sequestrants:** May interfere with the absorption of other drugs (digoxin, Coumadin, thiazides). Constipation and gas are common.
- **Niacin:** Cheap and effective, but facial flushing limits patient compliance.

> **Cardiovascular risk factors—**
>
> **CAD HDL**
> **C**igarettes
> **A**ge and sex
> **D**iabetes mellitus
>
> **H**ypertension
> **D**eath from MI in family
> **L**DL high and **L**ow HDL

Target LDL in patients with CAD < 100.

RISK FACTOR MODIFICATION (POSTMENOPAUSE)

Lifetime risks for a 50-year-old Caucasian woman:

- CAD 46%, hip fracture 15%, breast cancer 10%, endometrial cancer 3%.
- Leading causes of death in women 50–75: CAD > cancer > stroke.

Benefits of HRT:

- Reduction of CAD risk.
- Reduction of fracture risk (all fractures) by 50%.
- Possibly decreases colon cancer risk and stroke risk; delays onset of Alzheimer's.
- Minimizes vasomotor and genitourinary symptoms.

Risks of HRT:

- Endometrial cancer risk increased (reduced by giving progesterone).
- Increase in incidence of thromboembolic disease.

Management:

- HRT is currently recommended for postmenopausal women.
- Family or personal history of breast cancer is a relative contraindication.

Psychiatry

Depression has a prevalence of 5% and a lifetime risk of 20%. **Females** are affected twice as often as males. While socioeconomic status does not correlate with the likelihood of developing depression, **chronic illness** does. Up to 15% of patients with major depression commit suicide.

History/PE

Symptoms can be described by the mnemonic **SIG E CAPS** (see sidebar).

Differential

Medical illness *(Psych.31)*, bipolar disorder, substance-induced mood disorder, dysthymia *(Psych.32)*, dementia, schizophrenia, schizoaffective disorder.

Evaluation

In order to be diagnosed with depression, a patient must have five or more of the above symptoms for a two-week period with impairment in daily living.

Treatment

- **Selective serotonin reuptake inhibitors (SSRIs):** Relatively well tolerated and considered as first-line therapy for depression. Drawbacks include cost and high incidence of sexual dysfunction. Other potential side effects include agitation, anxiety, insomnia, GI distress, anorexia, and drug interactions.

- **Tricyclic antidepressants (TCAs):** Cheap and well studied but have significant side effects, including **anticholinergic effects, cardiac arrhythmias,** orthostatic hypotension, sexual dysfunction, and seizures. TCAs can be lethal in overdose. Check EKG before initiating therapy.

Symptoms of depression—
SIG E CAPS
Sleep, (↓ or ↑)
Interest
Guilt

Energy

Concentration
Appetite (↓ or ↑)
Psychomotor retardation
Suicidal ideations

TCAs are lethal in overdose.

Avoid cheese and red wine when taking an MAOI.

- **Monoamine oxidase inhibitors (MAOIs): Inexpensive** and the best drugs for atypical depression (hypersomnolence, hyperphagia), but have **dietary restrictions** and serious side effects, including **hypertensive crises** (tyramine or "cheese reaction"), headache, dizziness, and sleep abnormalities.
- **Electroconvulsive therapy:** Possibly the most effective therapy but reserved for refractory or catatonic depression (6–12 treatments are often needed). Adverse effects include postictal confusion, arrhythmias, and retrograde amnesia. Relative contraindications include intracranial mass, seizure disorder, and high anesthetic risk.
- **Others:** Venlafaxine, bupropion, trazodone, and nefazodone.

BIPOLAR I DISORDER

UCV *Psych.30*

Manic episodes with or without depressive episodes (mania is a prerequisite for diagnosis, but depression is not). Bipolar disorder has a prevalence of approximately 1% and affects males and females equally. The suicide rate of patients with bipolar disorder is 10–15%.

History/PE

The mnemonic **DIG FAST** describes the clinical presentation of mania (see sidebar). Patients may have a history of excessive spending, speeding tickets, or excessive sexual activity. Antidepressants may trigger manic episodes in patients with bipolar disorder.

Bipolar disorder—

DIG FAST
Distractibility
Insomnia
Grandiosity

Flight of ideas
Increase in goal-directed **A**ctivities/psychomotor **A**gitation
Pressured **S**peech
Thoughtlessness

Differential

Major depression, cyclothymic disorder, substance-induced mood disorder, schizophrenia, schizoaffective disorder, borderline personality disorder, and ADHD. Medical conditions such as metabolic derangements, CNS infections, or tumors may mimic bipolar disorder.

Evaluation

A manic episode must include **three of the above symptoms and must last at least one week** (less if hospitalization is necessary). Symptoms cannot be substance-related or due to a preexisting medical condition. Hypomanic episodes are similar but do not cause marked impairment in social or occupational functioning. Bipolar II disorder is characterized by a history of one or more major depressive episodes and at least one hypomanic episode.

Treatment

- **Acute mania:** Control mood (lithium, valproic acid); resolve psychosis (antipsychotics) and manage agitation (benzodiazepines).
- **Bipolar depression:** Mood stabilizers (lithium, valproic acid) +/– antidepressant. ECT may be used in cases that fail to respond to pharmacologic intervention.

Lithium levels should be monitored to prevent acute side effects (CNS findings, including seizures) as well as chronic side effects (renal insufficiency). **Valproic acid** may be associated with GI distress, sedation, hepatotoxicity, and thrombocytopenia. Monitor platelets and LFTs. **Carbamazepine,** a second-line agent, has been associated with aplastic anemia and Stevens–Johnson syndrome (monitor CBC).

POST-TRAUMATIC STRESS DISORDER (PTSD) — UCV *Psych.6*

Occurs after an individual is exposed to a traumatic event outside the realm of normal human experience (e.g., combat, natural disasters, physical/sexual assault, accidents). PTSD has a lifetime prevalence of 1–3%. Its prevalence in combat soldiers is as high as 60%.

History/PE

Patients reexperience traumatic events by having **intrusive thoughts** or **nightmares** and often have feelings of detachment, anhedonia, and amnesia. PTSD is associated with an increased state of arousal **(hypervigilance)** and leads to social and occupational impairment. Also watch for survivor guilt, personality change, substance abuse, depression, and suicidality.

Differential

Acute stress disorder (lasts < 1 month), adjustment disorder, depression, obsessive- compulsive disorder, anxiety disorder, borderline personality disorder.

Treatment

First-line agents include **antidepressants** and **mood stabilizers** (lithium, valproic acid, carbamazepine). Adjunctive agents to **target anxiety** include beta-blockers, benzodiazepines, and alpha 2-antagonists. **Cognitive-behavior therapy** and **support groups** may help.

Consider malingering in any case involving litigation or potential for secondary gain.

Anorexic patients deny any health risks associated with their behavior, making them resistant to treatment.

An eating disorder in which patients refuse to maintain a normal body weight and are > **15% below ideal body weight.** Patients either restrict themselves (fast, diet, and **exercise excessively**) or engage in binge-eating/purging behavior. Patients have a distorted body image (they **perceive themselves as fat**) and deny the potential medical consequences of their behavior. Ninety percent of cases of anorexia nervosa occur in females (1% prevalence in adolescent females).

History/PE

Amenorrhea, lanugo, cold intolerance, lethargy, excess energy, emaciation, bradycardia, hypotension, hypothermia, dry skin, electrolyte abnormalities, and hypercarotenemia. Patients are often preoccupied with food rituals, **intensely fear becoming fat,** and judge themselves by their weight.

Evaluation

Evaluation should include height and weight measurements, CBC, electrolytes, endocrine tests, EKG, and psychiatric evaluation.

Treatment

Early treatment centers on monitoring caloric intake to stabilize weight and then focuses on **weight gain.** Later treatment includes individual, family, and group **psychotherapy.** SSRIs may help treat comorbid depression. Mortality is as high as 5–10%.

Bulimic patients tend to be more disturbed by their behavior and consequently are more easily engaged in therapy.

An eating disorder in which patients are usually **ashamed of their eating behaviors,** tend to keep them secret, and often maintain **normal body weight.** Bulimia has a 3–5% prevalence rate among late adolescent girls and can be classified into purging and nonpurging types.

History/PE

Dental enamel erosion (from vomiting), **enlarged parotid glands, scars on the dorsal surfaces of their hands** (from inducing vomiting), menstrual irregularities, electrolyte abnormalities, and laxative dependence. Patients' self-esteem is overly dependent on body weight.

Evaluation

Diagnosis is based on recurrent episodes of **binge eating** and **recurrent compensatory behaviors** to prevent weight gain (**induced vomiting, laxative abuse,** diuretic use, enemas, fasting, and excessive exercise), occurring at least twice weekly for three months.

Treatment

Psychotherapy focuses on behavior modification and body self-image. **Antidepressants** are effective in both depressed and nondepressed patients.

SCHIZOPHRENIA
UCV *Psych.39*

Schizophrenia is characterized by psychotic symptoms that significantly impair social/occupational functioning. Schizophrenia has a prevalence of 1%, with males and females affected equally. Schizophrenia most commonly manifests itself in males 15–25 years of age and in females 25–35 years of age. Schizophrenics are at high risk for **suicide.**

Schizophrenic patients are at high risk for suicide.

History/PE

Positive symptoms include **delusions, auditory hallucinations,** thought alienation (thought broadcasting, withdrawal and insertion), and disorganization (of thought and behavior). **Negative symptoms** include **withdrawal,** apathy, and **flattened affect.**

Differential

Schizoaffective disorder, major depression, bipolar disorder, substance-induced psychotic disorder, drug withdrawal, and psychotic disorder due to a general medical condition (e.g., seizure disorder, CNS tumor, Cushing's syndrome, SLE).

Evaluation

In order to be diagnosed, patients must exhibit two or more of the above signs and symptoms with **an impaired level of social/occupational functioning for at least six months' duration.**

Treatment

Treat with **antipsychotics,** psychotherapy (supportive, group), and hospitalization during psychotic episodes. Negative symptoms are often more difficult to treat than positive symptoms. Prognosis is often directly proportional to the premorbid level of functioning. Paranoid schizophrenia has the best overall prognosis.

Lower-potency drugs have more anticholinergic side effects, whereas higher-potency drugs have more extrapyramidal side effects.

Traditional Antipsychotics

Antipsychotics block dopamine receptors (mostly D_2 and D_4 subtypes). High-potency drugs include haloperidol, droperidol, fluphenazine, and thiothixene. Medium-potency drugs include trifluoperazine and perphenazine. Low-potency drugs include thioridazine and chlorpromazine.

Side effects include the following:

- **Extrapyramidal symptoms:** Acute dystonia, akathisia (treat with propranolol or benzodiazepine), parkinsonism (tremor, rigidity, bradykinesia), and tardive dyskinesia (lip smacking, etc.).
- **Anticholinergic effects:** Dry mouth, urinary retention, constipation, sedation, orthostatic hypotension, etc.
- **Neuroleptic malignant syndrome:** Fever, rigidity, autonomic instability, clouding of consciousness. Withdraw neuroleptic; treat with dantrolene/bromocriptine and IV fluids (EM.39).
- **Hyperprolactinemia:** Amenorrhea, gynecomastia, galactorrhea.
- **Other:** Seizures, EKG changes.

Atypical antipsychotics have fewer anticholinergic and extrapyramidal side effects.

Atypical Antipsychotics

Atypical antipsychotics have fewer anticholinergic and extrapyramidal side effects. **Clozapine,** a first-generation drug, has a 0.5% incidence of **agranulocytosis** and requires weekly CBCs. Although clozapine is the most effective antipsychotic, its use is reserved for treatment-resistant psychosis due to the high incidence of agranulocytosis. Side effects of atypical agents include sedation, anticholinergic effects, drooling, weight gain, seizures, and arrhythmias. Newer agents (risperidone, olanzapine, sertindole, and quetiapine) do not cause agranulocytosis and may have fewer side effects.

Women are more likely to attempt suicide, whereas men are more likely to commit suicide.

SUICIDALITY　　　　　　　　　　**UCV** *EM.37*

Suicide is the **eighth-leading cause of death** in the United States and is the second-leading cause of death (after accidents) among 15- to 24-year-olds. Risk factors include depression, other major psychiatric disorders, a past history of suicide attempts, alcohol/substance abuse, a recent severe stressor, and a family history of suicide. Also at risk are single, divorced, and recently widowed individuals with poor social support; patients recovering from suicidal depression or from a first schizophrenic episode; and patients with a chronic medical condition (e.g., AIDS). Police officers and doctors are at increased risk compared to the general population, and whites commit suicide more frequently than blacks.

Evaluation

Look for an expressed desire to kill oneself, a **feasible plan,** a positive family history, a previous suicide attempt, ambivalence toward death, and feelings of hopelessness. **Ask directly about suicidal ideation, intent, and plan.** Look for available means of committing suicide; perform a mental status exam.

Treatment

Patients who express a desire to kill themselves, or those whom you believe may do so, require **emergent inpatient hospitalization,** even if it is against their wishes. ECT may be used for actively suicidal patients who are refractory to medication and psychotherapy. Note that the greatest risk for suicide is often in the first few weeks after antidepressant medication is started because a patient's energy often returns before the depressed mood lifts.

Always assess whether a patient has available means for committing suicide (e.g., a gun, prescription medication).

SUBSTANCE ABUSE/DEPENDENCE

Substance abuse/dependence has a 13% lifetime prevalence. Abuse is diagnosed if the patient's life has been disrupted by substance use. Dependence can be diagnosed if three of the following are observed over a one-year period: tolerance; withdrawal; desire to cut back; a significant amount of time involved in substance use; withdrawal from former activities; and persistent use despite awareness of these problems.

Differential

Differentiate from other axis I psychiatric disorders and delirium. The signs and symptoms of intoxication and withdrawal for some drugs are summarized in Table 2.16–1.

Evaluation

Tox screen, LFTs, breathalizer or serum ethanol level. Offer HIV testing (especially to IV drug users).

HIGH-YIELD FACTS

Psychiatry

TABLE 2.16–1. Signs and Symptoms of Substance Abuse.

Drug	Intoxication	Withdrawal
Alcohol	Disinhibition, emotional lability, incoordination, slurred speech, ataxia, coma, blackouts (retrograde amnesia).	Tremor, tachycardia, hypertension, malaise, nausea, seizures, delirium tremens (DTs), tremulousness, agitation, hallucinations.
Opioids *Psych.50*	CNS depression, nausea and vomiting, constipation, **pupillary constriction,** seizures, respiratory depression (overdose is life-threatening).	Anxiety, insomnia, anorexia, sweating, fever, rhinorrhea, piloerection, nausea, stomach cramps, diarrhea.
Amphetamines	Psychomotor agitation, impaired judgment, **pupillary dilation,** hypertension, tachycardia, euphoria, prolonged wakefulness and attention, cardiac arrhythmias, delusions, hallucinations, fever.	Post-use "crash," including anxiety, lethargy, headache, stomach cramps, hunger, severe depression, dysphoric mood, fatigue, insomnia/hypersomnia.
Cocaine *Psych.46*	Euphoria, psychomotor agitation, impaired judgment, tachycardia, **pupillary dilation,** hypertension, hallucinations (including tactile), paranoid ideations, angina, and sudden cardiac death.	Hypersomnolence, fatigue, depression, malaise, severe craving, suicidality.
PCP *Psych.51*	Belligerence, impulsiveness, fever, psychomotor agitation, **vertical and horizontal nystagmus,** tachycardia, ataxia, homicidality, psychosis, delirium.	Recurrence of symptoms due to reabsorption from lipid stores; sudden onset of severe, random, homicidal violence.
LSD *Psych.49*	Marked anxiety or depression, delusions, visual hallucinations, flashbacks.	
Marijuana *Psych.45*	Euphoria, anxiety, paranoid delusions, slowed time sense, impaired judgment, social withdrawal, increased appetite, dry mouth, persecutory delusions, hallucinations, amotivational syndrome.	
Barbiturates	Low safety margin, respiratory depression.	Anxiety, seizures, delirium, life-threatening cardiovascular collapse.
Benzodiazepines	Alcohol interactions, amnesia, ataxia, sleep, minor respiratory depression.	Rebound anxiety, seizures, tremor, insomnia, hypertension, tachycardia.
Caffeine	Restlessness, insomnia, diuresis, muscle twitching, cardiac arrhythmias.	Headache, lethargy, depression, weight gain.
Nicotine	Restlessness, insomnia, anxiety, arrhythmias.	Irritability, headache, anxiety, weight gain, craving, tachycardia.

Treatment

Management of substance intoxication is described in Table 2.16–2.

TABLE 2.16–2. Management of Substance Intoxication.

Drug	Management
Hallucinogens (e.g., LSD)	If severe, benzodiazepines; otherwise provide reassurance.
Cocaine/crack	Severe agitation is treated with haloperidol, benzodiazepines, anti-emetics, anti-diarrheals, and NSAIDs (for muscle cramps).
PCP	If severe, benzodiazepines; otherwise provide reassurance.
Amphetamines EM.42	Same as with cocaine/crack.

ALCOHOLISM

Alcohol is the most commonly abused substance (not counting tobacco and caffeine), and alcoholism has a lifetime prevalence of 6%. Males are affected almost four times as often as females, but the incidence of alcoholism among females is increasing. The highest prevalence is in males aged 21–34. Abuse and dependence criteria are similar to those of other substances.

Alcohol abuse is more common in men, but the incidence of alcoholism in females is increasing.

History/PE

Alcohol intoxication results in **euphoria, disinhibition, hypoglycemia, ataxia, impaired judgment and reflexes,** and CNS depression. Acute overdose can result in respiratory depression, coma, or death. See "Toxicology" for symptoms and signs of alcohol withdrawal.

DTs are a medical emergency with a mortality rate of 15–20%.

HIGH-YIELD FACTS

Psychiatry

Evaluation

Evaluation is similar to that of substance abuse. Screen with the CAGE questionnaire (see sidebar). Monitor vital signs in hospitalized patients to assess for signs of withdrawal.

Treatment

- Rule out medical complications.
- Start benzodiazepine taper for withdrawal symptoms.
- Give **thiamine, folate, and MVI;** correct electrolyte abnormalities.
- For patients with alcohol seizure history, give carbamazepine and avoid neuroleptics, which decrease seizure threshold.
- Alcohol dependence can be treated with group therapy (Alcoholics Anonymous), disulfiram, or naltrexone.

Complications

GI bleeding (gastritis, ulcers, varices, or Mallory–Weiss tears), **pancreatitis, liver disease,** susceptibility to infections, and electrolyte disturbances, delirium tremens *(Psych.47)*.

DELIRIUM   **UCV** *Psych.14*

A transient global disorder of consciousness. Etiologies include infectious disease, hypoxia, **ICU psychosis, "sundowning,"** CVA, endocrine causes, autoimmune disease, **uremia,** hepatic encephalopathy, Wilson's disease, electrolyte abnormalities, and drugs (alcohol withdrawal, **corticosteroids,** psychedelic drugs, acyclovir, amphotericin B, antihistamines, **anticholinergics,** TCAs, phenytoin, heavy metal poisoning, INH, rifampin, beta-blockers, digitalis, aminophylline, lithium, barbiturates, and benzodiazepines).

History/PE

Waxing and waning levels of consciousness and **perceptual disturbances** (hallucinations or illusions). Patients may be anxious, restless, paranoid, or combative and may have a short attention span, decreased short-term memory, and autonomic disturbances (tachycardia, diaphoresis).

Differential

Must be distinguished from dementia, schizophrenia, mania, psychotic depression, and substance abuse.

Evaluation

Check vitals, pulse oximetry, and glucose; conduct a thorough physical and neurological exam. Note recently started meds, overdose, alcohol use, previous history, concurrent medical problems, signs of organ failure, and signs of infection (occult UTI is common in the elderly). Laboratory studies include CBC, electrolytes, tox screen, UA, ABG, CXR, EKG, LP, and head CT.

Treatment

Treat the underlying cause; normalize fluid and electrolyte status. Use **antipsychotics** for agitation. **Benzodiazepines** may also be used. **Physical restraints** may be necessary to prevent patients from harming themselves or others.

DEMENTIA UCV *Psych.15*

A syndrome of global intellectual impairment. Dementia has its highest prevalence among those > 85 years old. The most common etiologies are **Alzheimer's disease** (70–80%), vascular dementia (10%), head trauma, alcohol use, and Huntington's and Parkinson's diseases (1–5% each). Less than 10% of dementias are reversible (e.g., normal pressure hydrocephalus). Other etiologies include hypothyroidism, B$_{12}$/folate deficiency, lead toxicity, Wilson's disease, CNS tumors, HIV dementia, chronic hypoxia, Creutzfeldt–Jakob disease, neurosyphilis, Down's syndrome, and multiple sclerosis.

De**mem**tia =
memory
impairment
Deli**rium** =
change in
senso**rium**

History/PE

Dementia is chronic and insidiously progressive, resulting in the **deterioration of cognitive functions.** Patients present with memory impairment, aphasia, apraxia, agnosia, and disturbances in abstract thought, planning, organizing, and sequencing. Symptoms typically occur in the presence of a clear sensorium.

Differential

Depression (pseudodementia), delirium, schizophrenia, amnestic disorder, mental retardation.

Evaluation

See "Alzheimer's Disease" (p. 236) for dementia workup.

Treatment

Treat reversible causes. Provide **environmental clues** and supportive intervention. Use low-dose, **antipsychotics** for agitation. **Avoid benzodiazepines,** as they will often worsen disinhibition and confusion.

HIGH-YIELD FACTS

Psychiatry

Personality disorders typically become evident by late adolescence or early adulthood. They tend to be stable over time and affect all facets of interpersonal relationships. Their prevalence is 10% in the general population, 30% among psychiatric outpatients, and 40% among psychiatric inpatients.

Evaluation

Differentiate from axis I disorders. Ask about attitudes toward self and others, moral and religious attitudes and standards, variability of mood, leisure activities and interests, fantasy life, and reaction patterns to stress. Consider psychological testing (Minnesota Multiphasic Personality Inventory [MMPI], Bender Gestalt, Rorschach) as an aid in diagnosis.

Treatment

Treat with **psychotherapy** and **pharmacotherapy.** Recognize and treat comorbid axis I disorders. For specific personality disorders, see Table 2.16–3.

TABLE 2.16–3. Signs and Symptoms of Personality Disorders.

Cluster	Examples	Characteristics	Clinical Dilemma	Clinical Strategy
Cluster A	Paranoid Schizoid Schizotypal	Eccentric, strange, fearful of social relationships, paranoid, suspicious, social isolation, odd beliefs, shy, withdrawn, impoverished personal relationships.	Patient is suspicious of doctor and does not trust doctor.	Use clear, honest attitude, noncontrolling, nondefensive, **no humor;** keep distance.
Cluster B	Borderline Histrionic Narcissistic Antisocial	Emotional, dramatic, erratic, self-indulgent, hostile, aggressive, exploitive relationships, attention seeking.	Patient will change rules on doctor. Clingy and demands attention. Feels that he or she is special. Will manipulate doctor and staff ("splitting").	Firm: **Stick to treatment plan** and don't waffle. Fair: Don't be punitive or derogatory. Consistent: Don't change the rules on them.
Cluster C	Obsessive-compulsive Avoidant Dependent Passive-aggressive	Fearful, anxious, adheres to rules and regulations, anxiety, repressed, unable to express affect.	Patient may subtly sabotage his or her own treatment. Very controlling.	**Avoid power struggles.** Give clear treatment recommendations, but do not push the patient into a decision.

Fears that are **persistent,** intense, and often out of proportion to the object feared, leading to **impairment** of daily living. Less than 1% of the population has a disabling phobic disorder. The disorder is classified as either a social phobia or as a specific phobia.

In phobias, the fear is often out of proportion to the object feared.

Treatment

Treatment includes **cognitive-behavior therapy,** relaxation training, and exposure-based techniques (systemic desensitization). Benzodiazepines, beta-blockers, SSRIs, and MAOIs may be used.

SEXUAL ABUSE

Sexual abuse has become more common in recent years; there is now an incidence of 200,000 cases per year in the U.S. The abuser is commonly known to the victim. Incidence is highest at ages 9–12 years. Risk factors include single-parent households, marital problems, substance abuse, sick mothers, and crowded living conditions.

History/PE

Precocious sexual behavior, **genital or anal trauma, STDs,** or UTIs. Sexual abuse may predispose patients to psychiatric problems, including anxiety, phobias, and depression.

Treatment

When sexual abuse is suspected, the physician must intervene to protect the abused and **report the case to the appropriate authority.**

HIGH-YIELD FACTS

Psychiatry

HIGH-YIELD FACTS

Psychiatry

Pulmonary Medicine

SINUSITIS

Infection of the sinuses due to an undrained collection of pus. Risk factors include barotrauma, allergic rhinitis, viral infection, asthma, and nasal decongestant overuse. Acute sinusitis (symptoms lasting < 1 month) is most commonly associated with **Streptococcus pneumoniae, H. flu, Moraxella catarrhalis,** and viral infection, while chronic sinusitis is often due to anaerobic infections.

History/PE

Fever, facial pain that can **radiate to the upper teeth,** nasal congestion, and **headache. Tenderness,** erythema, swelling over the affected area and **purulent discharge** may be noted. Febrile ICU patients may have **occult sinusitis,** especially if they are intubated or have NG tubes.

Always consider occult sinusitis in febrile ICU patients.

Evaluation

Sinusitis is a **clinical** diagnosis. Clouding of sinuses may be observed on **transillumination;** air-fluid levels may be seen on maxillary sinus **radiographs** (Figure 2.17–1). Obtain a coronal CT if complications are suspected.

Treatment

- **Acute: Amoxicillin** or another appropriate antibiotic for 2–3 weeks and symptomatic therapy (e.g., decongestants).
- **Chronic:** 6–12 weeks of antibiotic treatment.

Complications

Osteomyelitis, mucocele, meningitis, epidural abscess, subdural empyema, orbital cellulitis, cavernous sinus thrombosis.

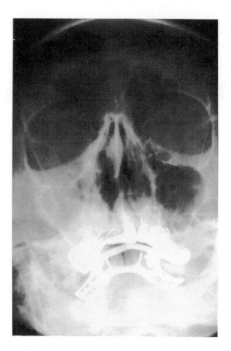

FIGURE 2.17–1. Sinusitis. Compare the opacified right maxillary sinus and normal air-filled left sinus on this sinus x-ray.

PNEUMONIA   UCV *IM2.23, 24*

Rust-colored sputum =

  Pneumococcus

Currant jelly sputum =

  Klebsiella

An infection of the bronchoalveolar unit with an inflammatory exudate. Causes include bacteria, viruses, atypical organisms (e.g., mycobacteria, mycoplasma), parasites, and fungi.

History

Productive cough (purulent yellow or green sputum, or hemoptysis), dyspnea, fever/chills, night sweats, and **pleuritic chest pain.**

PE

Decreased or bronchial breath sounds, crackles, wheezing, dullness to percussion, egophony, and tactile fremitus.

Evaluation

A good sputum sample (i.e., not contaminated with oropharyngeal flora) has many PMNs and few epithelial cells.

- **CBC: Leukocytosis** and **left shift** (bands > 5% and/or immature WBCs).
- **Sputum Gram stain and culture:** Identifies pathogenic organism and the organism's antibiotic susceptibilities (Figures 2.17–2 to 2.17–4). A good sputum sample (i.e., one not contaminated by oropharyngeal flora) has many PMNs and few epithelial cells.
- **Blood culture:** If patient appears very ill, suspect sepsis due to pneumonia.

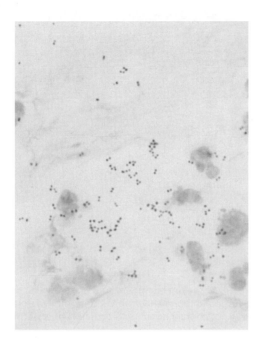

FIGURE 2.17–2. *Staphylococcus aureus.* These clusters of gram-positive cocci were isolated from the sputum of a patient with pneumonia.

- **ABGs:** Ill patients will have poor oxygen saturation and acid-base disturbances.
- **CXR:** Look for lobar consolidation and patchy infiltrates.

Treatment

In uncomplicated cases, treat community-acquired pneumonia on an outpatient basis with oral antibiotics (e.g., macrolides). Patients > 65 years old,

Alcoholics: Klebsiella

Aspiration: anaerobes

COPD: H. flu

Young adults: Mycoplasma

Anyone: S. pneumoniae

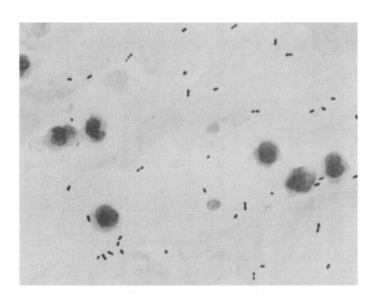

FIGURE 2.17–3. *Streptococcus pneumoniae.* This is a sputum sample from a patient with pneumonia. Note the characteristic lancet-shaped gram-positive diplococci.

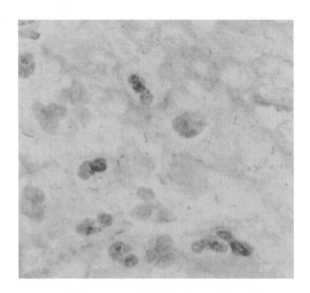

FIGURE 2.17–4. *Pseudomonas.* This sputum sample from a patient with pneumonia revealed gram-negative rods. The large number of neutrophils and relative paucity of epithelial cells indicates that this sample is not contaminated with oropharyngeal flora.

those with comorbidity (alcoholism, COPD, diabetes, malnutrition), immunosuppression, unstable vitals or signs of respiratory failure, altered mental status, and/or multilobar involvement require hospitalization with IV antibiotics. Table 2.17–1 summarizes recommended treatment for pneumonia. Ad-

TABLE 2.17–1. Initial Antibiotic Treatment of Pneumonia.

Category	Suspected Pathogens	Initial Coverage
Outpatient community-acquired pneumonia, < 60 years of age, otherwise healthy	*Streptococcus pneumoniae, Mycoplasma pneumoniae, Chlamydia pneumoniae, H. flu*, viral	Erythromycin, tetracycline. Consider clarithromycin or azithromycin in smokers to cover *H. flu.*
Greater than 60 or with comorbidity (COPD, heart failure, renal failure, diabetes, liver disease, EtOH abuse)	*S. pneumoniae, H. flu*, aerobic gram-negative rods (GNRs, including *E. coli, Enterobacter, Klebsiella*), *S. aureus*	Second-generation cephalosporin (cefuroxime), TMP/SMX, amoxicillin. Add erythromycin if atypicals (*Legionella, Mycoplasma, Chlamydia*) are suspected.
Community-acquired pneumonia requiring hospitalization	*S. pneumoniae, H. flu*, anaerobes, aerobic GNRs, *Legionella, Chlamydia*	Third-generation cephalosporin (ceftriaxone, cefoperazone). Add erythromycin if atypicals are suspected.
Severe community-acquired pneumonia requiring hospitalization (generally needs ICU care)	*S. pneumoniae, H. flu*, anaerobes, aerobic GNRs, *Mycoplasma, Legionella*	Erythromycin and third-generation cephalosporin (ceftriaxone, cefoperazone).
Nosocomial pneumonia—patient hospitalized > 48 hours	GNRs including *Pseudomonas, S. aureus, Legionella*	Third-generation cephalosporin and aminoglycoside (gentamicin).

HIGH-YIELD FACTS

Pulmonary Medicine

minister the **pneumococcal vaccine** in patients > 65 and those with chronic illnesses, immune compromise, asplenia, and sickle cell disease.

Most cases of pulmonary tuberculosis (TB) are due to reactivation of old infection rather than to primary disease. Risk factors include immunosuppression, alcoholism, preexisting lung disease, diabetes, advancing age, homelessness, malnourishment, and crowded living conditions; also at high risk are **immigrants** from developing nations and persons with "sick contacts."

History/PE

Cough, hemoptysis, dyspnea, **weight loss,** malaise, **night sweats,** and fever. Pulmonary TB is a common cause of FUO, and the kidney is the most common site of extrapulmonary infection.

TB is a common cause of FUO.

Differential

Pneumonia (bacterial, fungal, viral), other mycobacterial infections, HIV infection, UTI, lung abscess, lung cancer.

Evaluation

Pulmonary TB is presumptively diagnosed by a **positive sputum acid-fast stain,** since culture may take several weeks (Figure 2.17–5). CXR may show **apical fibronodular infiltrates** with or without cavitation. A positive PPD test indicates previous exposure (not necessarily active infection) to *Mycobacterium tuberculosis* and may not be present in immune-compromised individuals.

Immune-compromised individuals with TB may have a negative PPD (check anergy panel).

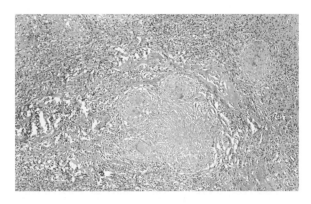

FIGURE 2.17–5. Tuberculosis (AFB smear). Note the red color of the tubercle bacilli on acid-fast staining of a sputum sample.

Treatment

Drugs for TB—

RESPIre
Rifampin
Ethambutol
Streptomycin
Pyrazinamide
INH

- **Respiratory isolation** (if TB is suspected) followed by **multidrug therapy** (usually INH, pyrazinamide, rifampin, and ethambutol).
- **Vitamin B$_6$ (pyridoxine)** is given with INH to prevent peripheral neuritis.
- **Prophylactic therapy** for PPD conversion without active symptoms is with INH for nine months.
- Many physicians choose to forgo INH prophylaxis in patients > 35 years old because the risk of INH-induced liver toxicity increases with age.

PURIFIED PROTEIN DERIVATIVE (PPD) PLACEMENT

PPD (0.5 mL) is injected intradermally on the volar surface of the arm. The transverse length of induration is measured at 48–72 hours. BCG vaccination typically renders a patient PPD positive for at least one year. The size of induration that indicates a positive test is as follows:

- Greater than **5 mm:** HIV or risk factors, close TB contacts, CXR evidence of TB.
- Greater than **10 mm:** Indigent/homeless, developing nations, IVDU, chronic illness, residents of health and correctional institutions.
- Greater than **15 mm:** Everyone else.

A negative reaction with **negative controls** implies anergy from immunosuppression, old age, or malnutrition and thus does not rule out TB.

PLEURAL EFFUSION

Abnormal accumulation of fluid in the pleural space. Pleural effusions are classified as **transudative** or **exudative.**

History

Often **asymptomatic,** but patients may present with **dyspnea** and **pleuritic chest pain.**

Consolidation = decreased breath sounds + increased fremitus.

Effusion = decreased breath sounds + decreased fremitus.

PE

Decreased breath sounds, dullness to percussion, and **decreased** tactile fremitus.

Differential

Transudative and exudative pleural effusions may be differentiated as follows:

	Pleural/serum protein	Pleural/serum LDH
Transudate	< 0.5	< 0.6
Exudate	> 0.5	> 0.6

- **Transudative effusion: Intact capillaries** lead to protein-poor pleural fluid. Common causes of pleural fluid transudates include **CHF, nephrotic syndrome, cirrhosis,** and protein-losing enteropathy.
- **Exudative effusion:** Inflammation leads to **leaky capillaries,** resulting in protein-rich pleural fluid. Common causes of exudative pleural effusions include **malignancy, TB,** bacterial **infection** (parapneumonic effusion and empyema), viral infection, pulmonary emboli with infarct, collagen vascular disease, pancreatitis, chylothorax, and traumatic tap.

Evaluation

CXR shows **blunting of the costophrenic angles.** A **decubitus CXR** will determine whether the fluid is free flowing or loculated. Definitive diagnosis is made by **thoracocentesis.** Send pleural fluid for CBC, differential, protein, LDH, pH, glucose, Gram stain, and possibly cytology.

Treatment

- **Transudative:** Treat the underlying condition. Perform therapeutic thoracocentesis if the patient is dyspneic.
- **Malignant:** Consider pleurodesis in symptomatic patients who are unresponsive to chemotherapy and radiation therapy. Alternatives include therapeutic thoracocentesis, pleuroperitoneal shunting, and surgical pleurectomy.
- **Parapneumonic:** Pleural effusion in the presence of **pneumonia.** If there is evidence of empyema (pH < 7.2, glucose < 50 mg/dL, positive Gram stain, LDH > 1000 IU/L), initiate **chest tube** drainage.
- **Hemothorax:** Chest tube.

Parapneumonic effusions require chest tube drainage.

PULMONARY THROMBOEMBOLISM
UCV EM.24, 40

Occlusion of the pulmonary vasculature by a blood clot. Ninety-five percent of emboli originate from DVTs in the deep leg veins. Pulmonary thromboembolism often leads to pulmonary infarction, right heart failure, and hypoxia. Risk factors for DVT and subsequent pulmonary thromboembolism include **Virchow's triad: stasis** (immobility, CHF, obesity, surgery), **endothelial injury** (e.g., trauma, surgery, recent fracture, previous DVT), and **hypercoagulable states** (e.g., pregnancy/postpartum, OCP use, and coagulation disorders such as protein C/protein S deficiency, factor V Leiden, malignancy, and severe burns).

History/PE

Presenting symptoms include dyspnea, **pleuritic chest pain, low-grade fever,** cough, anxiety, and, rarely, hemoptysis or syncope. Signs include **tachypnea; tachycardia;** erythematous, **edematous, tender, warm lower extremity;** and positive Homans' sign (calf pain on forced dorsiflexion; neither sensitive nor specific).

Evaluation

- ABGs reveal **respiratory alkalosis** (due to hyperventilation), with PO_2 < 80 mm (90% sensitive). Calculate alveolar-arterial gradient (may be elevated).
- CXR is usually normal but may show a pleural effusion, **Hampton's hump** (wedge-shaped infarct) or **Westermark's sign** (oligemia in the embolized lung zone). **Dyspnea, tachycardia, and a normal CXR** in a hospitalized and/or bedridden patient should raise suspicion of pulmonary thromboembolism.
- **V/Q scan** may reveal segmental area(s) of mismatch. Results are reported with a designated probability of pulmonary thromboembolism (low, medium, high) and interpreted based on clinical suspicion.
- **Pulmonary angiogram** is the gold standard but is more invasive (Figure 2.17–6).
- EKG is not diagnostic and will most often show **sinus tachycardia.** The "classic" pattern of acute right heart strain with an S in lead I and T-wave inversion in V3 is uncommon.

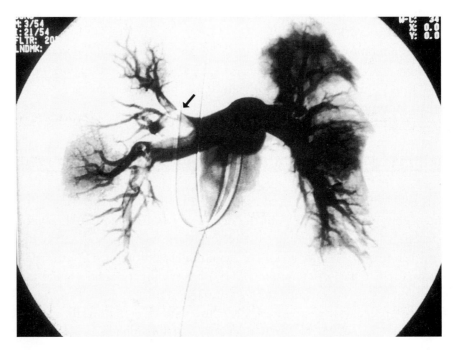

FIGURE 2.17–6. Pulmonary embolus. A large filling defect in the pulmonary artery (arrow) is evident on pulmonary angiogram.

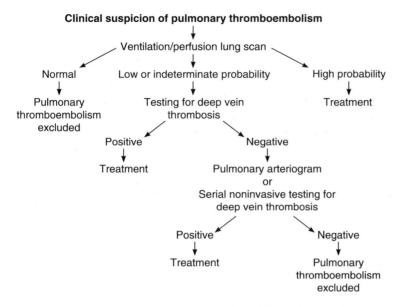

Clinical suspicion of pulmonary thromboembolism

Ventilation/perfusion lung scan

Normal → Pulmonary thromboembolism excluded

Low or indeterminate probability → Testing for deep vein thrombosis

High probability → Treatment

Testing for deep vein thrombosis:
Positive → Treatment
Negative → Pulmonary arteriogram or Serial noninvasive testing for deep vein thrombosis

Positive → Treatment
Negative → Pulmonary thromboembolism excluded

FIGURE 2.17–7. Diagnostic approach to pulmonary embolism.

Figure 2.17–7 describes the evaluation algorithm.

Treatment

- Treat with **heparin.** Start **warfarin** for long-term anticoagulation.
- A **Greenfield filter** is indicated if anticoagulation is contraindicated or if the patient has recurrent emboli while anticoagulated.
- **Thrombolysis** is indicated in severe cases.
- **Prevent DVTs** in bedridden and surgical patients with intermittent pneumatic compression of the lower extremities, **low-dose heparin,** and **early ambulation.**

PNEUMOTHORAX
UCV IM2.47, Surg.36

A collection of air in the pleural space that can lead to pulmonary collapse. **Spontaneous** (primary) pneumothorax occurs with the rupture of subpleural apical blebs (usually in tall, thin young males). **Secondary** causes of pneumothorax include COPD, TB, trauma, *Pneumocystis carinii* pneumonia, and iatrogenesis (thoracocentesis, subclavian line placement, positive-pressure mechanical ventilation, or bronchoscopy). **Tension** pneumothorax occurs when a pulmonary or chest wall defect acts as a one-way valve, drawing air into the pleural space during inspiration but trapping air during expiration. Tension pneumothorax is a life-threatening condition that proceeds to shock and death unless it is immediately recognized and treated.

History

Tension pneumothorax is a medical emergency.

Pleuritic chest pain and dyspnea.

PE

Tachypnea, **diminished/absent breath sounds, hyperresonance,** and **decreased tactile fremitus.** Suspect tension pneumothorax if you see respiratory distress, falling O_2 saturation, hypotension, distended neck veins, and **tracheal deviation.**

Differential

MI, pulmonary emboli, pneumonia, pericardial tamponade, pleural effusion.

Evaluation

CXR shows **lung retraction** from the chest wall (best seen in end-expiratory films; Figure 2.17–8).

Treatment

Small pneumothoraces may reabsorb spontaneously. Large, symptomatic pneumothoraces require **chest tube** placement and/or **pleurodesis** (injection of an irritant into the pleural cavity to scar the two pleural layers together).

Tension pneumothorax is an emergency requiring **immediate needle decompression** in the second intercostal space at the midclavicular line. Do not wait for a CXR! After initial decompression, insert a chest tube.

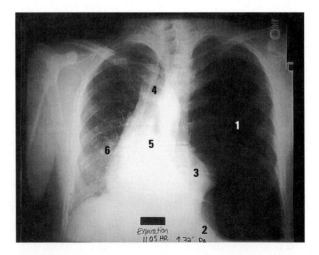

FIGURE 2.17–8. Tension pneumothorax. Note the hyperlucent lung field (1), hyperexpanded lower diaphragm (2), collapsed lung (3), tracheal deviation (4), mediastinal shift (5), and compression of the opposite lung (6) on anteroposterior chest x-ray.

Acute respiratory failure with refractory **hypoxemia, decreased lung compliance,** and **noncardiogenic pulmonary edema.** Its underlying pathogenesis is thought to be endothelial injury. ARDS commonly occurs in the setting of aspiration, infection, multiple blood transfusions, lung injury, shock, or sepsis.

ARDS occurs in the setting of aspiration, infection, shock, or sepsis.

History/PE

Acute onset (12–48 hours) of respiratory distress, tachypnea, fever, crackles, and rhonchi.

Differential

Cardiogenic pulmonary edema, pneumonia, bronchiolitis obliterans with organizing pneumonia.

Evaluation

Findings include **diffuse, bilateral pulmonary infiltrates** on CXR, hypoxemia refractory to oxygen therapy, **normal capillary wedge pressure,** and decreased lung compliance.

Treatment

Administer **mechanical ventilation with PEEP;** treat underlying disorder. Overall mortality is > 50%.

Reversible airway obstruction secondary to bronchial **hyperreactivity,** acute airway **inflammation, mucous plugging,** and smooth muscle hypertrophy of the airways. Triggers include allergens (dust, animal hair, odors), URIs, cold air, exertion, and stress.

Asthma triggers include allergens, URIs, cold air, exercise, and stress.

History

Cough, dyspnea, **episodic wheezing,** and/or chest tightness. Historical features suggesting severe asthma include a history of frequent ER visits, intubations, and PO steroid use.

PE

Tachypnea, tachycardia, **prolonged expiratory duration** (decreased I/E ratio), decreased O$_2$ saturation (late sign), decreased breath sounds, wheezing, hyperresonance, **accessory muscle use,** and possibly pulsus paradoxus.

HIGH-YIELD FACTS

Pulmonary Medicine

Differential

"All that wheezes is not asthma."

- **Children:** Aspiration, bronchiolitis, bronchopulmonary dysplasia, CF, GERD, vascular rings, pneumonia.
- **Adults:** CHF, COPD, GERD, pulmonary embolism, foreign body, tumor, sleep apnea, anaphylaxis.

Evaluation

Rising PaCO$_2$ may indicate fatigue and impending respiratory failure.

ABGs may reveal **mild hypoxia** and **respiratory alkalosis; acidosis indicates severe attack. Peak flow** is **diminished** during acute exacerbation. Spirometry demonstrates decreased 1-second forced expiratory volume (FEV$_1$). **CBC** may demonstrate **eosinophilia. CXR** shows **hyperinflation.** Definitive diagnosis (when patient is not acutely ill) can be made with the bronchial hyperresponsiveness (BHR) test with a **methacholine challenge.**

Treatment

- **Acute management** includes **oxygen, bronchodilators** (beta-agonist or ipratropium), and **steroids.**
- **Chronic management** includes avoidance of allergens, regularly inhaled **bronchodilators** or **steroids,** systemic steroids, **cromolyn,** or **theophylline.** New guidelines support the use of anti-inflammatory agents if the patient is symptomatic > 2 times per week or has nocturnal symptoms ≥ 2 times per month. **Zafirlukast** and other leukotriene antagonists are oral agents that may serve as adjuncts to inhalant therapy.

CHRONIC OBSTRUCTIVE PULMONARY DISEASE (COPD)   U©V *IM2.43, 44*

A disease characterized by airflow obstruction due to chronic bronchitis or emphysema. **Chronic bronchitis** is a productive cough lasting at least 3 months over a period of two years. **Emphysema** is a pathologic diagnosis of terminal airway destruction. Most patients have components of both, and **nearly all are smokers.**

History/PE

- **Emphysema ("pink puffer"):** Decreased breath sounds, minimal cough, dyspnea, pursed lips, hypercarbia/hypoxia late, barrel chest.
- **Chronic bronchitis ("blue bloater"):** Rhonchi, productive cough, mild dyspnea, hypercarbia/hypoxia early.

Differential

Asthma, bronchiectasis, CF, lung cancer.

Evaluation

CXR classically shows decreased markings with flat diaphragms, **hyperinflated lungs,** and a thin mediastinum; parenchymal **bullae** or subpleural **blebs** may be noted (Figure 2.17–9). Peak flows are decreased, total lung capacity and residual volumes are increased, and DLCO is decreased. An ABG during an acute exacerbation will show **hypoxemia** with **acute respiratory acidosis** (↑ PCO_2; however, patients have baseline ↑ PCO_2). Obtain blood cultures if the patient is febrile or has a productive cough.

Treatment

- **Acute exacerbations: Oxygen, beta-agonists** (albuterol), **anticholinergics** (ipratropium), **steroids,** and **antibiotics.**
- **Chronic: Smoking cessation,** supplemental oxygen, beta-agonists (albuterol), anticholinergics (ipratropium), **pneumococcal and flu vaccines.**

"CO_2 retainers" occasionally do worse with supplemental O_2 because they lose their hypoxemic drive to breathe and acutely increase their PCO_2.

Complications

- **Chronic respiratory failure:** Chronic hypoxemia with a compensated respiratory acidosis (high PCO_2).
- **Cor pulmonale:** Secondary to pulmonary vascular obliteration. *IM1.5*
- **Pneumonia.**
- **Bronchogenic carcinoma.**

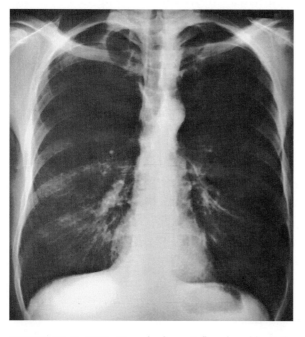
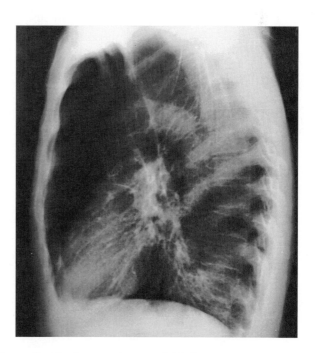

FIGURE 2.17–9. COPD. Note the hyperinflated and hyperlucent lungs, flat diaphragms, increased AP diameter, narrow mediastinum, and large upper lobe bullae on anteroposterior and lateral chest x-rays.

A systemic disease of unknown etiology characterized by **noncaseating granulomas.** Sarcoid is most common in **black females** and usually presents in the third or fourth decade of life.

History/PE

Fever, cough, malaise, weight loss, dyspnea, and **arthritis,** commonly of the knees and ankles. The lungs, liver, eyes, skin, nervous system, heart, and kidney may be affected.

Differential

TB, lymphoma, histoplasmosis, coccidioidomycosis, idiopathic pulmonary fibrosis, pneumoconioses, HIV, berylliosis.

Evaluation

Sarcoidosis is a **diagnosis of exclusion** (steroid treatment for sarcoid will exacerbate TB or other infections).

- CXR shows **bilateral hilar lymphadenopathy** and/or pulmonary infiltrates.
- Biopsy (transbronchial is best) of involved regions reveals noncaseating granulomas.
- PFTs show decreased volumes and diffusion capacity.
- Other findings may include **elevated serum ACE levels** (neither sensitive nor specific), **hypercalcemia,** hypercalciuria, elevated alkaline phosphatase (with liver involvement), and lymphopenia.
- Kveim skin test is often positive (performed by injecting protein from human sarcoid tissue).

Treatment

Systemic **corticosteroids.**

Features of sarcoid—

GRUELING
Granulomas
Rheumatoid arthritis
Uveitis
Erythema nodosum
Lymphadenopathy
Interstitial fibrosis
Negative TB test
Gammaglobulinemia

Renal

$$ANION\ GAP = Na^+ - Cl^- - HCO_3^-$$

RENAL TUBULAR ACIDOSIS (RTA)   UCV *IM2.38*

↓ H⁺ SECRETION
OR
↓ HCO₃⁻ ABSORPTION
⇓
NON ANION GAP
METABOLIC ACIDOSIS

A net decrease in tubular hydrogen secretion or bicarbonate reabsorption that produces a non-anion-gap metabolic acidosis. There are three main types:

- **Type 1:** Defective hydrogen ion secretion. ↑ urinary pH.
- **Type 2:** Decreased bicarbonate reabsorption. ↑ urinary pH until bicarbonate wasting reaches a steady state and no longer causes a rise in urinary pH.
- **Type 4:** Aldosterone resistance or deficiency impairs distal Na^+ reabsorption and K^+ secretion. Results in hyperkalemia. The most common type of RTA.

Table 2.18–1 further distinguishes the three main types of RTA.

TABLE 2.18–1. Types of RTA.

Variable	Type 1 (Distal)	Type 2 (Proximal)	Type 4 (Distal)
Defect	↓ H⁺ secretion	↓ HCO₃ reabsorption	Inadequate aldosterone
Serum K	Low GIVE K	Low GIVE K	High COMMON
Urinary pH	> 5.3	< 5.3	< 5.3
Etiology (most common)	Hereditary, amphotericin, collagen vascular disease, cirrhosis, nephrocalcinosis	Hereditary, sulfonamides, carbonic anhydrase inhibitors, Fanconi syndromes	Hyporeninemic hypoaldosteronism with diabetes, HTN, or chronic interstitial nephritis; aldosterone resistance
Treatment	HCO₃ + K	HCO₃ + K, thiazide	Fludrocortisone, K restriction, HCO₃ *MINERACORTICOID*

Etiologies are derived from multiple referenced articles in *Primary Care Pearls and References*, Blackwell Science, 1996, p. 225. Table format is derived from *Guide to Inpatient Medicine*, Williams & Wilkins, 1997, p. 225.

(handwritten top-left: 3.5 < K < 5)

Serum potassium > 5.0 mEq/L.   *(handwritten: Nₖ   ↓NEURO FXN)*

History/PE

Asymptomatic or present with nausea, vomiting, **intestinal colic, areflexia, weakness,** flaccid paralysis, and paresthesias. Causes include:

- **Spurious:** Hemolysis (e.g., during phlebotomy), fist clenching during blood draw, leukocytosis, thrombocytosis.
- **Decreased excretion:** Renal insufficiency, drugs (spironolactone, triamterene, **ACE inhibitors,** trimethoprim, NSAIDs), mineralocorticoid deficiency.
- **Cell shifts:** Tissue injury, acidosis, insulin deficiency, drugs (succinylcholine, digitalis, beta-agonists, arginine).
- **Iatrogenic**

Evaluation

EKG findings may include **tall peaked T waves,** PR prolongation followed by loss of P waves, and wide QRS complex that can progress to **torsades de pointes** (Figures 2.18–1 and 2.18–2).

Treatment

- First verify hyperkalemia with a **repeat blood draw** unless the suspicion was already very high.
- Values > 6.5–7.0 mEq/L and/or EKG changes require emergent treatment.
- Use **calcium gluconate** for cardiac membrane stabilization.
- Shift potassium into cells (an immediate, short-term solution) with **sodium bicarbonate, insulin + glucose,** or albuterol.
- **Kayexalate** and **loop diuretics** (furosemide) will remove potassium from the body.
- **Dialysis** is an option for patients with renal failure or in severe, refractory cases.

(margin note, italic) Verify hyperkalemia with a repeat blood draw.

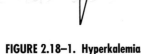

FIGURE 2.18–1. Hyperkalemia. Electrocardiographic manifestations include peaked T waves, PR prolongation, and a widened QRS complex.

(handwritten margin: ↓P ←QRS→ ↑T)

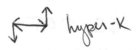
(handwritten: hyper-K)

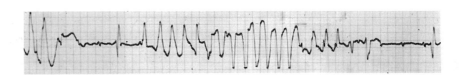

FIGURE 2.18–2. Torsades de pointes. The QRS axis gradually shifts so the complex appears as a twisting strip; this is a pleomorphic ventricular tachycardia often caused by QT prolongation from electrolyte abnormalities or drugs. *IM1.16*

HYPOKALEMIA

Serum potassium < 3.5 mEq/L.

History/PE

Fatigue, **muscle weakness,** and **muscle cramps** progressing to **ileus,** hyporeflexia, paresthesias, and flaccid paralysis if severe.

SIMILAR TO ↑K

Evaluation

EKG may show **T-wave flattening** and ST depression followed by AV block and then cardiac arrest. **U waves** may be present.

↓T ↓ST

↓ST ↓T hypo-K

Differential

Inadequate intake, diarrhea, alkalosis, drugs (diuretics, insulin, gentamicin, amphotericin, carbenicillin), RTA, mineralocorticoid excess, DKA.

TYPE I, II

Treatment

Treat the underlying disorder. Administer oral and/or IV **potassium replacement.** Magnesium deficiency will make potassium repletion more difficult.

Mg deficiency makes K repletion difficult.

HYPOCALCEMIA

Serum calcium < 8.5 mg/dL.

8.5 < Ca < 10.5

History

Abdominal/muscle cramps, dyspnea, tetany, and convulsions.

PE

Facial spasm with tapping over facial nerve (**Chvostek's sign**) and carpal spasm seen with arterial occlusion by a blood pressure cuff (**Trousseau's sign**). EKG may show a **prolonged QT interval** (a variety of drugs do this).

Serum calcium may be falsely low in hypoalbuminemia.

Differential

Hypoparathyroidism *(IM1.25)* (postsurgery, idiopathic), lack of vitamin D (nutrition, renal failure, short bowel), hypomagnesemia, acute pancreatitis, medullary thyroid cancer (excess calcitonin).

↓Ca ↑QT

corrected Ca
Ca = Ca meas + .8(4 - Alb)

↓PTH, ↓VIT D, ↓Mg, PANCREATITIS

HIGH-YIELD FACTS

Renal

Treatment

Treat underlying disorder. Administer oral **calcium supplements;** give IV calcium if symptoms are severe.

HYPERCALCEMIA

Serum calcium > 10.5 mg/dL and/or elevated ionized calcium. Most cases are caused by hyperparathyroidism or malignancy. The major causes can be remembered with the mnemonic **CHIMPANZEES:**

- **C**alcium supplementation
- **H**yperparathyroidism (common)
- **I**atrogenic (thiazides)/**I**mmobility
- **M**ilk alkali syndrome
- **P**aget's disease
- **A**ddison's disease/**A**cromegaly
- **N**eoplasm (common, especially squamous cell cancers, myeloma)
- **Z**ollinger–Ellison syndrome (MEN I)
- **E**xcess vitamin A
- **E**xcess vitamin D
- **S**arcoid

(Handwritten margin notes: ↑Ca, ↑PTH, I ATRO, MILK ALK)

(Handwritten note: TREAT ↑Ca WITH STEROIDS)

History/PE

Clinical presentation involves **"bones"** (fractures), **stones** (renal), abdominal **groans** (anorexia, vomiting, constipation), and psychic **overtones"** (weakness, fatigue, altered mental status).

Evaluation

Evaluation should include EKG (may show **short QT interval**), total/ionized calcium, albumin, phosphate, PTH (IRMA), vitamin D, and TSH.

(Handwritten margin note: ↑Ca ↓QT)

Treatment

Treat with **IV hydration** (watch for CHF) followed by **furosemide** diuresis. Calcitonin, pamidronate, etidronate, glucocorticoids, plicamycin, and dialysis are used in severe or refractory cases. **Avoid thiazide diuretics** (increase tubular reabsorption of calcium).

(Handwritten margin note: "Loops (furosemide) Lose calcium.")

(Handwritten note: Calcitonin ↓ Ca → BONE, INHIB OSTEOCLASTS)

Acute renal failure is an abrupt decrease in renal function leading to the retention of creatinine and BUN. Acute renal failure is categorized as **prerenal, intrinsic,** or **postrenal.** Prerenal failure is caused by decreased renal plasma flow. Intrinsic renal failure results from injury within the nephron unit. Postrenal failure is caused by urinary outflow obstruction. Table 2.18–2 outlines the causes of acute renal failure according to subtype.

[handwritten: PRERENAL VS. INTRINSIC VS. POSTRENAL]

History

Malaise, anorexia, and nausea secondary to **uremia.**

PE

Pericardial friction rub, asterixis, hypertension, or decreased urine output. Hypovolemia and orthostasis suggest a prerenal etiology. Findings in intrinsic failure vary depending on etiology. Patients with postrenal etiologies may have an enlarged prostate, weight gain, or pelvic mass.

[handwritten: OBVIOUSLY]

Evaluation

[handwritten: TO CALC FeNa]

Obtain **UA** (RBCs, casts, WBCs), **urine electrolytes,** and serum electrolytes. Always pass a urinary catheter to rule out obstruction. **Renal ultrasound** may rule out obstruction or chronic renal failure. Calculate the following:

$$FeNa = (U_{Na}/P_{Na}) / (U_{Cr}/P_{Cr})$$

A FeNa < 1%, U_{Na} < 20, or BUN/creatinine ratio > 20 suggests a prerenal etiology.

Table 2.18–3 lists the potential findings on microscopic urine examination.

FeNa < 1% suggests a prerenal etiology.

TABLE 2.18–2. Causes of Acute Renal Failure.

Prerenal	Renal (Intrinsic)	Postrenal
Hypovolemia (dehydration, hemorrhage)	Renal ischemia	Prostate disease
	Glomerulonephritis	Kidney stones
Cardiogenic shock	Nephrotic syndrome	Pelvic tumors
Sepsis	Nephrotoxic drugs (e.g., NSAIDs, aminoglycosides)	Recent pelvic surgery
Drugs (NSAIDs)		
Renal artery stenosis	Thromboembolism	

Adapted from Stobo et al., *Principles and Practice of Medicine*, 23rd ed., p. 383.

TABLE 2.18–3. Findings on Microscopic Urine Examination.

Urine Sediment (UA)	Etiology
Hyaline casts	Prerenal
Red cell casts, red cells	Glomerulonephritis (intrinsic)
White cells, white cell casts, +/– eosinophils	Allergic tubulointerstitial nephritis (intrinsic)
Granular casts, renal tubular cells	Acute tubular necrosis (intrinsic)

> **Indications for dialysis—**
>
> **AEIOU**
> **A**cidosis
> **E**lectrolyte abnormalities (K > 6.5 mEq/L)
> **I**ngestions
> **O**verload (fluid)
> **U**remic symptoms (pericarditis, encephalopathy)

Treatment

Fluid and electrolyte balance; adjust medication dosages; **dialyze** if indicated. Give **diuretics** and **IV hydration** for ATN; **discontinue offending medication** in interstitial nephritis; give **corticosteroids/cytotoxic agents** for glomerulonephritis.

NEPHROLITHIASIS   UCV EM.50

Nephrolithiasis most commonly occurs in males in the third and fourth decades of life. Risk factors include a positive family history, **low fluid intake,** gout, postcolectomy/ileostomy, specific enzyme disorders (e.g., glyoxylate carboxylase deficiency, xanthine oxidase deficiency), RTA, certain medications (e.g., acetazolamide, allopurinol, chemotherapeutic agents, calcium carbonate, methoxyflurane, loop diuretics, vitamin D), and hyperparathyroidism. Table 2.18–4 further details the various forms of nephrolithiasis.

History/PE

Acute-onset, colicky, severe flank pain that may radiate to the testes or vulva; nausea and vomiting. Patients move around and are unable to get comfortable (as opposed to those with an acute surgical abdomen).

Evaluation

Lab studies may show either gross or **microscopic hematuria** and an **altered urinary pH.** Obtain **plain film** of the abdomen and possibly **renal ultrasound.**

TABLE 2.18–4. Types of Nephrolithiasis.

Type	Frequency	Etiology/Characteristics
Calcium oxalate	75%	Most common cause is **idiopathic hypercalciuria.** Form in alkaline urine. Radiopaque.
Calcium phosphate	8%	Think **primary hyperparathyroidism.** Radiopaque. _↑Ca ↑Phos_
$Mg-NH_4-PO_4$ (struvite)	9%	Synonymous with struvite or triple phosphate stones. Associated with _Proteus, Pseudomonas, Providencia, Klebsiella_ **UTIs.** Form in alkaline urine. Radiopaque; **staghorn** calculi.
Uric acid	7%	The pH is < 5.5. Can be dissolved by alkalinizing urine. **Radiolucent.** Occur in gout and high purine turnover states. _Tx ALKALINIZE_
Cysteine	1%	Amino acid transport defect. COLA: cysteine, ornithine, lysine, arginine. Radiopaque; **staghorn** calculi.

An **IVP** can be used to confirm the diagnosis (it will show nonfilling of contrast; Figure 2.18–3). **Helical CT scans** may help diagnose other potential etiologies of flank pain.

Treatment

Hydration, analgesia. Further treatment is based on the size of the stone. Kidney stones < 5 mm in diameter can pass through the urethra. Kidney stones < 3 cm in diameter can be treated with **extracorporeal shock wave lithotripsy** or percutaneous nephrolithotomy. Preventive measures include **hydration** and **thiazide diuretics** for calcium stones.

Thiazide diuretics decrease calcium concentration in urine. _↑Ca REABSORPTION_

5mm → PASS

3cm or less LITHOTRIPSY

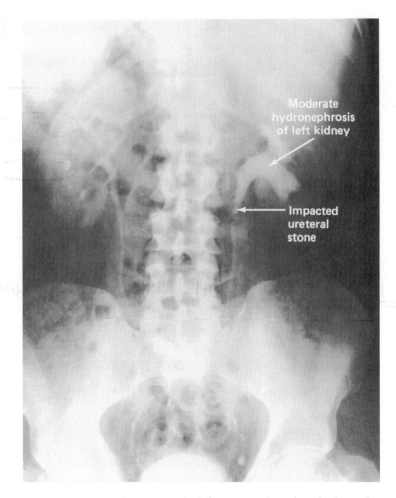

FIGURE 2.18–3. Nephrolithiasis. The stone in the left ureter and resulting hydronephrosis are evident on excretory urogram.

HYPONATREMIA

Serum sodium < 135 mEq/L.

History/PE

Asymptomatic or may present with confusion, muscle cramps, nausea, and **lethargy.** Hyponatremia can progress to seizures, status epilepticus, or coma.

Evaluation

Hyponatremia can be classified by serum osmolality, volume status, and urinary sodium. Osmolality can be further classified as:

- **High** (> 295): Hyperglycemia, hypertonic infusion.
- **Normal** (280–295): Pseudohyponatremia.
- **Low** (< 280): Hypotonic. See Table 2.18–5.

TABLE 2.18–5. Evaluation of Hypotonic Hyponatremia. *Low URINE osm (< 280)*

Varible	Hypervolemic	Euvolemic	Hypovolemic
Renal salt wasting, FeNa > 1%	Renal failure	SIADH, hypothyroidism, renal failure, drugs	Diuretics, RTA, adrenal insufficiency ↓MINERALOCORT
Renal salt conservation, FeNa < 1%	Nephrosis, CHF, cirrhosis	Polydipsia	Vomiting, diarrhea, third spacing
Treatment	Salt and water restriction	Salt and water restriction	Replete volume with normal saline

SIADH

UCV *IM1.30*

INAPPROPRIATE ADH   ↑H₂O RESORP → ↓Na|serum

An important cause of hyponatremia due to **nonosmotically stimulated ADH release.** SIADH is associated with CNS disease (head injury, tumor, nausea), pulmonary disease (e.g., sarcoid), ectopic tumor production/paraneoplastic syndrome (small cell carcinoma), or drugs (antipsychotics, antidepressants).

> *SIADH may be due to CNS disease, pulmonary disease, paraneoplastic syndromes, or drugs.*

Evaluation

Diagnosis is based on urine osmolality > 50–100 mOsm/kg in the setting of serum hyposmolarity. **Urinary sodium is ≥ 20 mEq/L.** A water-loading test can be performed to evaluate free water excretion.

Treatment

Treat with **fluid restriction.** If symptomatic, give saline plus furosemide.

Toxicology

Table 2.19–1 summarizes the major pathogens in food-borne illnesses.

TABLE 2.19–1. Food-borne Illnesses.

Pathogen	Source	Signs/Symptoms/Treatment
Staphylococcus aureus	Meats, **dairy** (mayonnaise). Pre-formed toxin.	Abrupt, intense vomiting within 1–8 hours. Self-limited.
Bacillus cereus	Reheated fried **rice.** Pre-formed toxin.	Abrupt vomiting (within 1–8 hours) followed by watery diarrhea (8–16 hours). Self-limited.
Clostridium perfringens	Rewarmed meat. Pre-formed toxin.	Abrupt, profuse, watery diarrhea (within 8–16 hours).
Clostridium botulinum IM2.11, Ped.27	Home-canned food (ingestion of toxin). Honey.	**Flaccid paralysis.** Onset in 1–4 days. May also occur in infants who are fed honey (ingest spores). Treat with IV antitoxin.
E. coli	Uncooked foods, fecal contamination.	Abrupt diarrhea; vomiting rare. "Traveler's diarrhea."
Vibrio cholera	Endemic areas. Toxin-mediated.	Severe, voluminous, **"rice water" diarrhea.** Treat with vigorous fluid and electrolyte replacement.
Vibrio parahaemolyticus	Contaminated **seafood.**	Self-limited unless immune compromised.
Campylobacter jejuni	Contaminated food, milk, and water.	Fever and inflammatory diarrhea (blood, pus). Usually self-limited. Ciprofloxacin if severe.
Shigella	Transmission by **F**ood, **F**lies, **F**ingers, **F**eces.	Abrupt inflammatory diarrhea, often with blood and mucus, lower abdominal cramps. Ciprofloxacin if severe.

TABLE 2.19–1. (continued) Food-borne Illnesses.

Pathogen	Source	Signs/Symptoms/Treatment
Salmonella	Raw/undercooked chicken.	Fever and inflammatory diarrhea, nausea/vomiting. Usually self-limited. Antibiotics may prolong carrier state and increase relapse rate.
Yersinia enterocolitica	Raw/undercooked pork.	Fever, abdominal pain, inflammatory diarrhea. Ciprofloxacin if severe.

COMMON DRUG SIDE EFFECTS

Table 2.19–2 below summarizes some major drug side effects.

TABLE 2.19–2. Drug Side Effects.

Drug	Side Effects
Penicillin/beta-lactams	Hypersensitivity reactions
Vancomycin	Nephrotoxicity, ototoxicity, "red man syndrome" (histamine release; not an allergy)
Aminoglycosides	Ototoxicity, nephrotoxicity
Tetracyclines	Tooth discoloration, photosensitivity, Fanconi's syndrome
Chloramphenicol	Aplastic anemia, gray baby syndrome
Fluoroquinolones	Cartilage damage in children
Metronidazole	Disulfiram reaction, vestibular dysfunction
INH	Neuropathies, hepatotoxicity, seizures with overdose
Rifampin	Induction of liver enzymes, orange body secretions
Amphotericin	Fever/chills, nephrotoxicity
–azoles (fluconazole, etc.)	Inhibition of liver p450 enzymes
Amantadine	Ataxia
AZT	Thrombocytopenia, anemia
Antipsychotics	Sedation, akathisia, tardive dyskinesia, neuroleptic malignant syndrome
Clozapine	Agranulocytosis
TCAs *Psych.53*	Sedation, anticholinergic effects, seizures and arrhythmias in overdose
SSRIs	Anxiety, sexual dysfunction
MAOIs *Psych.54*	Hypertensive crisis with tyramine (cheese and wine)
Benzodiazepines	Sedation, dependence

HIGH-YIELD FACTS

Toxicology

TABLE 2.19–2. (continued) Drug Side Effects.

Drug	Side Effects
Carbamazepine	Induction of p450, agranulocytosis, aplastic anemia
Phenytoin	Nystagmus, diplopia, ataxia, gingival hyperplasia, hirsutism
Valproic acid	Neural tube defects
Halothane	Hepatotoxicity
HCTZ	Hypokalemia, hyperuricemia, hyperglycemia
Furosemide	Ototoxicity, hypokalemia, nephritis
Clonidine	Dry mouth, severe rebound hypertension
Methyldopa	Positive Coombs' test
Reserpine	Depression
Prazosin	First-dose hypotension
Beta-blockers	Asthma exacerbation, masking of hypoglycemia, impotence
Hydralazine	Lupus syndrome
Calcium channel blockers	Peripheral edema, constipation, cardiac depression
ACE inhibitors	Cough, rash, proteinuria, angioedema, taste changes
Nitroglycerin	Hypotension, tachycardia, headache, tolerance
Digoxin	GI disturbance, yellow visual changes, arrhythmias
Quinidine	Cinchonism (headache, tinnitus), thrombocytopenia, dysrhythmias (e.g., torsades de pointes)
Amiodarone	Pulmonary fibrosis, peripheral deposition (bluish), arrhythmias, hypo/hyperthyroidism
Procainamide	Lupus syndrome
Bile acid resins	GI upset, malabsorption of vitamins and medications
HMG-CoA reductase inhibitors	Myositis, reversible ↑ LFTs
Niacin	Cutaneous flushing
Gemfibrozil	Myositis, reversible ↑ LFTs
Cyclophosphamide	Myelosuppression, hemorrhagic cystitis
Cisplatin	Nephrotoxicity, acoustic nerve damage
Doxorubicin	Cardiotoxicity
Corticosteroids	Mania (acute), immunosuppression, bone mineral loss, thin skin, easy bruising, myopathy (chronic)

HIGH-YIELD FACTS

Toxicology

Table 2.19–3 summarizes drug withdrawal symptoms and treatment.

HIGH-YIELD FACTS

Toxicology

TABLE 2.19–3. Management of Drug Withdrawal.

Drug	Withdrawal	Treatment
Alcohol	Tremor (6–12 hours), tachycardia, hypertension, agitation, seizures (within 48 hours), hallucinations, **delirium tremens** (severe autonomic instability, including tachycardia, hypertension, delirium, and death) within 2–7 days. Mortality is 15–20%.	Benzodiazepines, haloperidol for hallucinations. Thiamine, folate, and multivitamin replacement (will not affect withdrawal, but most alcoholics are malnourished).
Opioids	Anxiety, insomnia, anorexia, sweating/piloerection, fever, rhinorrhea, nausea, stomach cramps, diarrhea.	Clonidine and/or buprenorphine for moderate withdrawal. Methadone for severe symptoms. Naltrexone for patients drug-free for 7–10 days.
Cocaine/amphetamines	Depression, hyperphagia, hypersomnolence.	Bromocriptine.
Barbiturates	Anxiety, seizures, delirium, tremor.	Mainstay of treatment is with benzodiazepines.
Benzodiazepines	Rebound anxiety, seizures, tremor, insomnia.	Mainstay of treatment is with benzodiazepines (same as alcohol withdrawal). Watch out for delirium tremens.

Table 2.19–4 describes some common drug interactions.

TABLE 2.19–4. Drug Interactions.

Interaction/Reaction	Drugs
Induction of p450 enzymes	Barbiturates, phenytoin, carbamazepine, rifampin
Inhibition of p450 enzymes	Cimetidine, ketoconazole
Metabolism by p450 enzymes	Benzodiazepines, amide anesthetics, metoprolol, propranolol, nifedipine, phenytoin, quinidine, theophylline, warfarin, barbiturates
Raising of serum levels of digoxin	Quinidine, amiodarone, calcium channel blockers
Competition for albumin binding sites	Warfarin, aspirin, phenytoin
Blood dyscrasias	Ibuprofen, quinidine, methyldopa, chemotherapeutic agents
Hemolysis in G6PD-deficient patients	Sulfonamides, INH, aspirin, ibuprofen, primaquine
Gynecomastia	Cimetidine, ketoconazole, spironolactone
Stevens–Johnson syndrome	Ethosuximide, sulfonamides
Photosensitivity	Tetracycline, amiodarone, sulfonamides
Lupus-like syndrome	Procainamide, hydralazine, INH

HIGH-YIELD FACTS

Toxicology

345

Table 2.19–5 summarizes the treatment for various substance overdoses.

TABLE 2.19–5. Specific Antidotes.

Toxin	Antidote/Treatment
Acetaminophen	N-acetylcysteine
Anticholinesterases, organophosphates	Atropine, pralidoxime
Iron salts	Deferoxamine
Methanol, ethylene glycol (antifreeze)	Ethanol, tomepizole, dialysis
Lead	CaEDTA, dimercaprol, succimer
Arsenic, mercury, gold	Dimercaprol, succimer
Copper, arsenic, lead, gold	Penicillamine
Antimuscarinic, anticholinergic agents	Physostigmine
Cyanide	Nitrite, sodium thiosulfate
Salicylates	Alkalinize urine, dialysis
Heparin	Protamine
Methemoglobinemia	Methylene blue
Opioids	Naloxone
Benzodiazepines	Flumazenil
Tricyclic antidepressants	Sodium bicarbonate for QRS prolongation, diazepam or lorazepam for seizures, cardiac monitor for arrhythmias
Warfarin	Vitamin K, FFP
Carbon monoxide	100% O_2, hyperbaric O_2
Digitalis	Stop dig, normalize K, lidocaine, anti-dig Fab
Beta-blockers	Glucagon
tPA, streptokinase	Aminocaproic acid
PCP	Nasogastric suction
Theophylline/phenobarbital	Activated charcoal
Cocaine/amphetamines	Supportive, avoid beta-blockers

Table 2.19–6 summarizes the symptoms of vitamin deficiencies.

TABLE 2.19–6. Vitamin Deficiencies.

Vitamin	Deficiency	Comment
Vitamin A (retinol)	Night blindness, dry skin	A constituent of retinal pigments.
Vitamin B_1 (thiamine)	Beriberi, Wernicke–Korsakoff syndrome	Wet beriberi refers to high-output cardiac failure. Dry beriberi refers to associated peripheral neuropathies. Wernicke–Korsakoff syndrome includes ataxia, diplopia, amnesia, and confabulation.
Vitamin B_2 (riboflavin)	Angular stomatitis	Constituent of FAD.
Vitamin B_3 (niacin)	Pellagra (dermatitis, diarrhea, dementia)	Constituent of NAD.
Vitamin B_5 (pantothenate)	Dermatitis, enteritis, alopecia, adrenal insufficiency	Constituent of CoA.
Vitamin B_6 (pyridoxine)	Glossitis, cheilosis	Deficiency caused by INH; used in transamination reactions.
Biotin	Dermatitis, enteritis	Caused by antibiotic use, ingestion of raw eggs.
Folic acid	Macrocytic megaloblastic anemia, neural tube defects	Common. Seen in alcoholics and in elderly who do not eat fruits or vegetables. Supplement in pregnancy.
Vitamin B_{12} (cobalamin)	Macrocytic megaloblastic anemia, neuropathies	Usually seen in malabsorption syndrome (sprue, enteritis, postresection, *Diphyllobothrium latum*), pernicious anemia (no intrinsic factor).
Vitamin C (ascorbic acid)	Scurvy (bleeding, bruising, poor wound healing)	Necessary for collagen cross-linking.
Vitamin D *IM1.29*	Rickets, osteomalacia, hypocalcemic tetany	Increased intestinal absorption of calcium and phosphate.
Vitamin E	Increased RBC fragility, ataxia	Antioxidant.
Vitamin K	Increased PT	Necessary for synthesis of factors II, VII, IX, and X. Synthesized by intestinal flora; antagonized by warfarin.

Vitamins A, D, E, and K are fat-soluble. Expect deficiencies of these vitamins in fat malabsorption syndromes.

A **hypoxemic poisoning syndrome** seen in patients exposed to automobile exhaust, smoke inhalation, barbecues in poorly ventilated locations, or old appliances.

History/PE

Hypoxemia, flushed, **cherry-red skin,** confusion, and **headaches.** Coma or seizure occurs in severe cases. Chronic low-level exposure may mimic **flu-like symptoms** with generalized myalgias, nausea, and headaches. **Suspect smoke inhalation in the presence of singed nose hairs, facial burns, hoarseness, wheezing, or carbonaceous sputum.**

Evaluation

Pulse oximetry will be falsely elevated in CO poisoning.

Check ABG; normal serum carboxyhemoglobin level is < 5% in nonsmokers and < 10% in smokers. Look for evidence of smoke inhalation, including carbon deposits and mucosal edema on laryngoscopy or bronchoscopy. Check an EKG in the elderly and in patients with a history of cardiac disease.

Treatment

Treat with 100% oxygen (**hyperbaric oxygen** for pregnant patients and those with neurologic symptoms or severely elevated carboxyhemoglobin) to facilitate displacement of CO from hemoglobin. Patients with **smoke inhalation** may require early intubation, since upper airway edema can rapidly progress to complete obstruction.

Trauma

COMPARTMENT SYNDROME

Elevated pressure within a confined space that compromises nerve, muscle, and soft tissue perfusion, most often in the lower leg or forearm. Etiologies include fractures, crush injuries, burns, and reperfusion following arterial repair in an ischemic extremity.

History/PE

Pain out of proportion to physical findings; **pain with passive extension** of the finger/toes; **weakness and paresthesias;** tense compartment on palpation; **pulselessness** and **paralysis** (late findings); and **Volkmann's contracture** of the wrist and fingers secondary to vascular insufficiency (seen after supracondylar fractures).

Evaluation

This is a clinical diagnosis. Measure compartment pressures (which are usually elevated to > 30 mmHg) if diagnosis is uncertain.

Treatment

A **surgical emergency** that requires **immediate fasciotomy** to decrease compartmental pressures and restore tissue perfusion.

> **Signs of compartment syndrome—**
>
> **6P's**
> **P**ain
> **P**allor
> **P**ulselessness
> **P**aresthesias
> **P**aralysis
> **P**oikilothermia

Arterial pulses are often normal early in presentation.

AIRWAY MANAGEMENT IN TRAUMA

Evaluation/Treatment

Airway patency and adequacy of ventilation take precedence over other treatment (the A of the "ABCs" of CPR). Start with supplemental oxygen by

Intubate patients with apnea, inability to protect their airway, impending airway compromise, inadequate oxygenation.

nasal cannulae or face mask for conscious patients. Try a chin-lift or jaw-thrust maneuver to reposition the tongue (the most common cause of airway obstruction in an unconscious patient). An oropharyngeal airway (in unconscious patients) or a nasopharyngeal airway (in responsive patients) can aid bag mask ventilation. Intubate patients with apnea, decreased mental status (protect airway from aspiration of blood/vomitus), impending airway compromise (significant maxillofacial trauma, inhalation injury in fires), and severe closed head injury (to hyperventilate) or if there is failure to adequately oxygenate with a face mask. In traumas, patients should be immediately intubated if the patency of the airway is in doubt. A surgical airway (cricothyroidotomy) may be necessary in patients with significant maxillofacial trauma or who cannot be intubated. Remember to maintain C-spine stabilization in trauma patients, but **never allow this concern to delay airway management.**

PELVIC FRACTURES

Patients often present after a motor vehicle accident. Evaluate with x-rays of the hip and pelvis. Pelvic fractures should be discovered during the secondary trauma survey (after ABCs) and may present as instability when the pelvis is "rocked" or compressed. Hypotension and shock suggest **exsanguinating hemorrhage** requiring emergent operative therapy or embolization of bleeding vessels. MAST (Military Anti-Shock Trousers) can be used in the field to maintain adequate BP/perfusion. A stable pelvic hematoma found on CT should not be explored; follow with serial Hct/Hgb and clinical exams. Patients with uncontrolled pelvic hemorrhage require fracture stabilization with **external pelvic fixation.** If this fails to control hemorrhage, embolization of the injured pelvic vessels is necessary. Pelvic fractures may be associated with **bladder rupture** or urethral injury. Thus, if there is blood at the urethral meatus (do not insert a Foley catheter!), the next critical step in management is to obtain a **retrograde urethrogram** to rule out GU injury.

If there is blood at the urethral meatus, do not insert a Foley catheter.

AORTIC DISRUPTION

A **rapid deceleration injury** seen in high-speed motor vehicle accidents, falls from great heights, or ejection from vehicles. Since complete aortic rupture is rapidly fatal (85% of cases die at the scene), trauma patients with an aortic injury usually have a contained hematoma within the adventitia.

Evaluation/Treatment

Aortic disruption is often associated with first and second rib fractures.

Obtain an immediate CXR, which may reveal a, **widened mediastinum, pleural cap,** deviation of the trachea to the right, and obliteration of the aortic knob. Be suspicious if there are first/second rib fractures. Laceration usually occurs at the ligamentum arteriosum. **Aortography is the gold standard for evaluation.**

Evaluation via CT remains controversial, although spiral CT has improved the utility of CT. TEE should be performed on patients going to the OR.

Evaluation/Treatment

- **Neck:** Intubate early. Surgically explore penetrating injuries to **zone 2.** Evaluation can include aortography, tracheobronchoscopy, and esophagoscopy for zone 1/zone 3 injuries (see Figure 2.20–1).
- **Chest:** Unstable patients with penetrating thoracic injuries require immediate **intubation** and bilateral **chest tubes.** Thoracotomy may be necessary for patient in extremis or if a patient remains unstable despite resuscitative efforts. Leave any impaled objects in place until the patient is taken to the OR, since such objects may tamponade further blood loss. Beware of pneumothorax, hemothorax, cardiac tamponade, aortic disruption, diaphragmatic tear, and esophageal injury.
- **Abdomen:** Patients with a gunshot wound to the abdomen require an **exploratory laparotomy.** Patients with stab wounds who are hemodynamically unstable or who are demonstrating peritoneal signs or evisceration need an exploratory laparotomy. The remainder of patients with abdominal stab wounds should undergo local wound exploration, serial physical examinations, and diagnostic peritoneal lavage or abdominal CT. The **spleen is the most common abdominal organ injured in blunt trauma** (*Surg.35*).
- **Wound irrigation** and **tissue debridement,** not antibiotic therapy, is the most important step in the treatment of contaminated wounds.

Leave any impaled objects in place until the person is taken to the OR.

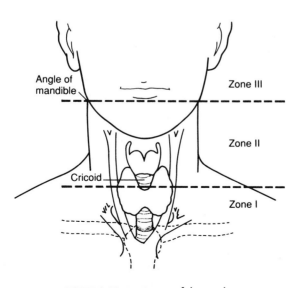

FIGURE 2.20–1. Zones of the neck.

Angle of mandible

Zone III

Zone II

Cricoid

Zone I

HIGH-YIELD FACTS

Trauma

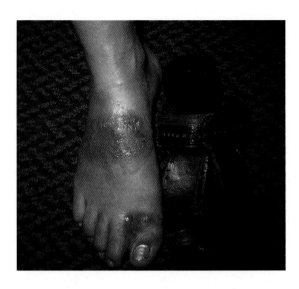

Contact dermatitis. Erythematous papules, vesicles, and serous weeping localized to areas of contact with the offending agent are characteristic.

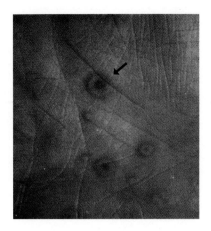

Erythema multiforme. The classic target lesion has a dull red center, pale zone, and darker outer ring (arrow). This acute self-limited reaction may occur with infection, antibiotic use, exposure to radiation or chemicals, or malignancy.

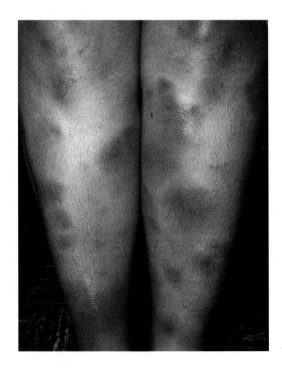

Erythema nodosum. The erythematous plaques and nodules are commonly located on pretibial areas. Lesions are painful and indurated and heal spontaneously without ulceration.

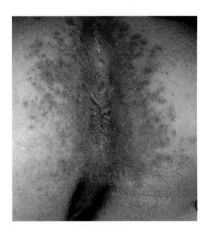

Candidial intertrigo. Erythematous areas surrounded by satellite pustules are restricted to warm, moist intertriginous areas.

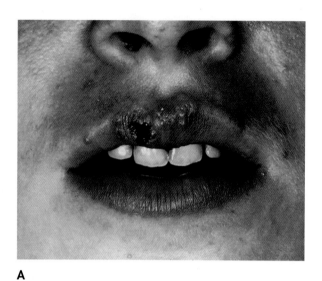
A

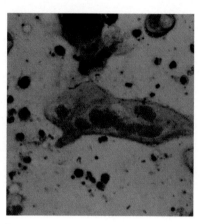
B

Herpes simplex. (A) Primary infection. Grouped vesicles on an erythematous base on the patient's lips and oral mucosa may progress to pustules before resolving. (B) Tzanck smear. The multinucleated giant cells from vesicular fluid provide a presumptive diagnosis of HSV infection. However, the Tzanck smear cannot distinguished between HSV and VZV infection.

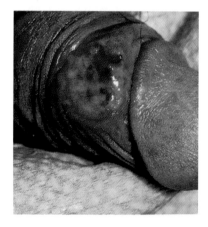

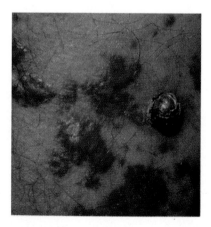

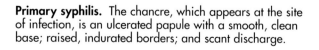

Primary syphilis. The chancre, which appears at the site of infection, is an ulcerated papule with a smooth, clean base; raised, indurated borders; and scant discharge.

Kaposi's sarcoma. Manifests as red to purple nodules and surrounding pink to red macules. The latter appear most often in immunosuppressed patients.

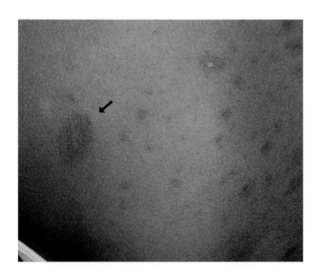

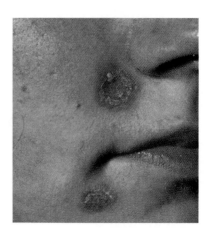

Pityriasis rosea. The round to oval erythematous plaques are often covered with a fine white scale ("cigarette paper") and are often found on the trunk ("Christmas tree distribution") and proximal extremities. The plaques are often preceded by a larger herald patch (arrow).

Impetigo. Dried pustules with superficial golden-brown crust are most commonly found around the nose and mouth.

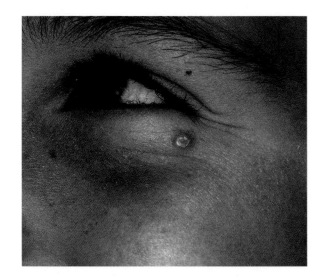

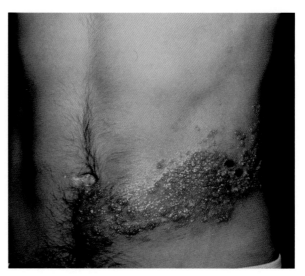

Molluscum contagiosum. The dome-shaped, fleshy, umbilicated papule on the child's eyelid is characteristic.

Herpes zoster. The unilateral dermatomal distribution of the grouped vesicles on an erythematous base is characteristic.

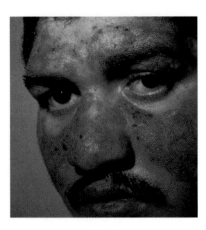

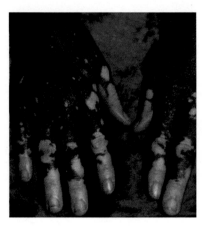

Malar rash of systemic lupus erythematosus. The malar rash is a red to purple continuous plaque extending across the bridge of the nose and to both cheeks.

Vitiligo. Depigmented macules and patches are sharply defined and nonscaling.

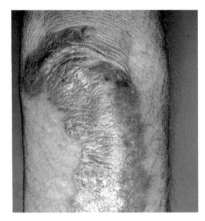

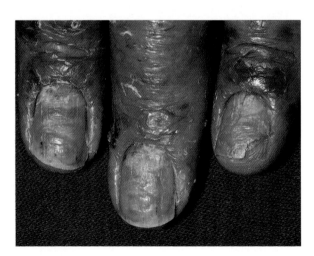

A

B

Psoriasis. (A) Skin changes. The classic sharply demarcated dark red plaques with silvery scale are commonly located on extensor surfaces (e.g., elbows, knees). (B) Nail changes. Note the pitting, onycholysis, and oil spots.

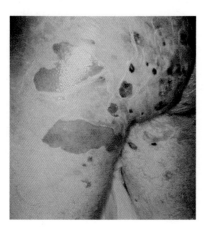

Toxic epidermal necrolysis. Blotchy erythema, burst bullae, and sloughing of epidermis are seen in this life-threatening variant of erythema multiforme.

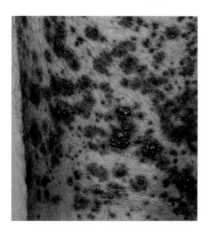

Palpable purpura. Round or oval pink to red macules or patches with overlying purple to red papules. Palpable purpura is associated with necrotizing vasculitides, including Henoch-Schönlein purpura, serum sickness, and essential mixed cyoglobulinemia.

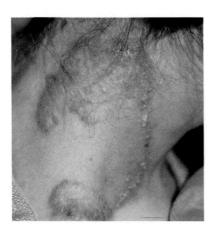

Tinea corporis. Ring-shaped, erythematous, scaling macules with central clearing are characteristic.

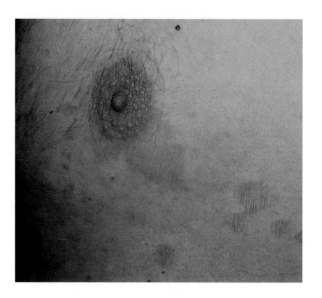

Tinea versicolor. These pinkish scaling macules commonly appear on the chest and back. Lesions may also be lightly pigmented or hypopigmented depending on the patient's skin color and sun exposure.

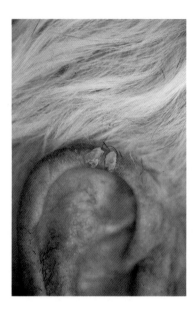

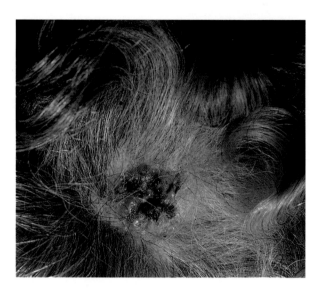

Actinic keratosis. The discrete patch has an erythematous base and rough white scaling. Actinic keratosis is a premalignant lesion that may progress to squamous cell carcinoma. It is most commonly found in sun-exposed areas.

Squamous cell carcinoma. Note the crusting and ulceration of this erythematous plaque. Most lesions are exophytic nodules with erosion or ulceration.

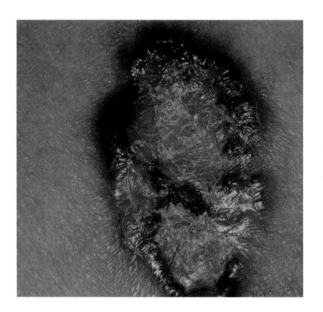

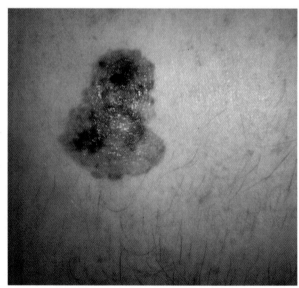

Basal cell carcinoma. Note the pearly, translucent surface (often covered with fine telangectasias), rolled border, and central ulceration.

Melanoma. Note the **a**symmetry, **b**order irregularity, **c**olor variation, and large **d**iameter of this plaque.

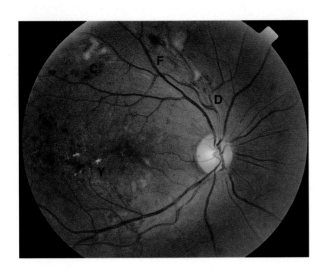

Nonproliferative diabetic retinopathy. Flame hemorrhages (F), dot-blot hemorrhages (D), cotton-wool spots (C), and yellow exudate (Y) result from small vessel damage and occlusion.

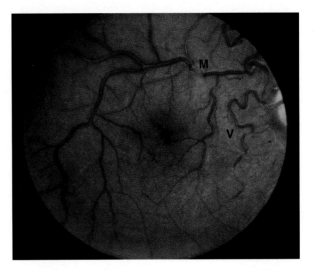

Hypertensive retinopathy. Note the tortuous retinal veins (V) and venous microaneurysms (M). Other findings include hemorrhages, retinal infarcts, detachment of the retina, and disk edema.

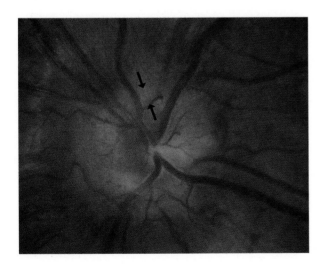

Papilledema. Look for blurred disk margins due to edema of the optic disk (arrows).

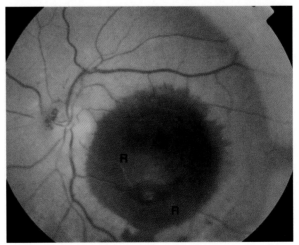

Subretinal hemorrhage. Note the preretinal blood (lighter red) and overlying retinal vessels (R). Subretinal hemorrhages may be seen in any condition with abnormal vessel proliferation (e.g., diabetes, hypertension).

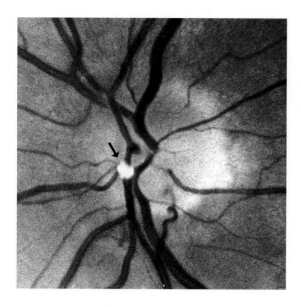

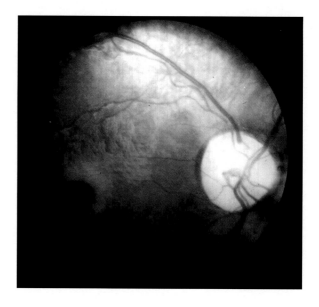

Cholesterol emboli. Cholesterol emboli (Hollenhorst plaque; arrow) usually arise in atherosclerotic carotid arteries and often lodge at the bifurcation of retinal arteries.

Tay-Sachs. Cherry-red spot. The red spot in the macula may be seen in Tay-Sachs disease, Niemann-Pick disease, central retinal artery occlusion, and methanol toxicity.

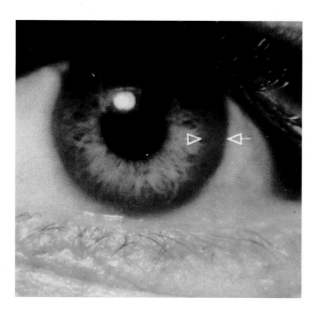

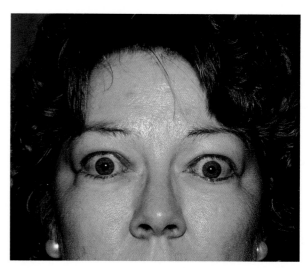

Kayser–Fleischer ring in Wilson's disease. The golden-brown corneal ring (arrows) is due to copper deposition in Descemet's membrane.

Graves' ophthalmopathy. Proptosis with lid retraction resulting from lymphocytic infiltration and edema of the extraocular muscles, which may progress to fibrosis with limited eye movement and blindness from optic nerve compression.

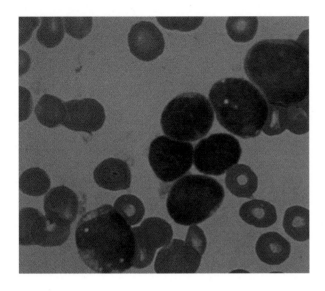

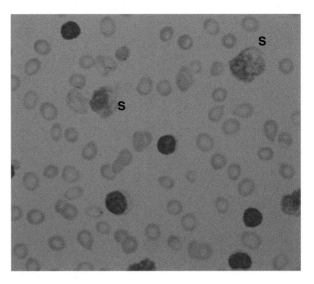

Acute lymphoblastic leukemia. Peripheral blood smear reveals numerous large, uniform lymphoblasts with fine granular cytoplasm and faint nucleoli.

Chronic lymphocytic leukemia. The numerous, small, mature lymphocytes and smudge cells (S; fragile malignant lymphocytes are disrupted during blood smear preparation) are characteristic.

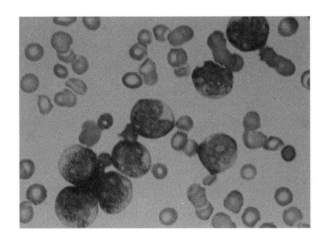

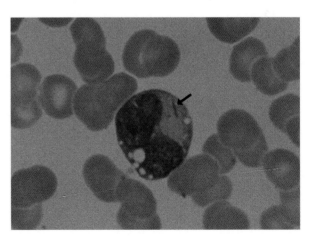

Acute myelocytic leukemia. Large, uniform myeloblasts with notched nuclei and prominent nucleoli are characteristic.

Auer rod in acute myelocytic leukemia. The red rod-shaped structure (arrow) in the cytoplasm of the myeloblast is pathognomonic.

Clinical Images

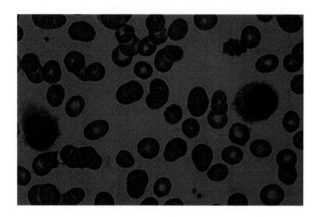

Hairy cell leukemia. Note the hairlike cytoplasmic projections from neoplastic lymphocytes.

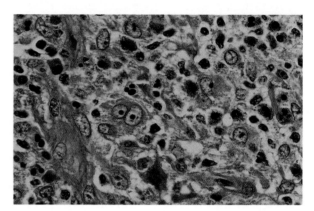

Hodgkin's disease (Reed-Sternberg cell). The characteristic cell of Hodgkin's disease (necessary but not sufficient for diagnosis) has abundant cytoplasm and binucleus with prominent owl-eye inclusion-like nucleoli.

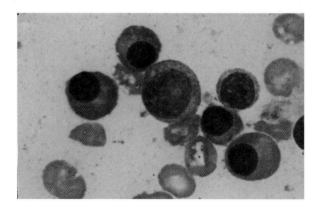

Multiple myeloma. Note the abundance of plasma cells. RBCs will often be in rouleaux formation.

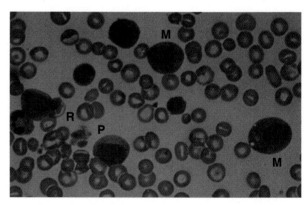

Myelofibrosis. Note the myeloblasts (M), nucleated RBCs (R), and giant platelets (P). Myelofibrosis is a myelodysplastic disorder characterized by fibrosis of the bone marrow and subsequent pancytopenia.

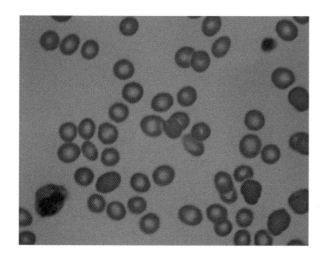

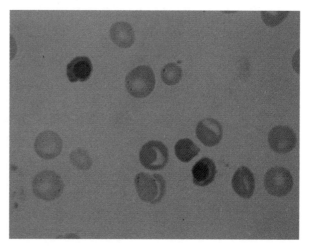

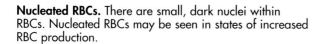

Nucleated RBCs. There are small, dark nuclei within RBCs. Nucleated RBCs may be seen in states of increased RBC production.

Polychromasia. The enlarged, basophilic, immature RBCs may be seen in states of increased RBC production.

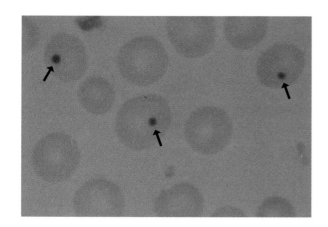

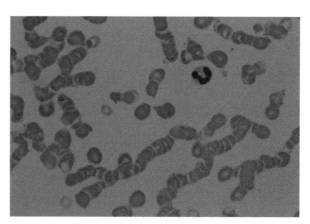

Howell-Jolly bodies. The nuclear fragments (arrow) in circulating red blood cells suggest asplenia.

Rouleaux. RBCs are stacked like poker chips. Rouleaux formation occurs in inflammatory states and multiple myeloma and is associated with a high ESR.

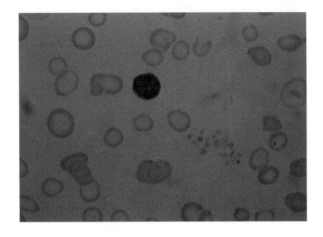

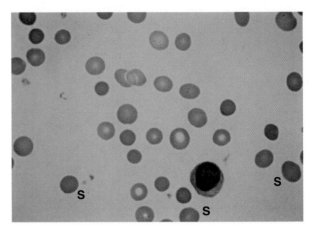

Iron deficiency anemia. Note the microcytic, hypochromic red blood cells ("doughnut cells") with enlarged areas of central pallor.

Spherocytes. These RBCs (S) lack areas of central pallor. Spherocytes are seen in autoimmune hemolysis and hereditary spherocytosis.

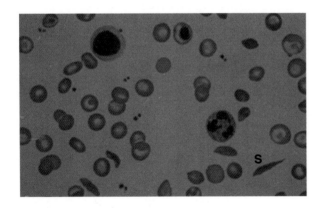

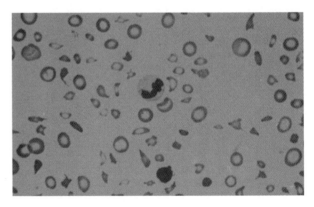

Sickle cells. Sickle-shaped RBCs (S) may appear during infection, dehydration, or hypoxia. Anisocytosis, poikilocytosis, target cells, and nucleated RBCs are also seen in sickle cell disease.

Schistocytes. These fragmented red blood cells may be seen in microangiopathic hemolytic anemia and mechanical hemolysis.

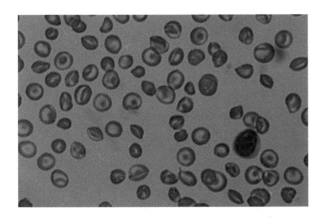

Target cells. The dense zone of hemoglobin in the RBC center is characteristic. Target cells are seen in hemoglobin C or S disease and thalassemia, or they may be an artifact.

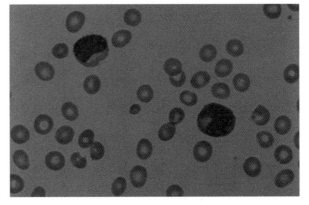

Mononucleosis. These lymphocytes, with enlarged nuclei and prominent nucleoli, are seen in EBV and CMV infections.

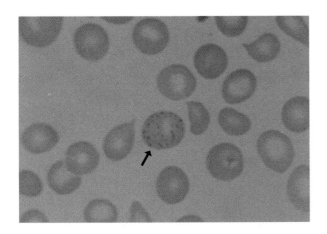
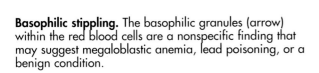

Basophilic stippling. The basophilic granules (arrow) within the red blood cells are a nonspecific finding that may suggest megaloblastic anemia, lead poisoning, or a benign condition.

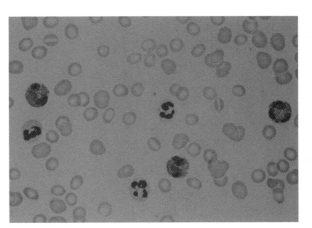

Eosinophilia. Eosinophils have red-staining cytoplasmic granules. Eosinophilia may be seen in allergic reactions, parasitic infections, collagen vascular diseases, malignancies such as Hodgkin's disease, and adrenal insufficiency.

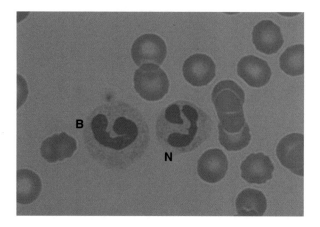

Neutrophil (N) and band (B). The more immature band form has a U-shaped rather than segmented nucleus.

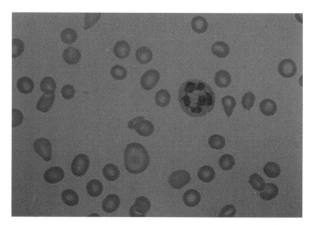

Hypersegmentation. The nucleus of this hypersegmented neutrophil has six lobes (six or more nuclear lobes are required). This is a characteristic finding of megaloblastic anemia.

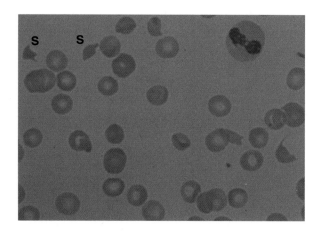

Thrombotic thrombocytopenic purpura (TTP). Note the schistocytes (S) and paucity of platelets. TTP is characterized by microangiopathic hemolytic anemia, thrombocytopenia, fever, neurologic abnormalities, and renal failure.

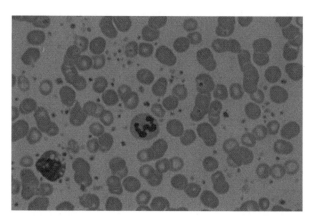

Thrombocytosis. Numerous clumps of platelets are seen in myeloproliferative disorders, severe iron deficiency anemia, acute bleeding, inflammation, malignancy, and postsplenectomy states.

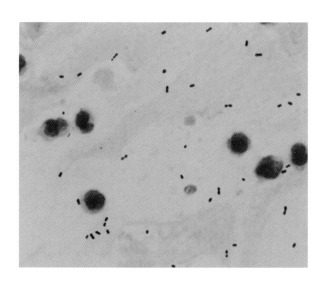

Streptococcus pneumoniae. This is a sputum sample from a patient with pneumonia. Note the characteristic lancet-shaped gram-positive diplococci.

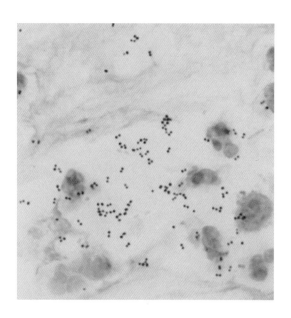

Staphylococcus aureus. These clusters of gram-positive cocci were isolated from the sputum of a patient with pneumonia.

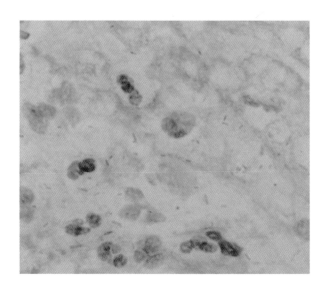

Pseudomonas aeruginosa. This sputum sample from a patient with pneumonia revealed gram-negative rods. The large number of neutrophils and relative paucity of epithelial cells indicates that this sample is not contaminated with oropharyngeal flora.

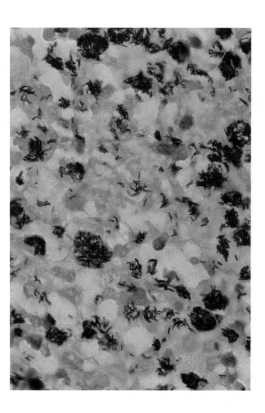

Tuberculosis (AFB smear). Note the red color of the tubercle bacilli an acid-fast staining of a sputum sample ("red snappers").

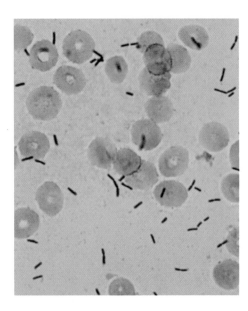

Listeria. These numerous rod-shaped bacilli were isolated from the blood of a patient with *Listeria* meningitis.

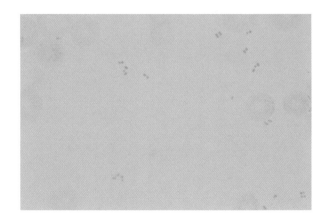

Neisseria. The small kidney-shaped gram-positive diplococci ("kissing kidneys") were isolated from the blood of a patient with meningococcemia.

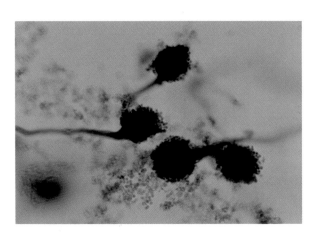

Aspergillosis. Note the characteristic appearance of *Aspergillus* spores in radiating columns.

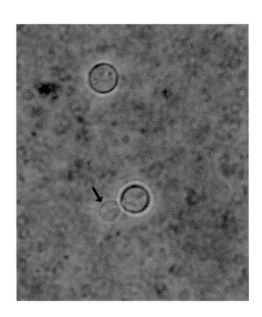

Cryptococcus. Note the budding yeast (arrow) and wide capsule of cryptococcus isolated from CSF.

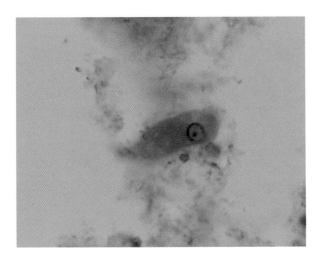

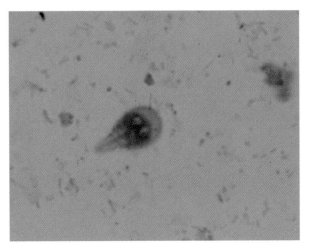

Entamoeba. *Entamoeba* cysts have large nuclei. This is a sample from diarrheal stool.

Giardia **trophozoite in stool.** The trophozoite exhibits a classic pear shape with two nuclei imparting an owl's-eye appearance.

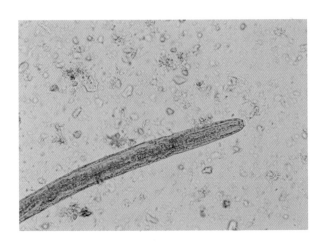

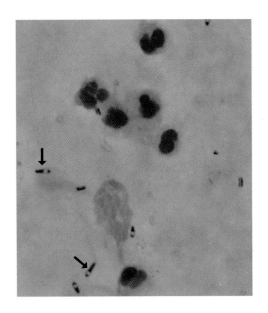

Strongyloides. These filarial larva were found in the stool of a patient watery diarrhea.

Clostridium **wound infection.** The lucency at the end of each gram-positive bacillus is the terminal spore (arrow). This sample was isolated from an infected wound site.

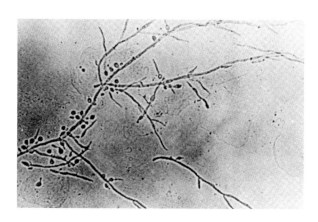

Candidal vaginitis. Branched and budding *Candida albicans* are evident on KOH preparation of vaginal discharge.

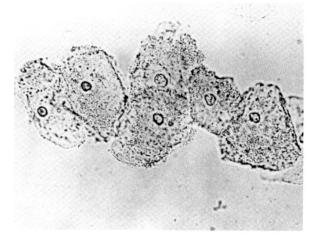

Gardnerella vaginalis. Saline wet mount of vaginal fluid reveals granulations on vaginal epithelial cells ("clue cells") due to adherence of *G. vaginalis* organisms to the cell surface.

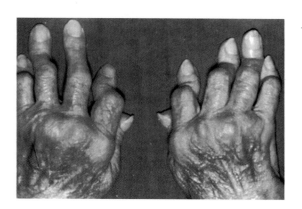

Rheumatoid arthritis. The swan-neck deformities of the digits and well as the severe involvement of the proximal interphalangeal joints is characteristic.

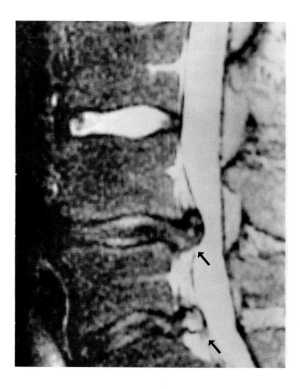

Disk herniation. MRI reveals herniations of the L4-L5 and L5-S1 (arrows).

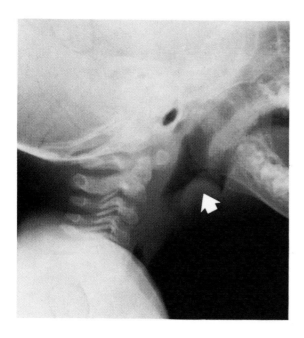

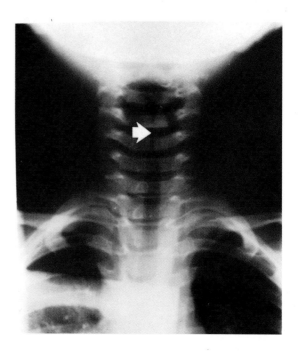

Epiglottitis. The classic swollen epiglottis ("thumbprint sign"; arrow) and obstructed airway are seen on lateral neck x-ray.

Croup. The x-ray shows marked subglottic narrowing of the airway (steeple sign; arrow).

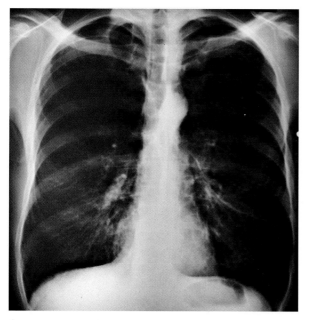

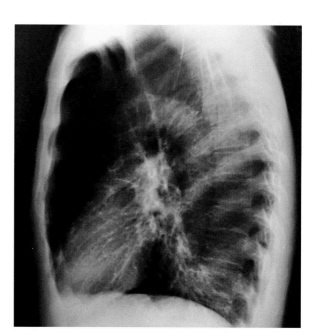

A

B

COPD. Note the hyperinflated and hyperlucent lungs, flat diaphrams, increased AP diameter, narrow mediastinum, and large upper lobe bullae on anteroposterior and lateral chest x-rays.

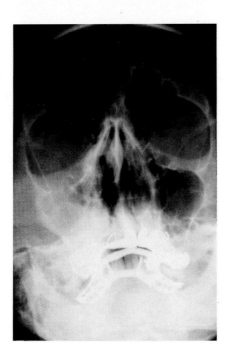

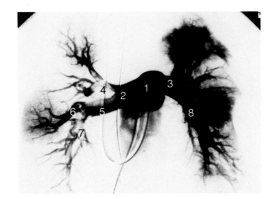

1. Main pulmonary artery
2. Right pulmonary artery
3. Left pulmonary artery
4. Large embolus straddling origin of right upper lobar artery
5. Interlobar artery with embolus
6. Right middle lobar artery
7. Right lower lobar artery and segmental branches filled with tubular emboli
8. Left lower lobar artery

Sinusitis. Compare the opacified right maxillary sinus and normal air-filled left sinus on sinus x-ray.

Pulmonary embolus. A large filling defect in the pulmonary artery is evident on pulmonary angiogram.

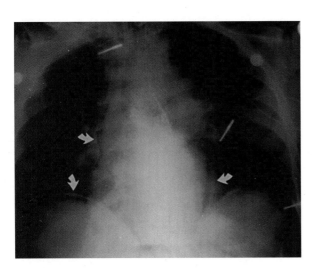

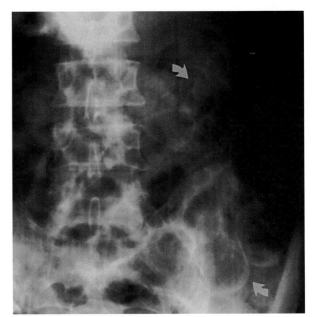

Pneumomediastinum. The lucency outlining the left heart border on chest x-ray suggests air in the mediastinum.

Pneumoperitoneum. The lucency outlining small bowel on abdominal x-ray indicated the abnormal presence of air.

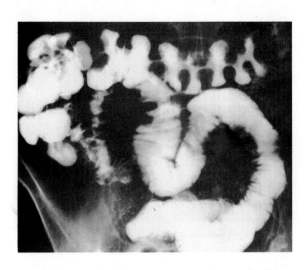

Crohn's disease. Barium enema x-ray reveals deep transverse fissures, ulcers, and edema of the bowel.

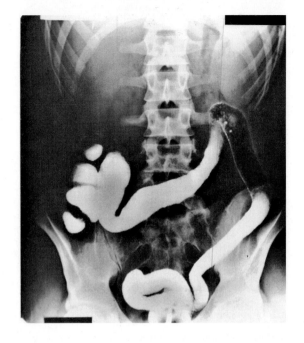

Ulcerative colitis. Barium enema x-ray demonstrates shortening of the colon, loss of haustra ("lead pipe" appearance), and fine serrations at the bowel edges from small ulcers.

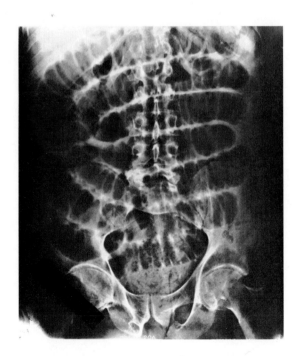

Small bowel obstruction. Supine abdominal x-ray reveals dilated loops of small bowel in a ladder-like pattern. Air-fluid levels may be apparent on an upright x-ray.

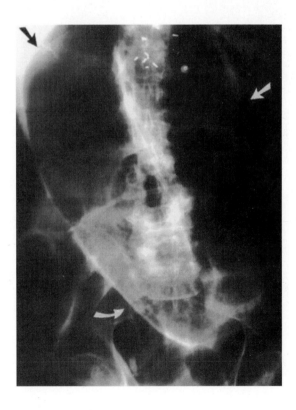

Sigmoid volvulus. Abdominal x-ray reveals the distinctive U-shaped appearance of the air-filled dilated sigmoid colon (arrows). Sigmoid volvulus is a common cause of large bowel obstruction.

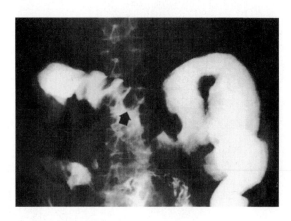

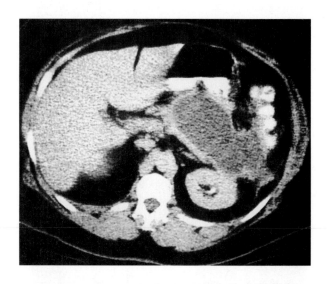

Ischemic colitis. The characteristic thumbprinting of the colonic mucosa is evident on barium x-ray.

Pancreatic pseudocyst. The large pseudocyst impinges on the posterior wall of the stomach (filled with contrast) on CT scan.

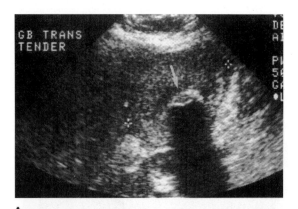

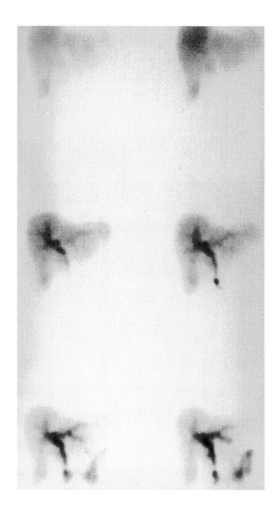

Acute cholecystitis, ultrasound. (A) Note the sludge-filled, thick-walled gallbladder with a hyperechoic stone (arrow) and acoustic shadow. (B) This patient exhibits sludge and pericholecystic fluid (arrow) but no gall-stones.

Acute cholecystitis, HIDA scan. Intravenous dye is taken up by hepatocytes, conjugated, and excreted into the common bile duct. The gallbladder is not visualized, although activity is present in the liver, common duct, and small bowel, suggesting cystic duct obstruction due to acute cholecystitis.

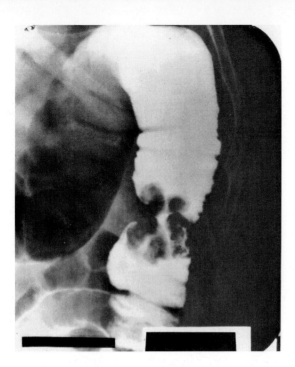

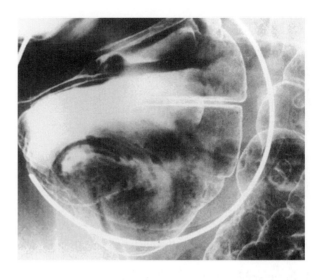

Colon carcinoma. The encircling carcinoma appears as an "apple core" filling defect in the descending colon on barium enema x-ray.

Familial adenomatous polyposis. Double-contrast barium enema x-ray reveals innumerable small polyps.

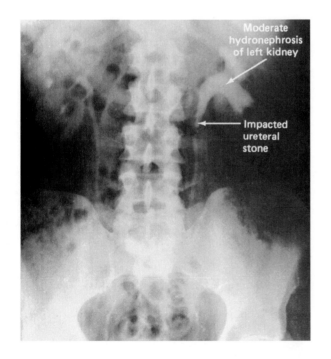

Moderate hydronephrosis of left kidney

Impacted ureteral stone

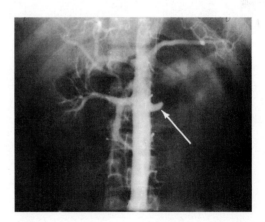

Nephrolithiasis. The stone in the left ureter and resulting hydronephrosis are evident on excretory urogram.

Renal artery thrombosis. Renal arteriogram reveals the loss of left renal vasculature (arrow) following blunt abdominal trauma.

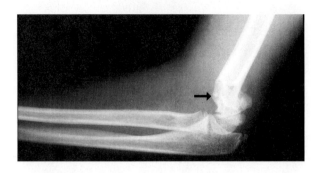

Supracondylar fracture of the humerus. The metaphyseal bone is fractured proximal to the elbow joint (arrow). The growth plate is not involved.

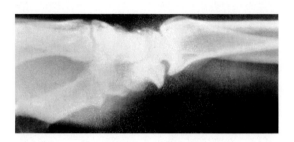

Lunate dislocation. The angle between the scaphoid and the radius is 90 degrees (the normal angle is 45 degrees). This injury is frequently overlooked and best seen on lateral x-ray.

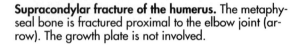

A

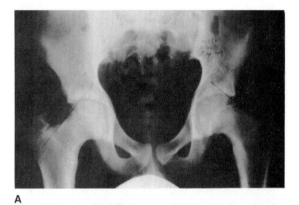

B

Slipped capital femoral epiphysis. (A) Anteroposterior x-ray. The medial displacement of the left femoral epiphysis is best seen with a line drawn up the lateral femoral neck. The abnormal epiphysis does not protrude beyond this line. (B) Frog-leg lateral x-ray. Posterior displacement of the femoral epiphysis is characteristic.

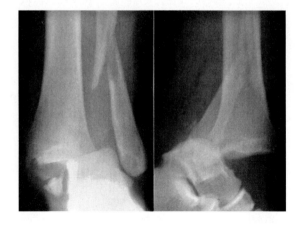

Fracture-dislocation of the ankle. Anteroposterior and lateral x-rays reveal fracture of the lower fibular shaft and medial malleolus. In addition, there is dislocation of the inferior tibiofibular and ankle joints.

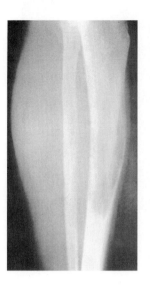
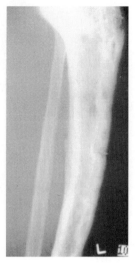

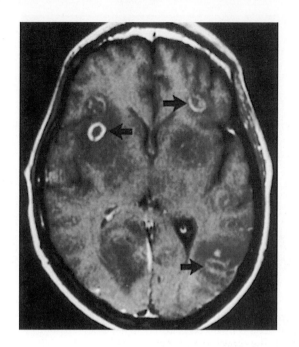

Paget's disease. (A) 45 years old. There are lytic changes in the proximal tibia associated with bulging of the anterior cortex. (B) 65 years old. There is increased cortical density of the tibia in this x-ray taken 20 years later.

CNS toxoplasmosis. This MRI with gadolinium was performed to evaluate an HIV-positive patient with seizures. Note the multiple ring-enhanced lesions (arrows) and surrounding edema. The lesions regressed after treatment with pyrimethamine, sulfadiazine, and leucovorin.

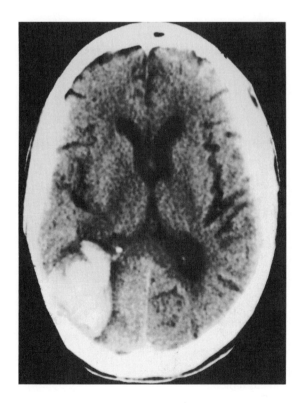

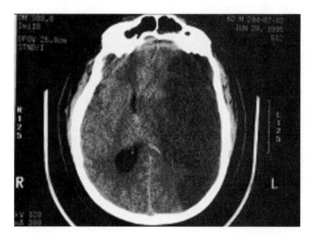

Intracerebral hematoma. Head CT without contrast reveals the irregularly shaped hyperdensity with midline shift of the choroid plexus.

Left MCA stroke. Note the ischemic brain parenchyma subtle midline shift to the right, and left lateral ventricles obliterated by edema. There is no visible hemorrhage.

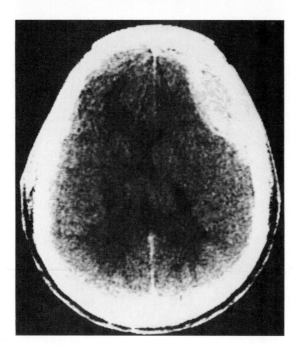

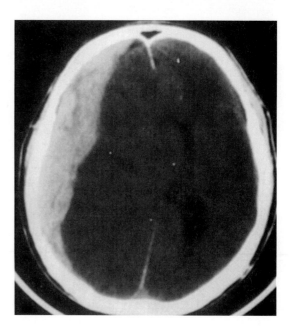

Epidural hematoma. CT scan without contrast reveals a convex, lens-shaped hyperdensity.

Subdural hematoma. The concave, crescent-shaped hyperdensity with shift of the lateral ventricles is evident on CT scan without contrast.

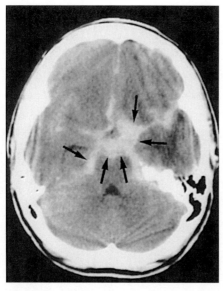

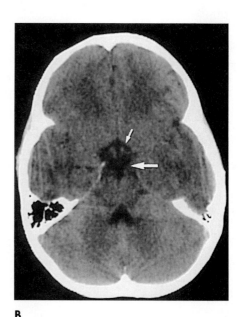

A   B

Subarachnoid hemorrhage. (A) CT scan without contrast reveals blood in the subarachnoid space at the base of the brain (arrows). (B) A normal noncontrast CT scan shows no density in this region.

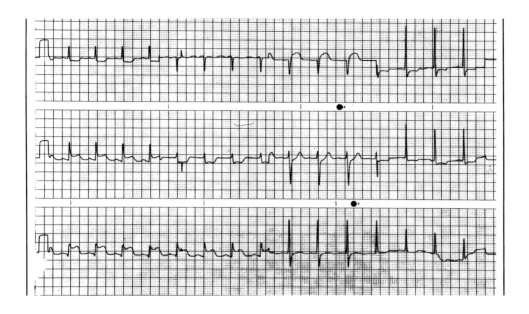

Inferior wall myocardial infarction. In this patient with acute chest pain, the EKG demonstrated acute ST elevation in leads II, III, and aVF.

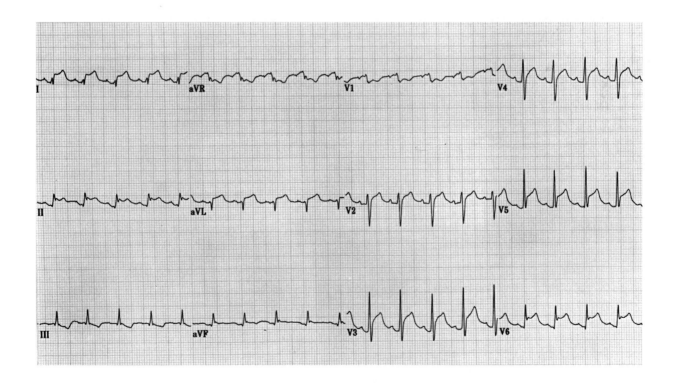

Pericarditis. There is characteristic ST elevation in all leads and PR depression in the precordial leads.

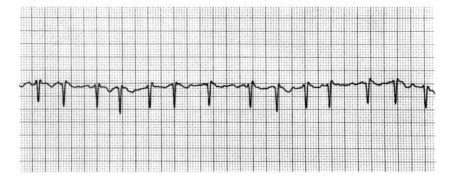

Atrial fibrillation. Note the absence of P waves and irregularly irregular ventricular rhythm.

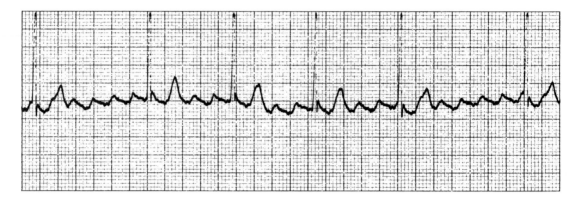

Atrial flutter. The sawtooth baseline of rapid but organized atrial activity (usually between 220 and 360 beats per minute) is characteristic.

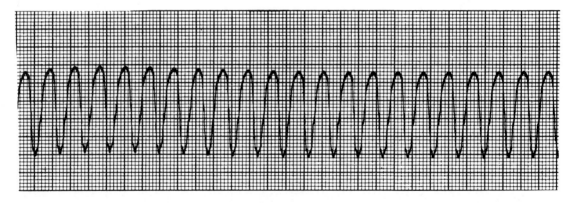

Monomorphic ventricular tachycardia. The widened QRS complex and rapid rate (usually 130-200 beats per minute) are characteristic.

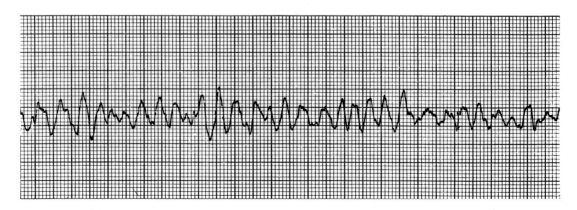

Ventricular fibrillation. Note the wavy baseline without recognizable P waves or QRS complexes.

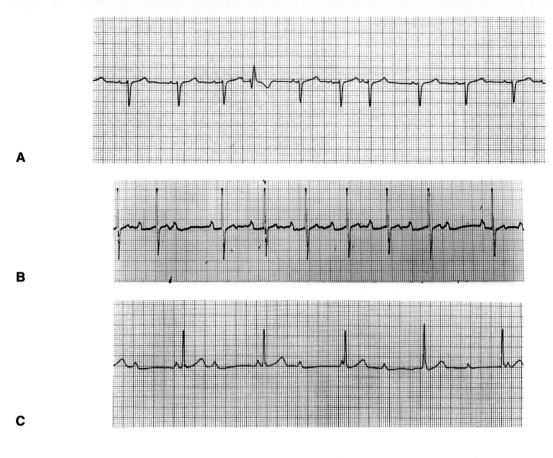

A

B

C

Atrioventricular (AV) block. (A) First-degree AV block is characterized by a prolonged PR interval. (B) Mobitz type I second-degree with Wenckebach phenomenon involves progressive lengthening of the AV interval leading to a dropped P wave. Look for "group beating." (C) Complete heart block. There is complete dissociation between the atrial and ventricular rhythms. The narrow complex rhythm at a heart rate of 40 suggests a junctional pacemaker.

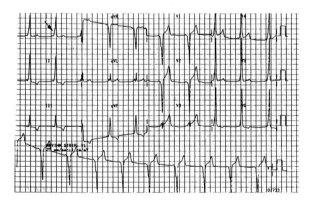

Wolff-Parkinson-White syndrome. The characteristic findings are a shortened PR interval and slurred QRS complex (delta wave; arrow) caused by preexcitation through the bypass tract.

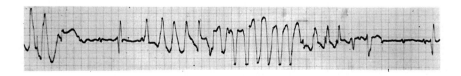

Torsades de pointes. The QRS axis gradually shifts so the complex appears as a twisting strip; this is a pleomorphic ventricular tachycardia that may follow QT prolongation caused by electrolyte abnormalities or drugs.

HIGH-YIELD FACTS

Clinical Images

Database of Clinical Science Review Resources

This section is a database of current clinical science review books, sample examination books, and commercial review courses marketed to medical students studying for the USMLE Step 2. At the end of this section there is a list of publishers and independent bookstores with addresses and phone numbers. For each book, we list the **Title** of the book, the **First Author** (or editor), the **Current Publisher,** the **Copyright Year,** the **Edition,** the **Number of Pages,** the **ISBN Code,** the **Approximate List Price,** the **Format** of the book, and the **Number of Test Questions.** Most entries also include Summary Comments that describe their style and utility for studying. Finally, each book receives a **Rating.** The books are sorted into a comprehensive section as well as into sections corresponding to the seven clinical disciplines (internal medicine, neurology, OB/GYN, pediatrics, preventive medicine, psychiatry, and surgery). Within each section, books are arranged first by Rating, then by Title, and finally by Author.

For this second edition of *First Aid for the USMLE Step 2*, the database of review books has been completely revised, with in-depth summary comments on nearly 100 books and software. A letter rating scale with ten different grades reflects the detailed student evaluations. Each book receives a rating as follows:

A+	Excellent for boards review.
A	Very good for boards review; choose among the group.
A–	
B+	
B	Good, but use only after exhausting better sources.
B–	
C+	
C	Fair, but many better books in the discipline, or low-yield subject material.
C–	
N	Not rated.

The **Rating** is meant to reflect the overall usefulness of the book in preparing for the USMLE Step 2 examination. This is based on a number of factors, including:

- The cost of the book.
- The readability of the text.
- The appropriateness and accuracy of the book.
- The quality and number of sample questions.
- The quality of written answers to sample questions.
- The quality and appropriateness of the illustrations (e.g., graphs, diagrams, photographs).
- The length of the text (longer is not necessarily better).
- The quality and number of other books available in the same discipline.
- The importance of the discipline on the USMLE Step 2 examination.

Please note that the rating does **not** reflect the quality of the book for purposes other than reviewing for the USMLE Step 2 examination. Many books with low ratings are well written and informative but are not ideal for boards preparation. We have also avoided listing or commenting on the wide variety of general textbooks available in the clinical sciences.

Evaluations are based on the cumulative results of formal and informal surveys of hundreds of medical students at many medical schools across the country. The summary comments and overall ratings represent a consensus opinion, but there may have been a large range of opinion or limited student feedback on any particular book.

Please note that the data listed are subject to change because:

- Publishers' prices change frequently.
- Individual bookstores often charge an additional markup.
- New editions come out frequently, and the quality of updating varies.
- The same book may be reissued through another publisher.

We actively encourage medical students and faculty to submit their opinions and ratings of these clinical science review books so that we may update our database. (See How to Contribute, p. xvii.) In addition, we ask that publishers and authors submit review copies of clinical science review books, including new editions and books not included in our database, for evaluation. We also solicit reviews of new books or suggestions for alternate modes of study that may be useful in preparing for the examination, such as flashcards, computer-based tutorials, commercial review courses, and World Wide Web sites.

Disclaimer/Conflict of Interest Statement

No material in this book, including the ratings, reflects the opinion or influence of the publisher. All errors and omissions will gladly be corrected if brought to the attention of the authors through the publisher. Please note that the *Underground Clinical Vignette* series are publications by the authors of this book.

A NMS Review for USMLE Step 2

$35.95   Test/900 q

NMSR

Lippincott Williams & Wilkins, 1999, 2nd ed., 470 pages, ISBN 0683302833

Comprehensive review book in question-and-answer format. **Pros:** The level of difficulty, content, and style of questions closely approximate those seen on the Step 2 exam. Clear, concise, excellent coverage of high-yield topics. Complete explanations. **Cons:** Lacks illustrations. **Summary:** Best single source of Step 2–style questions with appropriate format and content. Highly recommended.

A⁻ Advanced Life Support for the USMLE Step 2

$16.95   Review

Flynn

Lippincott Williams & Wilkins, 1997, 1st ed., 124 pages, ISBN 0397584369

Brief outline format, with high-yield topics described in tables or illustrations. **Pros:** Very quick, easy read. Includes many high-yield facts. Amusing, memorable cartoons highlight key facts. A great review the night before the exam. **Cons:** Not adequate for in-depth review. **Summary:** A quick review that covers the highest-yield topics. Worth the time and money to read through once before the exam.

B⁺ A & L's Flash Facts for the USMLE Steps 2 & 3

$26.50   Test/200 q

Kaiser

Appleton & Lange, 1998, 1st ed., 220 pages, ISBN 0838526063

More than 200 clinically based questions are presented on flashcards. Answers and discussions are on the reverse side of each card. **Pros:** Quick review. Covers high-yield topics in core specialties. Focuses on key aspects of management and diagnosis. Useful for on-the-go review. **Cons:** Style may not suit all students. Expensive for a limited number of topics. Awkward reference system. No index. **Summary:** Quick, concise, portable case-based approach with good emphasis on steps in diagnosis and management. High-quality material, but expensive and limited in scope. Use with other comprehensive resources.

B⁺ A & L's Review for the USMLE Step 2

$36.95   Test/1060 q

Chan

Appleton & Lange, 1999, 3rd ed., 400 pages, ISBN 0838503411

Review questions organized by specialty and two 150-question comprehensive practice exams. Review based on second edition. **Pros:** Overall question content is good, with broad coverage of high-yield topics. Well illustrated. **Cons:** Vignettes are brief. Questions often do not reflect Step 2 style and format. **Summary:** Good overall review questions on high-yield topics that lends itself well to focused specialty review. Good buy for the number of questions.

REVIEW RESOURCES

Comprehensive

B+ **Mosby's Ace the Boards: Specialty Clinical Sciences Step 3**   **$38.00**   Review/100+ q

Donnelly

Mosby-Year Book, 1997, 1st ed., 483 pages, ISBN 0815127561

General review for Step 3. Features questions in book and on disk. **Pros:** Well written and to the point. Appropriate emphasis on risk factors and management. **Cons:** Confusing icons and rampant boldfacing. Illustrations on insert separated from corresponding text. **Summary:** Well-written, above-average text review adequately suited to Step 2 preparation, complete with questions and illustrations.

B+ **NMS USMLE Step 2**   **$44.95**   Software/800 q

Lazo

Lippincott Williams & Wilkins, 1998, Version 2.0, ISBN 0683300962

Windows/Mac-based testing software. Features questions from *NMS Review for USMLE Step 2*. Organized as four comprehensive tests. **Pros:** Flexible test modes. Well-written questions with frequent clinical vignettes. **Cons:** Illustrations poorly reproduced. Does not accurately reflect CBT format. **Summary:** A good choice for computer-based testing with very good questions, although interface does not simulate CBT.

B+ **Rx: Prescription for the Boards USMLE Step 2**   **$29.95**   Review

Feibusch

Lippincott Williams & Wilkins, 1998, 2nd ed., 500 pages, ISBN 0781714273

Comprehensive text review based on the USMLE content outline. **Pros:** Comprehensive coverage of high-yield core and specialty topics, including outpatient medicine, dermatology, ophthalmology, ENT, and toxicology. Well-designed format. **Cons:** Some topics lack the necessary details. Facts outlining the next step in management are often not discussed. "Cram facts" at end are not very compact. Lengthy; not a quick review. **Summary:** Good single source for Step 2 review. Occasionally sparse coverage of topics. Requires time commitment.

B **A & L's Instant Exam Review of the USMLE Step 3**   **$34.95**   Review

Goldberg

Appleton & Lange, 1997, 2nd ed., 409 pages, ISBN 0838543375

General text review for USMLE Step 3. **Pros:** Organized review of many topics with emphasis on treatment. Nice dermatology illustrations. **Cons:** Dense text. Difficult to extract key points. Poorly illustrated except for dermatology. **Summary:** Complete but dense general review of clinical topics. Requires time commitment.

Comprehensive

B A & L's Outline Review for the USMLE Step 2

$36.95   Review

Goldberg

Appleton & Lange, 1999, 3rd ed., 749 pages, ISBN 0838503543
General outline of major clinical topics. **Pros:** Many classic photos. Covers most relevant topics. **Cons:** Coverage varies widely from topic to topic. Key facts are buried in text. Inadequate emphasis on management. Slow read at times. **Summary:** Big, well-illustrated book that is sometimes light on meaningful content.

B A&LERT USMLE Step 2

$65.00   Software/2200 q

Appleton & Lange

Appleton & Lange, 1997, 1st ed., ISBN 0838584470
Computerized test bank based on *Appleton & Lange's Review of the USMLE Step 2*. Users can take timed exams that are scored automatically. **Pros:** Quick way to review selected topics with use of search function and bookmarks. Allows user to simulate a timed exam. Questions and answers may be printed out. **Cons:** Some questions are too specific. Vignettes are relatively short and do not accurately reflect the length of questions on the exam. Interface does not reflect the new CBT. **Summary:** Good-quality questions, although interface is not reflective of the actual CBT.

B Medical Boards Step 2 Made Ridiculously Simple

$24.95   Review

Carl

MedMaster, 1997, 1st ed., 339 pages, ISBN 0940780283
General review of topics for Step 2 exam. Wide-ranging outline format with tables and brief discussions of topics. **Pros:** Quick review. Useful in areas that might otherwise be overlooked, e.g., ophthalmology, dermatology, ENT. **Cons:** Superficial review lacks substantive details. **Summary:** Highlights most high-yield topics. Should not be used as sole source for review.

B MEPC USMLE Step 2 Review

$32.95   Test/1000+ q

Jacobs

Appleton & Lange, 1996, 410 pages, ISBN 0838562701
Question-and-answer format with explanations. **Pros:** Relatively quick review. Numerous photographs of classic findings. Appropriate coverage of high-yield topics. Answers highlight key buzzwords. **Cons:** Discussions of answers are sometimes brief. Very brief vignettes do not reflect the current boards format. **Summary:** Fair source of additional questions that may be read quickly. Well illustrated.

Comprehensive

B **Passing the USMLE Case Clusters:**   **$30.00**   Test/500 q
Steps 2 & 3   **(each)**
Southland Staff
Southland Tutorials, 1996, 3rd ed., 163 pages, ISBN 1888628219
More than 70 clinical vignettes followed by 2–5 multiple-choice questions
with explanations. **Pros:** High-quality vignettes and questions similar to
Step 2. Detailed explanations. **Cons:** Expensive for the number of questions. No illustrations. **Summary:** Good but pricey collection of clinical-
vignette-style questions.

B **Passing the USMLE Step 2, Vols. 1–4**   **$30.00**   Test/500 q
                                                          (each)
Southland Staff
Vol. I: Southland Tutorials, 1996, 3rd ed., 189 pages, ISBN 1888628065
Vol. II: Southland Tutorials, 1996, 3rd ed., 237 pages, ISBN 1888628073
Vol. III: Southland Tutorials, 1996, 3rd ed., 207 pages, ISBN 1888628081
Vol. IV: Southland Tutorials, 1996, 3rd ed., 273 pages, ISBN 188862809X
General review of material for Step 2 in question format. Volumes 1 and 3
have questions in random order. Volumes 2 and 4 have questions organized by specialty. **Pros:** Questions accurately reflect style, format, and
length of Step 2. Virtually all clinical vignettes. Fairly complete explanations. **Cons:** Expensive for the number of questions. Some questions recur
in the same volume and within the series. Poorly illustrated. **Summary:**
Excellent questions with good explanations, but very expensive and lacks
illustrations.

B **USMLE Step 2 Clinical Sciences,**   **$14.00**   Test/315 q, 315 q,
Books 1, 2, 3, 4 & 5   **(each)**   315 q, 220 q
Luder
Book 1: Maval Medical Education, 1995, 74 pages, ISBN 1884083579
Book 2: Maval Medical Education, 1995, 67 pages, ISBN 1884083587
Book 3: Maval Medical Education, 1995, 63 pages, ISBN 1884083595
Books 4 & 5: Maval Medical Education, 1995, 62 pages, ISBN 1884083609
Individual mini-exam format with discussion of questions and answers.
Pros: Good clinical content with some clinical vignettes. Features many
classic pathologic images and radiographs. **Cons:** Many questions are too
easy and do not reflect boards format. Occasional factual mistakes and ty-
pographical errors are found in answer key. Some questions have letter answers only. Relatively expensive for the number of questions. **Summary:**
Good content review, but questions are too easy. Relatively expensive.

Comprehensive

B

USMLE Step 2, Clinical Sciences Book 6 $25.00   Test/540 q
Luder
Maval Medical Education, 1996, 128 pages, ISBN 1884083560
Individual mini-exam format with discussion of questions and answers.
Pros: Good clinical content with some clinical vignettes. Features many
classic pathologic images and radiographs. **Cons:** Many questions are too
easy and do not reflect boards format. Occasional factual mistakes and ty-
pographical errors are found in answer key. Some questions have letter an-
swers only. Relatively expensive for the number of questions. **Summary:**
Good content review, but questions are too easy.

B-

A & L's Review for the USMLE Step 3 $36.95   Test/1000 q
Jacobs
Appleton & Lange, 1997, 313 pages, ISBN 0838503055
Review questions organized by specialty in addition to two 150-question
comprehensive practice exams. **Pros:** Overall question content is good
with broad coverage of high-yield topics. Organized by specialty for focused review. Explanations are generally complete. Some classic illustrations. **Cons:** Vignettes are brief and few. Questions are frequently straight-
recall-oriented rather than clinically based. Not well illustrated. **Summary:** Average source of questions that do not reflect Step 2 style and
format.

B-

A&LERT USMLE Step 2 Deluxe $95.00   Software/3400 q
Appleton & Lange
Appleton & Lange, 1998, 1st ed., ISBN 0838503748
This question bank includes questions from *Appleton & Lange's Review of
the USMLE Step 2* and from A&L's MEPC series. Otherwise identical to
A&LERT: USMLE Step 2. Version 2.0 due in 2000. **Pros:** Large collection
of questions will keep you busy. **Cons:** Includes lower-yield "second-tier"
questions that do not accurately reflect USMLE style. **Summary:** Worth
considering if you need a large collection of computerized questions.

B-

Step 2 of the Boards Part A $129.00   Audio Review
Gold Standard Board Preparation Systems
Gold Standard, 1997–1999, 15 tapes
Audio review organized into the following topics: Differential Diagnosis,
Drugs of Choice, Urgent Care, Surgery, Pediatrics, OB/GYN, Advanced
Cardiac Life Support, Cardiology and EKGs, and Diabetes and Hypertension. Can be ordered at (740) 592-4124. **Pros:** Offers a novel study
method. Question-and-answer format keeps the listener engaged. **Cons:**
Lacks adequate emphasis on diagnosis and management. Focuses on low-
yield topics, sometimes overly simplistic. Disorganized, no outline to
search tapes for a particular topic. Expensive. **Summary:** Useful as supplemental review source but relatively expansive with some focus on low-
yield material.

B⁻ **Clinical Science Question Bank
for the USMLE Step 2** $28.00   Test/500 q

Zaslau
FMSG, 1997, 1st ed., 135 pages, ISBN 1886468168
Review-question book with five 100-question exams. Includes lengthy
clinical vignettes as well as figures and images. **Pros:** Questions focus on
high-yield topics. **Cons:** Questions are of variable quality and do not reflect boards style and format. Some questions lack explanations. Illustrations are not representative of Step 2. Relatively expensive. **Summary:**
Covers appropriate topics, but many questions are poorly written.

B⁻ **Mosby's Ace the Boards:
General Clinical Sciences Step 2** $37.00   Review/1000+ q

Bollet
Mosby-Year Book, 1996, 1st ed., 530 pages, ISBN 0815107234
General, detailed review of Step 2. Features questions in book and on
disk. **Pros:** Comprehensive review of most major Step 2 topics. Explanations to questions are generally complete. **Cons:** Very dense, overly detailed text makes for difficult reading. Few clinical vignette questions in
non-boards style. Poorly illustrated. **Summary:** Comprehensive review is
too dense and detailed for boards review or wards preparation.

B⁻ **Passing the USMLE Photo Diagnosis:
Steps 1, 2, & 3, Vols. 1 & 2** $30.00   Test/100 q
                                                          (each)

Southland Staff
Southland Tutorials, 1996, 3rd ed., 77 pages, ISBN 1888628235
Color images of selected topics. A short case or question is presented with
each image. **Pros:** Offers a quick and entertaining way to review classic
images in medicine. **Cons:** Very expensive for 100 images. **Summary:** Expensive collection of classic exam images. Worth checking out from the
library.

B⁻ **REA's Interactives Flashcards USMLE Step 2** $8.95   Flashcard

Fogiel
REA, 1998, 1st ed., 500 pages, ISBN 0878911685
"Flashcard" review in book format. **Pros:** Cheap. Has fill-in-the-blank format. **Cons:** Cannot remove pages to use as flashcards. Fairly random questions. Some picky and low-yield questions. **Summary:** Not very helpful
given non-boards-style questions and emphasis on low-yield topics.

B⁻   **Rypin's Clinical Sciences Review**   **$32.95**   Review/408 q
Frohlich
Lippincott-Raven, 1997, 17th ed., 376 pages, ISBN 0397515448
General, highly detailed review text of all of the clinical sciences, with
few diagrams or charts. Review questions at the end of each chapter. **Pros:**
Single, detailed source of all topics with discussion of clinical presenta-
tion, management, and treatment. Well organized and thorough. **Cons:**
Very detailed; requires considerable motivation and time commitment to
complete. Text-heavy format makes for monotonous reading. Poorly illustrated. **Summary:** A dense single-source review requiring significant motivation and time commitment. Compare with *Rx: Prescription for the
Boards*.

B⁻   **Step 2 Virtual Reality**   **$28.00**   Test/320 q
Zaslau
FMSG, 1998, 1st ed., 170 pages, ISBN 1886468249
Two practice exams are provided with discussions of correct and incorrect
responses. **Pros:** Lengthy question stems approximate those of Step 2.
Questions also reflect emphasis on management and treatment decisions.
Generally good-quality content. **Cons:** Relatively expensive given the
amount of material covered. Explanations of incorrect answers are very su-
perficial. **Summary:** Relatively expensive for a limited number of good-
quality questions.

C⁺   **The Medical Student's Guide to Top
Board Scores: USMLE Steps 1 and 2**   **$15.95**   Review
Rogers
Lippincott-Raven, 1996, 2nd ed., 146 pages, ISBN 0316754366
General review for Steps 1 and 2. Information is presented in tables, lists,
and mnemonics for many high-yield topics covered on both Step 1 and
Step 2. **Pros:** Mnemonics may be of benefit to readers who can learn in
this fashion. **Cons:** Some of the information is more relevant to Step 1
than to Step 2. **Summary:** Limited review for Step 1 and Step 2 that covers neither exam well.

C⁺   **Step 2 Success**   **$38.00**   Test/720 q
Zaslau
FMSG, 1995, 1st ed., 224 pages, ISBN 1886468060
Simulated full-length exam for Step 2. **Pros:** Many clinical vignettes.
Cons: Questions are generally too easy. Some focus on low-yield topics.
Some weak explanations. Poorly illustrated. Expensive for the number of
questions. **Summary:** Below-average questions that do not reflect boards
style and format.

Comprehensive

USMLE Success
Zaslau

$38.00   Review/540 q

FMSG, 1996, 3rd ed., 280 pages, ISBN 1886468095

General overview of information for Steps 1, 2, and 3 in outline format. Contains simulated exams for both Step 1 and Step 2. **Pros:** Many clinical vignette questions with appropriate emphasis on diagnosis and management. Quick read. **Cons:** Scanty facts; outdated book recommendations. Poor explanations. Few illustrations. Expensive for amount and quality of material. **Summary:** Inadequate source for any Step review. Questions may be helpful, but explanations are poorly written.

Clinical Science Review Success
Zaslau

$28.00   Review

FMSG, 1997, 1st ed., 132 pages, ISBN 188646815X

General overview of core clinical rotations. Notes are printed straight from the author's PowerPoint presentation. There is added information on the Match and residency. **Pros:** Overview of high-yield topics may be quickly reviewed. "Most common" list may be useful for quick cramming. **Cons:** Mostly superficial coverage. PowerPoint printout is difficult to read. **Summary:** Inadequate, superficial, poorly formatted content review with an expensive price tag.

NEW BOOKS—COMPREHENSIVE

A & L's Practice Tests: USMLE Step 2
Goldberg

$36.95   Test/900 q

Appleton & Lange, 1999, 1st ed., 350 pages, ISBN 0838503721

Classic Presentations and Rapid Review for USMLE Step 2
O'Connell

$25.00   Review

J & S, 1999, 215 pages, ISBN 1888308052

Medical Student Pearls of Wisdom USMLE Parts II & III
Plantz

$32.00   Review

Boston Medical Publishing, 1998, 1st ed., 331 pages, ISBN 1890369101

Not yet reviewed. Compact short question/short answer format is easy to read and designed for self-testing.

USMLE Step 2 Starter Kit
Kaplan

$29.95   Test/360 q

Appleton & Lange, 1999, 1st ed., 200 pages, ISBN 083858666X

REVIEW RESOURCES

Comprehensive

A⁻ **Blueprints in Medicine**   **$27.95** Review
Young
Blackwell Science, 1998, 1st ed., 247 pages, ISBN 086542537X
Text review of internal medicine organized by common diseases and common symptoms. No questions. **Pros:** Well-organized, concise review. En-
gaging, easy reading. Symptom approach is helpful for boards review.
Good charts and diagrams. **Cons:** Poorly illustrated—no photographs; no
radiographic studies. Has some superfluous details. **Summary:** Very good
primary boards review text for internal medicine though poorly illustrated.

B⁺ **A & L's Review of Internal Medicine**   **$34.95** Test/1100+ q
Goldlist
Appleton & Lange, 1999, 2nd ed., 260 pages, ISBN 0838503551
General review with questions and answers divided by subspecialty. **Pros:**
Well-written vignette questions reflect boards format. Representative of
the content of the boards. Complete explanations. Well illustrated. **Cons:**
Questions are shorter and some non-vignette questions are more straight-
forward than those on the exam. **Summary:** Very good source of questions
that accurately reflect the multi-step nature of boards questions.

B⁺ **High-Yield Internal Medicine**   **$18.95** Review
Nirula
Lippincott Williams & Wilkins, 1997, 1st ed., 197 pages, ISBN
0683180444
Core review of internal medicine in outline format, with few tables, clinical images, and diagrams. **Pros:** Focus is on high-yield diseases and symptoms. Quick and easy read. **Cons:** Some mistakes in formulas. Needs more
illustrations. No index. **Summary:** Good, fast review presented in a format
that allows for quick and repetitive readings.

B **NMS Medicine**   **$30.00** Review/500 q
Myers
Lippincott Williams & Wilkins, 1997, 3rd ed., 752 pages, ISBN
068318105X
Comprehensive review of internal medicine in outline format. Twenty
questions follow each chapter and there is a 140-question exam at the end
of the book. Eight case studies with discussions are also included at the
end of the book. **Pros:** Well-organized, thorough text. Covers the major
clinical entities. Doubles as wards text. **Cons:** Poor coverage of outpatient
topics. Very dense and very long. **Summary:** Too long and dense for effective review.

REVIEW RESOURCES

Internal Medicine

B⁻ Step 2 of the Boards Part B

$199.00   Audio Review

Gold Standard Board Preparation Systems

Gold Standard, 27 tapes

Audio review of internal medicine with tapes into Pulmonary, Hematology, Genitourinary, Heart Failure, Cardiac Arryhmias, Gastrointestinal, and Endocrinology. Can be ordered at (740) 592-4124. **Pros:** Offers a novel way to review medicine. Question-and-answer style of tapes makes listening interactive. Tapes well organized with specific subject labels. **Cons:** Expensive relative to other options for internal medicine review. Focuses on some low-yield topics while neglecting some important material. Requires time commitment. **Summary:** Expensive audio review with some focus on low-yield topics.

B⁻ Internal Medicine: Rypin's Intensive Reviews

$19.95   Review/231 q

Frohlich

Lippincott Williams & Wilkins, 1996, 1st ed., 320 pages, ISBN 0397515480

General-outline text format with few tables and no diagrams. Questions with short explanations. **Pros:** Clean layout with good use of boldfacing. Detailed, well-written text. Relatively inexpensive. **Cons:** Text heavy with no illustrations, charts, or diagrams. Minimal emphasis on management. Few vignette-type questions with brief explanations. **Summary:** Thorough but text-heavy review. Slow read.

B⁻ PreTest Medicine

$18.95   Test/400 q

Berk

McGraw-Hill, 1997, 8th ed., 170 pages, ISBN 0070525277

Question-and-answer format organized by medical subspecialty. **Pros:** Organization by subspecialty helps pinpoint weak areas. Detailed explanations. **Cons:** Questions are more difficult than those of the boards. Few vignette questions. Few illustrations. **Summary:** Solid source of challenging review questions.

C⁺ Oklahoma Notes Family Medicine

$19.95   Review/100 q

Hirsch

Springer-Verlag, 1996, 2nd ed., 189 pages, ISBN 0387946381

Outline review of family medicine. **Pros:** Quick read. Relatively inexpensive. **Cons:** Incomplete text with some errors. No emphasis on risk factors or management. Few tables and diagrams. Questions are really hokey (trust us). Letter answers only. **Summary:** Poor review for family medicine with inadequate details and poorly written (but entertaining) questions.

Oklahoma Notes Internal Medicine

$19.95   Review/358 q

Jarolim

Springer-Verlag, 1996, 2nd ed., 424 pages, ISBN 0387946365

General topics in internal medicine reviewed in brief outline format typical of this series. **Pros:** Inexpensive. Broad coverage of topics. Includes questions. **Cons:** Very little emphasis on treatment and management. No tables or illustrations. Questions at the end of the book have letter answers only without explanations. **Summary:** Mediocre medicine review text.

PreTest Physical Diagnosis

$18.95   Test/500 q

Cobb

McGraw-Hill, 1997, 3rd ed., 177 pages, ISBN 0070525315

General review questions for physical diagnosis organized by organ system. **Pros:** Many clinical vignettes. **Cons:** Questions are of variable length and quality. Covers many low-yield topics. **Summary:** Not a necessary book for the boards, as pertinent physical diagnosis information is covered in most quality Step 2 reviews.

NEW BOOKS—INTERNAL MEDICINE

Underground Clinical Vignettes: Emergency Medicine

$17.95   Review

Bhushan

S2S Medical, 1999, 1st ed., ISBN 1890061271

Concise clinical cases illustrating approximately 50 frequently tested diseases in emergency medicine. Cardinal signs, symptoms, and buzzwords are highlighted. Expected April 1999.

Underground Clinical Vignettes: Internal Medicine, Vol. I

$17.95   Review

Bhushan

S2S Medical, 1999, 1st ed., ISBN 1890061204

Concise clinical cases illustrating approximately 50 frequently tested diseases in internal medicine. Cardinal signs, symptoms, and buzzwords are highlighted. Expected April 1999.

Underground Clinical Vignettes: Internal Medicine, Vol. II

$17.95   Review

Bhushan

S2S Medical, 1999, 1st ed., ISBN 1890061255

Concise clinical cases illustrating approximately 50 frequently tested diseases in internal medicine. Cardinal signs, symptoms, and buzzwords are highlighted. Expected April 1999.

REVIEW RESOURCES

Internal Medicine

PreTest Neurology

$18.95 Test/500 q

Lechtenberg

McGraw-Hill, 1997, 3rd ed., 244 pages, ISBN 0070525285

Question-and-answer review of neurology. **Pros:** Thorough coverage of neurology topics with some clinical vignettes. **Cons:** Many questions are too picky. Some errors. Some explanations are incomplete. Poorly illustrated. **Summary:** Below-average source of neurology questions. Questions do not reflect boards style.

Oklahoma Notes Neurology & Clinical Neuroscience

$19.95 Review/100 q

Brumback

Springer-Verlag, 1996, 2nd ed., 186 pages, ISBN 0387946357

General topics in clinical neurology reviewed in brief outline format. **Pros:** Some illustrations. Inexpensive. Easy read. **Cons:** Outline has poor coverage of risk factors and management. Clinical vignette questions are too easy. **Summary:** Limited review of neuroscience topics with no emphasis on differential diagnosis, risk factors, or management.

Underground Clinical Vignettes: Neurology

$17.95 Review

Bhushan

S2S Medical, 1999, 1st ed., ISBN 1890061263

Concise clinical cases illustrating approximately 50 frequently tested diseases in neurology. Cardinal signs, symptoms, and buzzwords are highlighted. Expected April 1999.

A⁻ **Blueprints in Obstetrics and Gynecology** $26.95 Review

Callahan

Blackwell Science, 1998, 1st ed., 207 pages, ISBN 0865425051

Text review with tables and illustrations. **Pros:** Strong emphasis on high-yield topics with concise text, clear diagrams, and many classic illustrations. Easy read. **Cons:** Some overly detailed material included. **Summary:** Overall, very good choice for boards and wards preparation, although some low-yield material is included.

B **NMS Obstetrics and Gynecology** $30.00 Review/500 q

Beck

Lippincott Williams & Wilkins, 1997, 4th ed., 510 pages, ISBN 0683180150

Detailed outline review of OB/GYN with few tables and diagrams. **Pros:** Comprehensive review for both wards and boards. Final exam is relatively good with complete explanations. **Cons:** Dense and long OB/GYN review. Many questions do not reflect boards format. Lacks illustrations. **Summary:** Complete review with questions and discussion. May be too long for exam prep unless it is also used in clerkship.

B **PreTest Obstetrics & Gynecology** $18.95 Test/500 q

Evans

McGraw-Hill, 1997, 8th ed., 223 pages, ISBN 0070525293

Question-and-answer review with detailed explanations for OB/GYN. **Pros:** Organization by subtopic may be useful for studying weak areas. Good content emphasis. Some questions are well illustrated. **Cons:** Some questions are too difficult. Vignette-based questions are shorter and fewer as compared to Step 2. Some questions are too detailed. **Summary:** Decent source of questions that do reflect current Step 2 style and format.

B⁻ **BRS Obstetrics and Gynecology** $26.95 Review/500 q

Sakala

Lippincott Williams & Wilkins, 1997, 1st ed., 389 pages, ISBN 0683074989

General review text with questions at the ends of chapters and a comprehensive exam at the end of the book. **Pros:** Appropriate content for boards and wards study. **Cons:** Some sections are overly detailed with few diagrams. Slow reading. Questions are too short with few clinical vignettes. **Summary:** Appropriate content review, but more helpful for wards than for boards preparation.

B⁻ **MEPC Obstetrics and Gynecology** $19.95   Test/765 q

Ross

Appleton & Lange, 1997, 411 pages, ISBN 0838563287

Question-and-answer format with discussion. **Pros:** Another source of questions that may be quickly reviewed. Content of questions is appropriate for Step 2. Most explanations are thorough and well written. **Cons:** Very few vignette-based style questions. Few illustrations. **Summary:** Average source of additional questions that may be read quickly. Appropriate content emphasis, but questions do not reflect boards-style format.

B⁻ **Obstetrics and Gynecology:** $25.00   Test/530 q
Review for the New National Boards

Kramer, J & S Reviews

J & S, 1996, 1st ed., 190 pages, ISBN 0963287397

General review of OB/GYN in question-and-answer format. **Pros:** Good ultrasounds and fetal heart tracings. Appropriate depth of coverage. **Cons:** As many as 40 questions per vignette stem with corresponding multiple-page explanations. Focuses on some low-yield topics. **Summary:** Below-average source of questions. Does not reflect Step 2 format or style.

C⁺ **A & L's Review of Obstetrics & Gynecology** $34.95   Test/1600+ q

Vontver

Appleton & Lange, 1999, 6th ed., 400 pages, ISBN 0838503233

Detailed review of OB/GYN in question-and-answer format. **Pros:** Some high-yield sections such as clinical endocrinology. **Cons:** Overall emphasis is not appropriate for Step 2 preparation. May be more appropriate for specialty preparation. **Summary:** Far more detailed than required for Step 2.

C **Oklahoma Notes Obstetrics and Gynecology** $19.95   Review/104 q

Miles, Oklahoma Notes

Springer-Verlag, 1996, 2nd ed., 218 pages, ISBN 0387946322

General text review of OB/GYN. **Pros:** Relatively inexpensive. **Cons:** Low emphasis on high-yield topics (e.g., risk factors, management). Very few diagrams or tables. Questions lack clinical vignettes or discussions. **Summary:** Limited review of OB/GYN that does not reflect Step 2 content.

N **Underground Clinical Vignettes: OB/GYN**   **$17.95**   Review

Bhushan

S2S Medical, 1999, 1st ed., ISBN 1890061239

Concise clinical cases illustrating approximately 50 frequently tested diseases in OB/GYN. Cardinal signs, symptoms, and buzzwords are highlighted. Expected April 1999.

REVIEW RESOURCES / **Pediatrics**

A & L's Review of Pediatrics

$34.95   Test/1000+ q

Lorin

Appleton & Lange, 1997, 5th ed., 222 pages, ISBN 0838503039

Question-and-answer review of pediatrics with detailed explanations (next edition expected late 1999). **Pros:** Questions are focused on boards-relevant content. One hundred and twenty excellent vignette-based questions in last chapter. Thorough, well-written explanations. Nice primer on test-taking strategies. **Cons:** Non-vignette-based questions are shorter and more straightforward than those on Step 2. Needs more vignette-style questions. Some questions may be too detailed for Step 2 preparation. Poorly illustrated. **Summary:** Excellent, concise review with appropriate content and good discussions, although the majority of questions do not reflect Step 2 style.

PreTest Pediatrics

$18.95   Test/500 q

Yetman

McGraw-Hill, 1997, 8th ed., 241 pages, ISBN 0070525307

Question-and-answer review with detailed discussion. **Pros:** Organization by organ system is useful for pinpointing weaknesses. Strong, thorough explanations. Well illustrated. **Cons:** Many questions are too picky. Too few vignette-style questions. **Summary:** Good source of questions and review for pediatrics. Appropriate content with good illustrations, although questions do not follow Step 2 style and format.

Blueprints in Pediatrics

$26.95   Review

Marino

Blackwell Science, 1998, 1st ed., 258 pages, ISBN 0865425043

Text review of pediatrics with tables and diagrams. **Pros:** Appropriate focus on high-yield topics. **Cons:** Relatively dense text with few illustrations. Overly detailed. **Summary:** Good for the motivated student.

MEPC Pediatrics

$19.95   Test/700 q

Hansbarger

Appleton & Lange, 1995, 9th ed., 248 pages, ISBN 083856223X

Question-and-answer format with brief discussion. **Pros:** Appropriate content emphasis. Quick read. **Cons:** Few vignette questions. Scanty explanations. Poor illustrations. **Summary:** Below-average source of questions with poor discussion.

B− **NMS Pediatrics** $30.00 Review/475 q

Dworkin

Lippincott Williams & Wilkins, 1996, 3rd ed., 679 pages, ISBN
068306245X

General review of pediatrics in outline format with questions at end of
each chapter. **Pros:** Very thorough and detailed review of pediatrics. Outline format highlights key points. Short vignette questions with detailed
explanations. **Cons:** Too long and dense for Step 2 review. Lacks illustrations. **Summary:** Thorough review, but inappropriate for Step 2 review
unless used on clerkships.

B− **Oklahoma Notes Pediatrics** $19.95 Review/126 q

Puls

Springer-Verlag, 1996, 2nd ed., 390 pages, ISBN 0387946349

General outline format of pediatrics. **Pros:** Well organized by system.
Good tables. **Cons:** Poorly illustrated. Incomplete explanations. Focuses
on some low-yield topics. Questions lack clinical vignettes or explanations. **Summary:** Below-average review of pediatrics with incomplete text.
Above average for series.

C+ **Pediatrics: Rypin's Intensive Reviews** $19.95 Review/200 q

Heagarty

Lippincott Williams & Wilkins, 1997, 1st ed., 319 pages, ISBN
0397515561

Text outline review of pediatrics with few tables. **Pros:** Inexpensive for
amount of material. **Cons:** Very text heavy. Lacks illustrations and tables.
Some sections are overly detailed. Poorly written questions with scanty
explanations. **Summary:** Dense, low-yield review of pediatrics with inadequate practice questions. Typical for the series.

C **STARS Pediatrics: A Primary Care Approach** $35.00 Text

Berkowitz

Saunders, 1996, 525 pages, ISBN 0721656234

Text review of pediatrics. **Pros:** Comprehensive review. Has illustrative
case vignettes. **Cons:** Dense and overly detailed text and tables. Covers
many low-yield topics. Poorly illustrated. **Summary:** Inappropriate for
boards review. Difficult read for wards.

Underground Clinical Vignettes: Pediatrics $17.95   Review
Bhushan
S2S Medical, 1999, 1st ed., ISBN 1890061212
Concise clinical cases illustrating approximately 50 frequently tested diseases in pediatrics. Cardinal signs, symptoms, and buzzwords are highlighted. Expected April 1999.

REVIEW RESOURCES

Pediatrics

B+ **PreTest Preventive Medicine & Public Health** $18.95   Test/500 q
Ratelle
McGraw-Hill, 1997, 8th ed., 206 pages, ISBN 007052534X
Question-and-answer review of epidemiology, biostatistics, and preventive
medicine. **Pros:** Majority of test questions appropriately simulate boards
content and difficulty. Good explanations. **Cons:** Some questions are too
heavy on calculations. Biostatistics chapter is too detailed. Very few vignettes. **Summary:** Good question-and-answer review for a low-yield
topic.

B− **MEPC Preventive Medicine and Public Health** $21.95   Review/700 q
Hart
Appleton & Lange, 1996, 265 pages, ISBN 0838563198
Question-and-answer review with discussions. **Pros:** Appropriate level of
biostatistics review. **Cons:** Few clinical vignettes. Many questions are too
picky. Brief explanations with poor detail. **Summary:** Adequate content
review, but questions do not follow boards format and explanations are
poor.

C+ **NMS Clinical Epidemiology & Biostatistics** $27.00   Review/300 q
Knapp
Lippincott Williams & Wilkins, 1992, 435 pages, ISBN 0683062069
Detailed outline review of epidemiology and biostatics. **Pros:** Exhaustive
coverage. **Cons:** Too much detail for a small subject area. Very slow read.
Questions focus on low-yield topics. **Summary:** Inappropriate for Step 2
review. Better suited for an epidemiology student.

C+ **STARS Epidemiology, Biostatistics, and Preventive Medicine Review** $21.95   Review/350 q
Katz
Saunders, 1997, 249 pages, ISBN 0721640842
Detailed text review of epidemiology and biostatistics with questions and
answers. **Pros:** Good tables and diagrams. **Cons:** Small print makes for difficult reading. Text too detailed for quick review. Questions do not reflect
boards style and format. Discussions of questions are too detailed. Requires
time commitment. **Summary:** Too detailed and too slow for Step 2 review.

C **NMS Preventive Medicine & Public Health** $27.00   Review/450 q
Cassens
Lippincott Williams & Wilkins, 1992, 2nd ed., 497 pages, ISBN
068306262X
Detailed review of preventive medicine and public health. **Pros:** Very
comprehensive review. Questions have thorough explanations. **Cons:** Too
long and detailed for boards review. Too much low-yield material. **Summary:** Inappropriate for Step 2 review. Better suited for a public health
student.

A⁻ High-Yield Psychiatry

$18.95   Review

Fadem

Lippincott Williams & Wilkins, 1998, 1st ed., 151 pages, ISBN
0683302035

Brief outline-format review of psychiatry. **Pros:** Quick read with clinical
vignettes scattered throughout. Concise tables. **Cons:** Not enough detail
for in-depth review. **Summary:** Excellent, quick review of psychiatry; may
lack depth.

B⁺ Blueprints in Psychiatry

$22.95   Review

Murphy

Blackwell Science, 1998, 1st ed., 80 pages, ISBN 0865425035

Brief text review of psychiatry with DSM-IV criteria. **Pros:** Clear, concise
review of psychiatry with helpful tables. Good coverage of high-yield topics. Quick read. **Cons:** Relatively expensive for amount of material. **Summary:** Fast review with appropriate coverage of high-yield topics.

B⁺ NMS Psychiatry

$30.00   Review/500 q

Scully

Lippincott Williams & Wilkins, 1996, 3rd ed., 318 pages, ISBN
0683062638

General review of topics in outline format with questions at end of each
chapter and a comprehensive final exam. **Pros:** Well-written text with
concise disease discussions. Questions test appropriate content and have
complete explanations. Good companion text for clerkship. **Cons:** Not
enough vignette-style questions. Requires time commitment. **Summary:**
Detailed review that requires time commitment. Good single choice for
clerkship study and boards review.

B⁺ PreTest Psychiatry

$18.95   Test/500 q

Woods

McGraw-Hill, 1997, 8th ed., 194 pages, ISBN 0070525323

Question-and-answer review of topics in psychiatry. **Pros:** Questions are
well written and organized. Most questions have appropriate content
level. Good explanations. **Cons:** Too few vignette-type questions. Some
questions are too detailed. **Summary:** Good source of questions and review for psychiatry. Questions do not reflect Step 2 style.

REVIEW RESOURCES

Psychiatry

B | **A & L's Review of Psychiatry** | $34.95 | Test/900+ q

Easson

Appleton & Lange, 1998, 5th ed., 178 pages, ISBN 0838503705

General review of psychiatry with questions and answers (next edition due in 2000). **Pros:** Includes one hundred and fourteen vignette-style questions appropriate for boards review. Appropriate content emphasis. Thorough explanations. **Cons:** Questions are shorter and more straightforward than those of boards. **Summary:** Decent boards review for psychiatry, although does not reflect boards format.

B | **Behavioral Science/Psychiatry: Review for the New National Boards** | $25.00 | Test/521 q

Frank

J & S, 1998, 248 pages, ISBN 1888308001

General review of psychiatry in question-and-answer format. **Pros:** Includes some vignette-based questions with complete explanations. **Cons:** Does not emphasize high-yield topics. Does not follow boards format or style. Some questions are too short and easy. **Summary:** Mixed-quality questions with generally complete explanations.

B | **BRS Psychiatry** | $26.95 | Review/250 q

Shaner

Lippincott Williams & Wilkins, 1997, 1st ed., 378 pages, ISBN 0683076744

Outline review with questions and answers for psychiatry. **Pros:** Clearly written, comprehensive text. Good boards-style questions with complete explanations. **Cons:** Overly detailed in some areas. Long read for boards review. **Summary:** Good review, especially if used on wards. Excellent questions. Requires time commitment.

B− | **MEPC Psychiatry** | $19.95 | Test/700 q

Chan

Appleton & Lange, 1995, 10th ed., 259 pages, ISBN 0838557805

Question-and-answer format organized by topics in psychiatry. **Pros:** Last chapter has many good clinical vignette questions. **Cons:** Most questions are not vignette-based. Some questions are picky and focus on low-yield topics. Many explanations are brief. **Summary:** Below-average source of review questions.

C+ | **Oklahoma Notes Psychiatry** | $19.95 | Review/103 q

Shaffer

Springer-Verlag, 1996, 2nd ed., 247 pages, ISBN 0387946330

Outline-format review of clinical psychiatry. **Pros:** Inexpensive, quick read. **Cons:** Haphazard text lacks tables and details. Questions do not reflect Step 2 format or content. **Summary:** Below-average review of psychiatry.

Psychiatry & Behavioral Medicine: Rypin's Intensive Reviews

$19.95   Review

Deckert

Lippincott Williams & Wilkins, 1997, 178 pages, ISBN 0397515545

Text-outline review of psychiatry with few diagrams. **Pros:** Some vignette-based questions. **Cons:** Lacks tables. Overly simplistic with focus on low-yield topics. No DSM-IV criteria. Questions do not reflect Step 2 format. **Summary:** Low-yield review for Step 2.

NMS Behavioral Sciences in Psychiatry

$27.00   Review/300 q

Wiener

Lippincott Williams & Wilkins, 1995, 3rd. ed., 375 pages, ISBN 0683062034

Outline review of behavioral science in psychiatry. **Pros:** Clear outline format. Case studies highlight differential diagnosis and management. **Cons:** Focuses on many low-yield topics with little emphasis on clinical syndromes. **Summary:** Poor choice for psychiatry Step 2 review. Lacks adequate clinical emphasis for wards.

NEW BOOKS—PSYCHIATRY

Underground Clinical Vignettes: Psychiatry

$17.95   Review

Bhushan

S2S Medical, 1999, 1st ed., ISBN 1890061247

Concise clinical cases illustrating approximately 50 frequently tested diseases in psychiatry. Cardinal signs, symptoms, and buzzwords are highlighted. Expected April 1999.

A− **Blueprints in Surgery**   **$25.95**   Review

Karp

Blackwell Science, 1998, 1st ed., 113 pages, ISBN 0865425469

Short text review of general surgery with tables and diagrams. **Pros:** Well organized. Easy to read with strong focus on high-yield topics. Clear diagrams. **Cons:** Some sections are overly detailed (e.g., anatomy). Relatively expensive. **Summary:** Concise review of surgery with appropriate emphasis on high-yield topics.

B+ **A & L's Review of Surgery**   **$34.95**   Test/950+ q

Wapnick

Appleton & Lange, 1998, 3rd ed., 280 pages, ISBN 0838502458

General review of surgery with questions and answers. **Pros:** Good clinical emphasis. Many vignette-style questions. Explanations are thorough. **Cons:** Questions are shorter and style does not reflect that of the Step 2 exam. Questions are highly variable in difficulty. Few illustrations. **Summary:** Good content review for exam, although some questions are too picky.

B+ **Churchill's Surgery 1**   **$30.00**   Review/120 q

Lavelle-Jones

Churchill Livingstone, 1997, 1st ed., 207 pages, ISBN 0443051720

Text review of general surgery with illustrations and questions. **Pros:** Concise, well-organized text. Excellent illustrations and radiographs. Illustrative case vignettes. **Cons:** Need *Surgery 2* to complete review of surgery. Questions are not boards style. **Summary:** Excellent review with classic illustrations, but incomplete without *Surgery 2* title.

B+ **Surgery: Review for the New National Boards**   **$25.00**   Test/562 q

Geelhoed

J & S, 1995, 1st ed., 246 pages, ISBN 0963287354

Question-and-answer review of surgery. **Pros:** Good focus on high-yield topics. Very good explanations. Classic illustrations. **Cons:** Lacks the lengthy clinical vignette style typical of Step 2. **Summary:** Appropriate review of Step 2–relevant content, but questions do not reflect Step 2 format.

B **MEPC Surgery**   **$21.95**   Test/700 q

Metzler

Appleton & Lange, 1995, 11th ed., 317 pages, ISBN 0838561950

Question-and-answer self-examination for surgery. **Pros:** Questions have appropriate focus. Good explanations. Well illustrated. **Cons:** Questions do not reflect current boards format. **Summary:** Adequate source of questions for review, although it does not follow boards format.

REVIEW RESOURCES

Surgery

NMS Surgery   **$30.00**   Review/418 q
Jarrell
Lippincott Williams & Wilkins, 1996, 3rd ed., 647 pages, ISBN
0683062719
Detailed outline review of surgery. **Pros:** Good content coverage for Step
2 exam. Appropriate vignette-style questions at end of each chapter with
thorough explanations. **Cons:** Slow read. Lacks illustrations and diagrams.
Some questions are too picky. **Summary:** Too long for boards review unless used on clerkship as well.

B-

Oklahoma Notes General Surgery   **$19.95**   Review/168 q
Jacocks
Springer-Verlag, 1996, 2nd ed., 189 pages, ISBN 0387946373
Outline format for surgery. **Pros:** Inexpensive, quick read. **Cons:** Text
lacks high-yield details and illustrations. Questions lack vignettes and ex-
planations. **Summary:** Below average for this subject.

B-

Sabiston's Review of Surgery   **$41.00**   Test/900+ q
Sabiston
Saunders, 1997, 2nd ed., 280 pages, ISBN 0721686710
Question-and-answer review of surgery. **Pros:** Thorough discussion imme-
diately follows questions, promoting retention. **Cons:** Questions do not
reflect boards style or format. Poorly illustrated. Few clinical vignettes.
Summary: Overly detailed, non-Step 2-specific review of surgery.

B-

Surgery: Rypin's Intensive Reviews   **$19.95**   Review/192 q
Chari
Lippincott Williams & Wilkins, 1996, 205 pages, ISBN 0397515510
Text review of general surgery. **Pros:** Quick read for a text review. Questions test appropriate content. **Cons:** Does not highlight management and
differential. Poorly illustrated. Questions do not reflect boards style. Some
meager explanations. **Summary:** General review of surgery in a style that
does not emphasize high-yield topics.

C+

PreTest Surgery   **$18.95**   Test/500 q
Geller
McGraw-Hill, 1997, 8th ed., 305 pages, ISBN 0070525331
Question-and-answer-format review of topics in general surgery. **Pros:**
Well organized by subspecialty. Well illustrated. **Cons:** Many questions are
too picky or esoteric. Questions do not follow boards style. Some explana-
tions are overly detailed. **Summary:** Questions are too difficult for Step 2
preparation. May be more appropriate for surgical boards preparation.

N ## Underground Clinical Vignettes: Surgery

$17.95 Review

Bhushan

S2S Medical, 1999, 1st ed., ISBN 1890061220

Concise clinical cases illustrating approximately 50 frequently tested diseases in surgery. Cardinal signs, symptoms, and buzzwords are highlighted. Expected April 1999.

Commercial Review Courses

Commercial preparation courses can be helpful for some students, but these courses are expensive and require significant time commitment. They are usually effective in organizing study material for students who feel overwhelmed by the volume of material. Note that the multiweek courses may be quite intense and may thus leave limited time for independent study. Also note that some commercial courses are designed for first-time test takers while others focus on students who are repeating the examination. Some courses focus on foreign medical graduates who want to take all three steps in a limited amount of time. Student experience and satisfaction with review courses are highly variable. We suggest that you discuss options with recent graduates of the review courses you are considering. Course content and structure can change rapidly. Some student opinions can be found in discussion groups on the World Wide Web. Below is contact information for some Step 2 commercial review courses.

Compass Medical Education Network
820 W. Jackson Boulevard, Suite 550
Chicago, IL 60607
1-800-818-9128
csimek@arcventures.com
www.compass-meded.com

Kaplan Medical/National Medical School Review
888 7th Avenue
New York, NY 10106
1-800-KAP-TEST
1-800-533-8850
www.kaplan.com/usmle
nmsr@nmsr.com
www.nmsr.com

Northwestern Learning Center
4700 S. Hagadorn Suite #200
East Lansing, MI 48823
800-837-7737
517-332-0777
testbuster@aol.com or northwestern@voyager.net
www.northwesternlearning.com/nw

Postgraduate Medical Review Education
407 Lincoln Road, Suite 12E
Miami Beach, FL 33139
800-ECFMG-30
PMRE@aol.com
www.PMRE.com

The Princeton Review
St. Leonard's Court
39th and Chestnut, Suite 317
Philadelphia, PA 19107
800-USMLE84
www.review.com

Youel's Prep, Inc.
701 Cypress Green Circle
Wellington, FL 33414
800-645-3985
561-795-1555
Fax: 561-795-0169
YouelsPrep@aol.com
www.youelsprep.com

Publisher Contacts

If you do not have convenient access to a medical bookstore, consider ordering directly from the publisher.

Appleton & Lange
P.O. Box 120041
Stamford, CT 06912
(800) 423-1359
(203) 406-4690
Fax: (203) 406-4602
www.appletonlange.com

Blackwell Science
350 Main Street
Malden, MA 02148
(800) 759-6102
(781) 388-8250
Fax: (781) 388-8255
www.blacksci.com

Churchill Livingstone
300 Lighting Way
Secaucus, NJ 07094
(800) 553-5426
(973) 319-9800
Fax: (201) 319-9659

FMSG c/o IMP
100 Sylvan Pkwy
Amherst, NY 14228
(800) 443-4194
(716) 689-6000
Fax: (716) 689-6187
impltd@worldnet.att.net
www.intlmedicalplacement.com

Gold Standard Board Preparation Systems
6374 Long Run Road
Athens, OH 45701
(740) 592-4124
Fax: (740) 592-4045

J&S Publishing
1300 Bishop Lane
Alexandria, VA 22302
(703) 823-9833
Fax: (703) 823-9834
jandspub@ix.netcom.com
www.jandspub.com

Lippincott Williams & Wilkins
P.O. Box 1580
Hagerstown, MD 21741
(800) 777-2295
Fax: (301) 824-7390
www.lww.com

Maval Medical Education
567 Harrison St.
Denver, CO 80206
(303) 320-1835
www.maval.com

McGraw-Hill Customer Service
P.O. Box 545
Blacklick, OH 43004
(800) 262-4729
Fax: (614) 759-3644
www.mghmedical.com

MedMaster, Inc.
P.O. Box 640028
Miami, FL 33164
(800) 335-3480
(305) 653-3480
Fax: (954) 962-4508
mmbks@aol.com

Mosby-Year Book
11830 Westline Industrial Drive
St. Louis, MO 63146
(800) 325-4177 ext. 5017
Fax: (800) 535-9935
www.mosby.com

Southland Tutorials
(310) 475-5711

Springer-Verlag, NY Inc.
PO Box 2485
Secaucus, NJ 07096
(800) 777-4643
Fax: (201) 348-5405
www.Springer-NY.com
orders@Springer-NY.com

W.B. Saunders
6277 Sea Harbor Drive
Orlando, FL 32887
(800) 545-2522
Fax: (800) 874-6418

Abbreviations and Symbols

Abbreviation	Meaning
Ab	antibody
ABCs	airway, breathing, circulation
ABG	arterial blood gas
ACE	angiotensin-converting enzyme
ACh	acetylcholine
ACTH	adrenocorticotropic hormone
AD	autosomal dominant
ADH	antidiuretic hormone (vasopressin)
ADHD	attention-deficit hyperactivity disorder
AFP	alpha-fetoprotein
Ag	antigen
AIDS	acquired immunodeficiency syndrome
ALL	acute lymphocytic leukemia
ALS	amyotrophic lateral sclerosis
ALT	alanine aminotransaminase
AML	acute myelogenous leukemia
ANA	antinuclear antibody
ARDS	acute respiratory distress syndrome
ASD	atrial septal defect
ASO	antistreptolysin O
AST	aspartate aminotransaminase
AV	atrioventricular
AVM	arteriovenous malformation
AXR	abdominal x-ray
AZT	azidothymidine
β-HCG	β-human chorionic gonadotropin
BAL	British anti-Lewisite (dimercaprol)
BP	blood pressure
BPH	benign prostatic hyperplasia
BPPV	benign paroxysmal positional vertigo
BUN	blood urea nitrogen
CABG	coronary artery bypass grafting
CAD	coronary artery disease
CAST	computer-adaptive sequential testing
CBC	complete blood count
CBT	computer-based testing
CD	cluster of differentiation
CDC	Centers for Disease Control
CEA	carcinoembryonic antigen
CF	cystic fibrosis
CFTR	cystic fibrosis transmembrane regulator
CHF	congestive heart failure
CIN	cervical intraepithelial neoplasia
CIS	carcinoma in situ
CJD	Creutzfeldt–Jakob disease
CK	creatine phosphokinase
CLL	chronic lymphocytic leukemia
CML	chronic myelogenous leukemia
CMT	Computerized Mastery Test
CMV	cytomegalovirus
CN	cranial nerve
CNS	central nervous system

Abbreviation	Meaning
COPD	chronic obstructive pulmonary disease
CP	cerebral palsy
CPK-MB	creatine phosphokinase, MB fraction
Cr	creatinine
CSA	Clinical Skills Assessment (exam)
CSF	cerebrospinal fluid
CT	computed tomography
CV	cardiovascular
CXR	chest x-ray
D&C	dilation and curettage
DCIS	ductal carcinoma in situ
ddC	dideoxycytidine
DEA	Drug Enforcement Agency
DES	diethylstilbestrol
DI	diabetes insipidus
DIC	disseminated intravascular coagulation
DIP	distal interphalangeal
DKA	diabetic ketoacidosis
DMD	Duchenne muscular dystrophy
DNI	do not intubate
DNR	do not resuscitate
DPOA	durable power of attorney
DSM	Diagnostic and Statistical Manual
DTP	diphtheria-tetanus-pertussis
DTR	deep tendon reflex
DTs	delirium tremens
DVT	deep venous thrombosis
EBV	Epstein–Barré virus
ECFMG	Educational Commission for Foreign Medical Graduates
ECT	electroconvulsive therapy
EEG	electroencephalogram
EKG	electrocardiogram
ELISA	enzyme-linked immunosorbent assay
EMG	electromyogram
EPS	extrapyramidal symptoms
ER	emergency room
ERCP	endoscopic retrograde cholangiopancreatography
ESR	erythrocyte sedimentation rate
EtOH	ethanol
FAP	familial adenomatous polyposis
FDA	Food and Drug Administration
FEV	forced expiratory volume
FFP	fresh frozen plasma
FLEX	Federal Licensing Examination
FMG	foreign medical graduate
FOBT	fecal occult blood test
FSH	follicle-stimulating hormone
FSMB	Federation of State Medical Boards
FTA-ABS	fluorescent treponemal antibody—absorbed

Abbreviation	Meaning	Abbreviation	Meaning
5-FU	5-fluorouracil	MAC	*Mycobacterium avium–intracellulare* complex
FUO	fever of unknown origin	MAOI	monoamine oxidase inhibitor
FVC	forced vital capacity	MCA	middle cerebral artery
GBS	Guillain-Barré Syndrome	MCV	mean corpuscular volume
GERD	gastroesophageal reflux disease	MD	muscular dystrophy
GFR	glomerular filtration rate	MEN	multiple endocrine neoplasia
GI	gastrointestinal	MGUS	monoclonal gammopathy of unknown significance
GnRH	gonadotropin-releasing hormone	MHC	major histocompatibility complex
HAV	hepatitis A virus	MI	myocardial infarction
Hb	hemoglobin	MMPI	Minnesota Multiphasic Personality Inventory
HBsAG	hepatitis B surface antigen	MMR	measles, mumps, rubella
HBV	hepatitis B virus	MRI	magnetic resonance imaging
hCG	human chorionic gonadotropin	MS	multiple sclerosis
HCV	hepatitis C virus	MTP	metatarsophalangeal
HDL	high-density lipoprotein	NBME	National Board of Medical Examiners
HDV	hepatitis D virus	NCHS	National Center for Health Statistics
HEV	hepatitis E virus	NG	nasogastric
HHS	Department of Health and Human Services	NIDA	National Institute on Drug Abuse
HHV	human herpesvirus	NIDDM	non-insulin-dependent diabetes mellitus
HIDA	hepato-iminodiacetic acid	NPO	nil per os (nothing by mouth)
HIV	human immunodeficiency virus	NPV	negative predictive value
HLA	human leukocyte antigen	NSAID	nonsteroidal anti-inflammatory drug
HMG-CoA	hydroxymethylglutaryl-CoA	OCP	oral contraceptive pill
HNPCC	hereditary nonpolyposis colorectal cancer	OPV	oral polio vaccine
HPV	human papillomavirus	PAN	polyarteritis nodosa
HR	heart rate	PCP	*Pneumocystis carinii* pneumonia; phencyclidine hydrochloride
HRT	hormone replacement therapy	PCR	polymerase chain reaction
HSV	herpes simplex virus	PDA	patent ductus arteriosus
5-HT	5-hydroxytryptamine (serotonin)	PFTs	pulmonary function tests
HTN	hypertension	PG	prostaglandin
IBD	inflammatory bowel disease	PID	pelvic inflammatory disease
ICP	intracranial pressure	PIH	pregnancy-induced hypertension
ICU	intensive care unit	PIP	proximal interphalangeal
IDDM	insulin-dependent diabetes mellitus	PML	progressive multifocal leukoencephalopathy
IFN	interferon	PMN	polymorphonuclear leukocyte
Ig	immunoglobulin	PMR	polymyalgia rheumatica
IL-1, -2, -3, -4, -5	interleukin-1, 2, 3, 4, 5	PPD	purified protein derivative (of tuberculin)
IM	intramuscular	PPV	positive predictive value
IMG	international medical graduate	PSA	prostate-specific antigen
INH	isonicotine hydrazine (isoniazid)	PT	prothrombin time
INS	Immigration and Naturalization Service	PTCA	percutaneous transluminal coronary angioplasty
IPV	inactivated polio vaccine	PTH	parathyroid hormone
ITP	idiopathic thrombocytopenic purpura	PTSD	post-traumatic stress disorder
IUD	intrauterine device	PTT	partial thromboplastin time
IUGR	intrauterine growth retardation	PUD	peptic ulcer disease
IV	intravenous	RBC	red blood cell
JRA	juvenile rheumatoid arthritis	RDS	respiratory distress syndrome
LAD	left anterior descending	RLQ	right lower quadrant
LBO	large bowel obstruction	RPR	rapid plasma reagin
LCA	left coronary artery	RR	respiratory rate
LCIS	lobular carcinoma in situ	RSV	respiratory syncytial virus
LCME	Liaison Committee on Medical Education	RTA	renal tubular acidosis
LDH	lactate dehydrogenase	RUQ	right upper quadrant
LDL	low-density lipoprotein	RV	residual volume; right ventricle; right ventricular
LES	lower esophageal sphincter	RVH	right ventricular hypertrophy
LFT	liver function test	RVRR	renal vein renin ratio
LH	luteinizing hormone	SA	sino-atrial
LLQ	left lower quadrant		
LP	lumbar puncture		
LPS	lipopolysaccharide		
LUQ	left upper quadrant		
LV	left ventricle; left ventricular		
LVH	left ventricular hypertrophy		

Abbreviation	Meaning
SAH	subarachnoid hemorrhage
SBO	small bowel obstruction
SC	sickle cell, subcutaneous
SCFE	slipped capital femoral epiphysis
SCID	severe combined immunodeficiency disease
SIRS	systemic inflammatory response syndrome
SLC	Sylvan Learning Center
SLE	systemic lupus erythematosus
SRP	sponsoring residency program
SRS-A	slow-reacting substance of anaphylaxis
SSRI	selective serotonin reuptake inhibitors
STC	Sylvan Testing Center
STD	sexually transmitted disease
SVC	superior vena cava
SVT	supraventricular tachycardia
TAT	thematic apperception test
TB	tuberculosis
TCA	tricyclic antidepressant
TGV	transposition of great vessels
TIBC	total iron binding capacity
TIPS	transjugular intrahepatic portosystemic shunt
TM	tympanic membrane
TMP-SMX	trimethoprim-sulfamethoxazole
TNM	tumor, node, metastasis
ToRCHeS	toxoplasmosis, rubella, CMV, herpes, syphilis
tPA	tissue plasminogen activator

Abbreviation	Meaning
TSH	thyroid-stimulating hormone
TTN	transcient tachypnea of the newborn
TTP	thrombotic thrombocytopenic purpura
TV	tidal volumeTXA thromboxane
UA	urinalysis
UMN	upper motor neuron
URI	upper respiratory infection
USMLE	United States Medical Licensing Examination
UTI	urinary tract infection
VDRL	Venereal Disease Research Laboratory
VMA	vanillylmandelic acid
V/Q	ratio of ventilation to perfusion
VSD	ventricular septal defect
VWF	Von Willebrand factor
VZV	varicella-zoster virus
WBC	white blood cell

Symbol	Meaning
$\uparrow$	increase(s)
$\downarrow$	decrease(s)
$\rightarrow$	leads to
$1°$	primary
$2°$	secondary
$3°$	tertiary
$\approx$	approximately; homologous

Index

C

CA-125, 61, 185
CABG, 89, 90
CAD, 89, 301–302
CaEDTA, 346t
Caffeine, 310t
Calcitonin, 334
Calcium
  channel blockers, 70, 81, 343t, 345t
  gluconate, 332
  hypercalcemia, 53, 180t, 330, 334
  nephrolithiasis, 337t
  osteoporosis, 211
California and postgraduate training, 39
Campylobacter, 157, 239, 341t
C-ANCA, 65
Cancer. *See also* Oncology; Tumor(s)
  basal cell carcinoma, 106–107
  breast, 177–178
  cervical, 186–187
  colon, 140, 161t, 182–184, 299
  Crohn's disease, 143t
  endometrial, 268
  epidemiology, 62
  esophageal adenocarcinoma, 138
  hepatocellular carcinoma, 156
  hereditary nonpolyposis colorectal, 182
  Hodgkin's and non-Hodgkin's lymphoma,
    191
  invasive, 178
  leukemias
    acute lymphocytic, 191–192
    acute myelogenous, 192–194
    children, most common type of cancer
      in, 191
    chronic lymphocytic, 194–195
    chronic myelogenous, 195–196
    general considerations, 63
  lung, 64, 180–181
  lymphoma, 191
  melanoma, 62, 107–108
  ovarian, 185
  prostate, 178–179
  rectal, 184
  screening, 299t
  skin, 62, 106–107
  squamous cell carcinoma, 105–106, 210
  ulcerative colitis, 143t
Candidal intertrigo, 115–116
Candidal vaginitis, 262f, 262t
Captopril, 70
Carbamazepine, 231, 232, 257t, 305, 343t,
  345t
Carbimazole, 122
Carbon monoxide, 346t, 348
Carcinoembryonic antigen (CEA), 61
Carcinoid tumor, 64
Carcinoma in situ (CIS), 178. *See also* Cancer; Oncology; Tumor(s)
Cardiovascular system. *See also* Pulmonary
    medicine
  angina pectoris, 88–89
  aorta
    aneurysm, 86–87
    aortography, 350
    coarctation of the, 82, 276–277
    disruption, 350–351
    dissection, 87–88
    regurgitation, 65
    stenosis, 65

atrial fibrillation, 91–93
cardiac tamponade, 95–96
cardiomyopathies, 65
carditis, 84
congestive heart failure, 93–94
diabetes, 120
endocarditis, 85–86
enzymes, cardiac, 88
hypertension, primary
  complications, 81
  defining, 79
  measurements, classification and inter-
    pretation of blood pressure, 80
  medications, 81
hypertension, secondary, 82
hypertensive urgency, 83–84
output variables, cardiac, 72
paraneoplastic syndromes in lung cancer,
  180t
pericarditis, 94–95
rheumatic fever/heart disease, 84–85
shock, cardiogenic, 335t
stress testing, cardiac, 84
ventricular septal defect, 273–274
Caribbean people and hemoglobinopathy
  screens, 298t
Case control study, 131
Catecholamines, 68
Catheterization, coronary, 88
Cauda equina syndrome, 215, 216
CD4 lymphocytes, 199
Cefamandole, 67
Cefoperazone, 320t
Cefotaxime, 67, 198t, 204t
Ceftriaxone
  epiglottitis, 294
  gonorrhea, 67, 264
  Lyme disease, 206
  meningitis, 198t, 204t
  pneumonia, 320t
Cefuroxime, 320t
Cellulitis, 110
Cephalexin, 110
Cephalosporin, 67, 320t
Cerebellar tremor, 47
Cerebral edema, 203
Cerebral palsy (CP), 289
Cervical cancer, 186–187
Cervical motion tenderness (CMT), 264
Cesarean section, indications for, 254, 256
Chandelier sign, 264
Charcoal, activated, 346t
Cheilosis, 52
Chemical peel, 105
Chemotherapy, 108, 190. *See also* Cancer;
  Oncology
Chest, penetrating wounds to the, 351
Chest tubes, 351
Chest x-rays. *See* Cardiovascular system; Pe-
  diatrics; *individual diseases/disorders*
Children. *See also* Obstetrics; Pediatrics
  abuse of, 285–287
  asthma, 328
  death, leading causes of, 297
  diabetes, gestational, 244–245
  diarrhea, 157, 158
  infectious disease, 197
  insulin-dependent diabetes mellitus,
    119–120
  intracranial tumors, 228
  leukemias, 191
  molluscum contagiosum, 114–115
  screening measures, 298t

seizures, 231t
syphilis, 208
vaccinations, 300
Chlamydia, 263, 264, 320t
Chloramphenicol, 207, 294, 342t
Chocolate cysts, 269
Cholangiogram, intraoperative, 148
Cholangitis, 148–150
Cholecystectomy, 147, 148
Cholecystitis, acute, 147–148, 149f
Cholelithiasis, 146–147
Cholesterol, 301
Cholestyramine, 158
Chorea, 47, 84
Chédiak-Higashi disease, 58
Chronic atrophic gastritis, 61
Chronic bronchitis, 328
Chronic diarrhea, 156–158
Chronic granulomatous disease, 58
Chronic hepatitis, 155–156
Chronic hydroxyurea, 175
Chronic hypoxia, 168
Chronic lymphocytic leukemia (CLL), 63,
  194–195
Chronic mucocutaneous candidiasis, 58
Chronic myelogenous leukemia (CML), 63,
  195–196
Chronic obstructive pulmonary disease
  (COPD), 328–329
Chronic osteomyelitis, 209
Chronic pancreatitis, 145, 146f
Chronic renal failure, 73
Chronic transfusion therapy, 125
Chvostek's sign, 333
Cimetidine, 345t
Ciprofloxacin, 205
Cirrhosis, 61, 63
Cisplatin, 343t
Clarithromycin, 139, 200t, 320t
Clavicular fracture, 285t
Clavulanic acid, 241, 295
Clerkships, proximity to, 18
Clindamycin, 200t
Clinical Skills Assessment (CSA)
  international medical students
    administration of test, 30
    applying for the, 31–32
    communication score, 31
    definition, 29
    do's and don'ts, 30
    location of test site, 32
    need to take the, determining, 31
    preparing for the, 32
    scoring, 30–31
Clinical trial, 132
Clomiphene citrate, 271
Clomipramine, 69
Clonidine, 158, 343t, 344t
Clostridia, 54
Clostridium
  botulinum, 341t
  difficile, 54, 157
  perfringens, 54, 57, 341t
  tetani, 54
Clozapine, 308, 342t
Cluster headache, 230
Coarctation of the aorta, 82, 276–277
Cobalamin, 53, 347t
Cocaine, 68, 310t, 311t, 344t, 346t
Cognitive-behavior therapy, 305, 315
Cohort study, 131–132
Colchicine, 217, 218

D

Haloperidol, 344t
Halothane, 69, 343t
Hamartoma, 182
Hampton's hump, 324
Hartnup disease, 52
Hashimoto's thyroiditis, 122
HAV, 154
HBV, 154–156
H1B visa for international medical students, 38–39, 41–42
β-HCG
  abdomen, acute, 159
  amenorrhea, 266
  appendicitis, 142
  endometriosis, 269
  pelvic inflammatory disease, 265
  preeclampsia and eclampsia, 248
  tumor markers, 61
HCTZ, 343t
HCV, 154–156
HDV, 154, 156
Headache, 223, 226, 229–230
Health and Human Services, U.S. Department of (HHS), 36
Health care/lab workers and hepatitis B vaccine, 300
Health care screening, 298t
Heartburn, 137
Heart disease, 271, 272. See also Cardiovascular system
Heberden's nodes, 214
Height and health care screening, 298t
Helical CT scans, 337
Helicobacter pylori, 55, 138
HELLP syndrome, 245
Helmet cells, 165f
Hemarthroses, 173
Hematogenous seeding, 209
Hematology
  anemia
    aplastic, 305
    differential, 163–164
    evaluation, 164
    G6PD deficiency, 167
    history, 163
    iron deficiency, 165f, 183
    lung cancer, 180t
    megaloblastic, 53
    microangiopathic hemolytic, 170t
    PE, 163
    pernicious, 61
    renal failure, 73
    treatment, 165–166
  disseminated intravascular coagulation, 172–173
  G6PD deficiency, 167
  hemophilia, 173
  idiopathic thrombocytopenic purpura, 171–172
  paraneoplastic syndromes in lung cancer, 180t
  polycythemia vera, 168
  sickle cell disease, 174–175
  thalassemia, 166–167
  thrombotic thrombocytopenic purpura, 169–171
  transfusion
    chronic transfusion therapy, 125
    exchange, 280
    reactions, 168–169
  von Willebrand's disease, 173–174
Hemiballismus, 47
Hemochromatosis, 125–126
Hemoglobinopathy screens, 298t

Hemolytic-uremic syndrome, 170
Hemophilia, 173
Hemorrhage. See also Bleeding; Hematology
  exsanguinating, 350
  parenchymal, 227
  postpartum, 258–259
  stroke, 234
  subarachnoid, 225–227
  tumors, 62
Heparin, 172, 210, 235, 325, 346t
Heparinization, 89
Hepatic encephalopathy, 151
Hepatitis
  acute, 155
  alcoholic, 202
  chronic, 155–156
  types of, 154
  vaccine for hepatitis B, 300
Hepatocellular carcinoma, 156
Hepatorenal syndrome, 151
Herald patch, 100
Hereditary nonpolyposis colorectal cancer (HNPCC), 182
Hereditary spherocytosis, 60
Herpes
  acyclovir, 264
  simplex, 101–102
  symptoms, 263
  zoster, 104, 200t
HEV, 154
HIDA scan, 148, 149f
High-grade squamous intraepithelial lesion, 186
Hip dislocation, 220t, 282
Hip fracture, 221t
Histrionic personality disorder, 314t
HIV (human immune deficiency virus), 173, 199–200, 207–208, 297, 300
HMG-CoA reductase inhibitors, 343t
Hodgkin's lymphoma, 191
Homosexual men and hepatitis B vaccine, 300
Hormonal abnormalities, 119
Hormone replacement therapy (HRT), 211, 269, 272
Horner's syndrome, 180, 230
Hot flashes, 271
HSV, 200t, 208
Humerus fracture, 221t
Hutchinson's triad, 208
Hyaline membrane disease, 295–296
Hydatidiform mole, 251–252, 254
Hydralazine, 343t, 345t
Hydration, 175, 336, 337
Hydrocortisone, 99, 122, 204
Hydroxyurea, chronic, 175
Hyperactivity, 290
Hyperaldosteronism, 70, 74, 82, 127–128
Hyperbilirubinemia, 51, 167, 279
Hypercalcemia, 53, 180t, 330, 334
Hypercortisolism, 124
Hyperglycemia, 125
Hyperinflated lungs, 329
Hyperkalemia, 70, 73, 331, 332
Hyperparathyroidism, 123
Hyperprolactinemia, 267f–268f, 308
Hypersegmentation, 164
Hypersensitivity reactions. See Dermatology
Hypertension
  aortic dissection, 87
  β-blockers, 68
  diabetes, gestational, 245t
  eclampsia, 247t
  hypertensive urgency, 83–84

portal, 63, 150–151
pregnancy-induced, 245
primary
  complications, 81
  defining, 79
  measurements/classification/interpretation of blood pressure, 80t
  medications, 81
  retinopathy, 80f
  secondary, 82
Hyperthyroidism, 121–122
Hypertrophic cardiomyopathy, 65
Hypocalcemia, 333–334
Hypochondriasis, 50
Hypoglycemia, 244, 245t
Hypogonadism, 59
Hypokalemia, 82, 125, 333
Hyponatremia, 203, 338–339
Hypothyroidism, 122
Hypotonic hyponatremia, 339t
Hypovolemia, 335t
Hypoxemia, 329
Hypoxia, chronic, 168
Hysterectomy, 187, 269

I

IAP 66, 33–34
Ibuprofen, 345t
Idiopathic thrombocytopenic purpura (ITP), 171–172
Ileus, 152–153
Imaging, questions that include, 22
Imipramine, 69, 290
Immediate fasciotomy, 349
Immediate needle decompression, 326
Immigration and Naturalization Service (INS), 33
Immune deficiencies, 58
Immunoglobulin, 239
Immunologic reactions to transfused blood, 168
Immunosuppressants, 239
Impetigo, 116–117
Impulsivity, 290
Indomethacin, 274
Infants, 49. See also Obstetrics; Pediatrics
Infectious disease
  abortion, septic, 249t
  blood transfusions, 168
  congenital infections, 207–208
  fever of unknown origin, 202
  herpes simplex, 101–102
  HIV (human immune deficiency virus), 199–200
  Lyme disease, 205–206
  meningitis, 56, 200t, 202–204
  nosocomial infections, 57
  otitis externa, 204
  pneumonia
    antibiotics, 320t
    common causes of, 56
    history/PE/evaluation, 318
    solitary pulmonary nodule, 182
    treatment, 319–321
  Rocky Mountain spotted fever, 206–207
  rotavirus, 157
  sepsis, 197–198
  streptococcal pharyngeal, 85
  syphilis, 200–202
  urinary tract infection, 205
  varicella, 102–104
Infertility, 185, 269–272, 294
Inflammatory bowel disease (IBD), 142–143

397

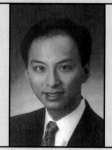
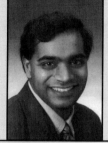
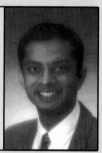

Tao Le, MD   Chirag Amin, MD   Vikas Bhushan, MD

About the Authors

Tao Le, MD

Tao earned his medical degree from UCSF. He has been involved in major writing and editing projects over the past six years including leading the completions of *First Aid for the Wards*, *First Aid for the Match* and the thoroughly revised *First Aid for the USMLE Step 2*. As a medical student he was editor-in-chief of *Synapse*, a campus-wide student-run newspaper with a weekly circulation of 5000. He is a senior resident in internal medicine at Yale-New Haven Hospital. Fortunately, Tao is happily married, so this won't be mistaken for a personal ad. He can be reached at taotle@aol.com

Chirag Amin, MD

Chirag graduated from medical school at the University of Miami and is a resident in orthopedic surgery at Orlando Regional Medical Center and plans on pursuing a spine fellowship. Chirag has been involved extensively in teaching and in writing books. He led the completion of *Jump Start MCAT: A High-Yield Student-to-Student Guide* (Williams & Wilkins). Chirag lives in Orlando, Florida. He can be reached at chiragamin@aol.com

Vikas Bhushan, MD

Vikas earned his medical degree from UCSF and trained in diagnostic radiology at UCLA. He is currently working very part-time *locum tenens* in radiology while focusing on writing and traveling. As a Reformer-Perfectionist (see p.135), he conceived the original *First Aid for the USMLE Step 1* in 1992 and the *Underground Clinical Vignettes* series in 1998. He is active in medical education, digital radiology and the Indo-American cultural community. His latest project is producing an art book of qawwali music translations in Urdu, Punjabi and English dedicated to the late Nusrat Fateh Ali Khan. Vikas is still single and resides in the Westside of Los Angeles. He can be reached at vbhushan@aol.com

Ross Berkeley, MD

Ross earned his medical degree from the University of California at San Francisco in 1997 and is currently a resident in emergency medicine at the University of Pittsburgh Medical Center. He was an editor and coordinator of *First Aid for the Wards* and a contributing author for the 1996 revision of *First Aid for the USMLE Step 1*. He remains dedicated to medical education and is currently writing *Underground Clinical Vignettes: Emergency Medicine*. Ross is single and lives in Pittsburgh. He can be reached at emergdoc@aol.com.

Ross Levine

Ross is a fourth year medical student at the Johns Hopkins University School of Medicine. He was the student editor of the 1997 revision of *First Aid for the USMLE Step 1*. He will train in internal medicine after graduation and has an interest in molecular biology.

Diego Ruiz

Diego is a fourth year medical student at the University of California at San Francisco. He plans to become an academic radiologist. He was a contributing author for *First Aid for the Wards* and numerous Underground Clinical Vignettes books. He has a special place in his heart for animals and an irrational love of spicy food.

Praise for the 1ST Ed *UNDERGROUND CLINICAL VIGNETTES* series...

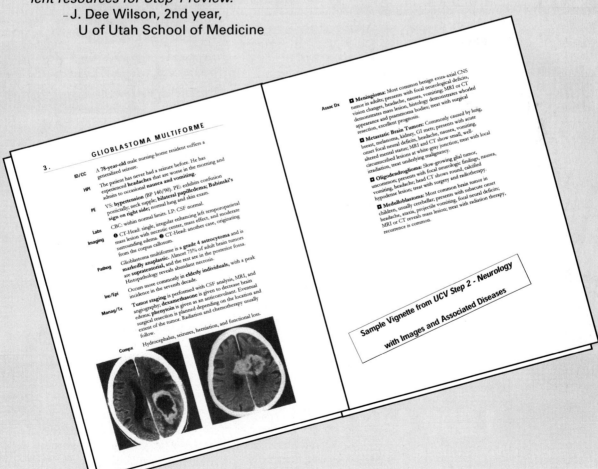

Sample Vignette from UCV Step 2 - Neurology with Images and Associated Diseases

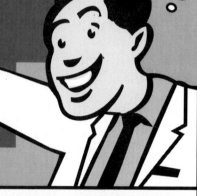
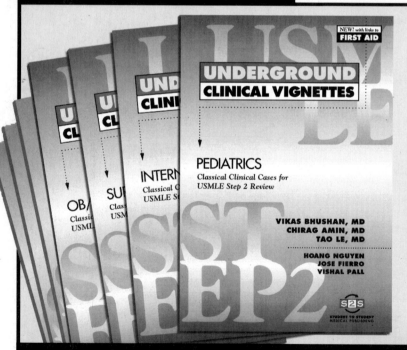